Clinical Problem Solving in Dentistry

Commissioning Editor: *Alison Taylor*
Development Editor: *Janice Urquhart, Louisa Welch*
Project Manager: *Shereen Jameel*
Designer/Design Direction: *Stewart Larking*
Illustration Manager: *Bruce Hogarth*
Illustrator: *Robert Britton*

CLINICAL **PROBLEM SOLVING** IN DENTISTRY
SERIES

THIRD EDITION

Clinical Problem Solving in Dentistry

Edited by
Edward W. Odell

Professor and Honorary Consultant in Oral Pathology and Medicine, King's College London Dental Institute, Guy's Hospital, London, UK

CHURCHILL LIVINGSTONE
ELSEVIER

Edinburgh London New York Oxford Philadelphia St Louis Sydney Toronto 2010

Clinical Problem Solving in Dentistry, 3e
Odell

CHURCHILL LIVINGSTONE
An imprint of Elsevier

Original ISBN: 978-0443-0678-46

This edition of **Clinical Problem Solving in Dentistry, 3ed** by **Edward W. Odell** is published by an arrangement with Elsevier Ltd.

Indian Reprint ISBN: 978-81-312-2928-6
First Printed in India 2011
Reprinted 2012, Repinted 2013

[redacted]

Notice

Medical Knowledge is constantly changing. Standard safety precautions must be followed, but as new research and clinical experience broaden our knowledge, changes in treatment and drug therapy may become necessary or appropriate. Readers are advised to check the most current product information provided by the manufacturer of each drug to be administered, to verify the recommended dose, the method and the duration of administration, and the contraindications. It is the responsibility of the practitioner, relying on their own experience and knowledge of the patient, to determine dosages and the best treatment for each individual patient. Neither the Publisher nor the Authors assume any liability for any injury and/or damage to persons or property arising from this publication.

The Publisher

Published by Elsevier, a division of Reed Elsevier India Private Limited.

Registered Office: 305, Rohit House, 3, Tolstoy Marg, New Delhi 110 001.
Corporate Office: 14th Floor, Building No. 10B, DLF Cyber City, Phase-II, Gurgaon-122 002, Haryana, India.
Printed and bound in India at Shree Maitrey Printech, Pvt. Ltd., Noida.

Contents

CONTENTS

Preface

The fact that a third edition of this book has been produced so soon after the last is testimony to the appeal of the problem solving format. I said in the preface to both previous editions that problem solving is a practical skill that cannot be learnt from textbooks. This book is designed to help the reader reorganize their knowledge into a clinically useful format. It cannot teach you to solve problems unless you supplement it with clinical experience, for which there is no substitute.

This third edition includes ten completely new problems, making it almost twice as long as the first edition. All the chapters have been completely revised. Despite the short interval since the last edition it is surprising how many have had to be extensively rewritten to account for new national guidance, changes in legislation and advances in treatment. Topics of the new sections range through basic dentistry, special care topics and child protection to name a few. We hope you enjoy them and find them useful.

I am indebted to the many friends and colleagues who have contributed. As before, many of these chapters are team efforts with input from people who are not acknowledged. It is difficult for a reader to appreciate how much effort the many authors have expended and the time they have given up to produce this book. Without them, and the patience and support of my wife Wendy and children, this book would never have been written.

EW Odell

Contributors

Dr Avijit Banerjee BDS FDS MSc PhD
Senior Lecturer and Hon Consultant in Restorative Dentistry, King's College London Dental Institute, London, UK

Professor David W. Bartlett, BDS PhD MRD FDSRCS (Rest. Dent.)
Professor of Prosthodontics, King's College London Dental Institute, London, UK

Ms Wendy Bellis BDS MSc
Senior Dental Officer in Paediatric Dentistry, Islington & Camden Primary Care Trust, London, UK

Mrs Jackie Brown BDS MSC FDSRCPS DDRRCR
Consultant and Honorary Senior Lecturer in Dental Radiology, King's College London Dental Institute, London, UK

Dr Shahid I. Chaudhry BDS MBBS FDS MRCP(UK)
Specialist Registrar/Honorary Lecturer in Oral Medicine, UCL Eastman Dental Institute, London, UK

Dr David C. Craig BA BDS MMedSci MFGDP
Consultant in Sedation and Special Care Dentistry, King's College London Dental Institute, London, UK

Dr Alexander Crighton BDS MBChB FDSRCS (Oral Med) FDSRCPS
Consultant in Oral Medicine, Hon Clinical Senior Lecturer in Medicine in Relation to Dentistry, Glasgow Dental Hospital & School, Glasgow, UK

Mr Chris Dickinson BDS MSc MFDS DDPH RCS DipDSed
Consultant in Special Care Dentistry, Guy's and St Thomas' NHS Foundation Trust, London, UK

Dr Michael Escudier BDS FDSRCS FDSRCS (Oral Med) MD FFGDP
Lecturer/Hon Consultant in Medicine in Relation to Oral Disease, King's College London Dental Institute, London, UK

Dr Anna Gibilaro BDS DDS MSc DOrth MOrth FDSCRCS FDSRCS (Orthodontics)
Consultant in Orthodontics, Guy's and St Thomas' NHS Foundation Trust, London, UK

Mr Nicholas M. Goodger PhD FRCS (OMFS) FDSRCS FFD DLORCS
Consultant Oral and Maxillofacial Surgeon, East Kent Hospitals NHS Trust and Honorary Senior Lecturer in Maxillofacial Surgery, University of Kent, Canterbury, UK

Mrs Jennifer C. Harris BDS MSc FDSRCS
Specialist in Paediatric Dentistry, Sheffield Salaried Primary Dental Care Service, Sheffield, UK

Mr Mike G. Harrison BDS FDSRCS (Paed. Dent) MPhil MScD
Consultant in Paediatric Dentistry, Guy's and St Thomas' NHS Foundation Trust, London, UK

Miss Emma K. Mahoney BDS MSc SND, MSND RCS
Senior Dental Officer in Special Care Dentistry, Islington and Camden Primary Care Trust, London, UK

Mr Robert M. Mordecai BDS FDSRCS DOrth MOrth
Formerly Senior Lecturer and Honorary Consultant in Orthodontics, King's College London Dental Institute, London, UK

Professor Edward W. Odell BDS FDSRCS MSc PhD FRCPath
Professor of Oral Pathology and Medicine, King's College London Dental Institute, London, UK

Mr Guy D. Palmer BDS MSc MRD
Consultant in Special Care Dentistry, King's College Hospital NHS Foundation Trust, London, UK

Professor Richard M. Palmer BDS FDSRCS PhD
Professor of Implant Dentistry and Periodontology, King's College London Dental Institute, London, UK

Dr David R. Radford BDS PhD FDSRCS MRD
Senior Lecturer and Honorary Consultant, King's College London Dental Institute, London, UK

Professor Tara F. Renton BDS FDSRCS FRACDS (OMS) PhD
Professor of Oral Surgery, King's College London Dental Institute, London, UK

Professor David Ricketts BDS MSc PhD FDSRCS FDS (Rest. Dent.)
Professor of Cariology and Conservative Dentistry and Honorary Consultant in Restorative Dentistry, Dundee Dental Hospital and School, Dundee, UK

Mr Paul D. Robinson MBBS BDS FDSRCS PhD
Specialist Oral Surgeon, Formerly Department of Oral and Maxillofacial Surgery, Guy's Hospital, London, UK

Dr Evelyn Sheehy BDSc PhD FDSRCS (Paed. Dent.)
Consultant in Paediatric Dentistry, Guy's and St Thomas' Hospitals NHS Foundation Trust, London, UK

Dr Martyn Sherriff BSc PhD MRSC MIMMM ANCRT FSS
Reader in Dental Materials Science, King's College London Dental Institute, London, UK

Mrs Penelope J. Shirlaw BDS FDSRCS
Consultant in Oral Medicine, Guy's and St Thomas' Hospitals NHS Foundation Trust, London, UK

Carol Tait BDS MSc MFDS MRD
Senior Clinical Teacher in Endodontology, Dundee Dental Hospital and School, Dundee, UK

Dr Anwar R. Tappuni LDSRCS MRACDS(OM) PhD
Clinical Senior Lecturer in Oral Medicine, Bart's and the London School of Medicine and Dentistry, London, UK

Professor Wanninayaka M. Tilakaratne BDS MS FDSRCS FRCPath
Professor and Consultant in Oral Pathology, University of Peradeniya, Sri Lanka

Dr Michael J. Twitchen FFD LMSSA
General Medical Practitioner, West Sussex, UK

Mr Eric Whaites MSc BDS FDS RCS FRCR DDRRCR
Senior Lecturer and Honorary Consultant in Dental Radiology, King's College London Dental Institute, London, UK

Case 1

A high caries rate

SUMMARY

A 17-year-old sixth-form college student presents at your general dental surgery with several carious lesions, one of which is very large. How should you stabilize his condition?

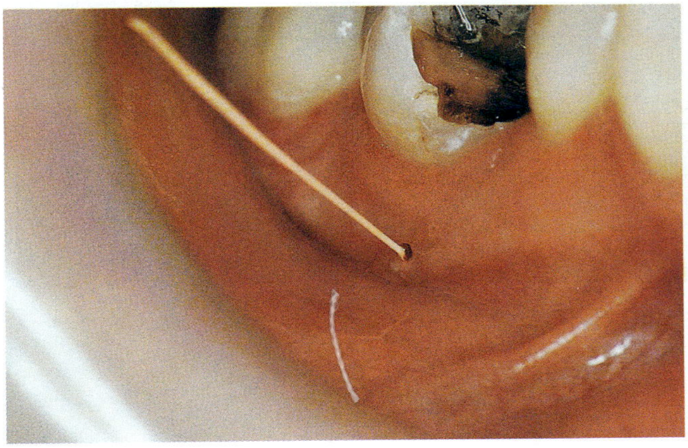

Fig. 1.1 The lower right first molar. The gutta percha point indicates a sinus opening.

History

Complaint

He complains that a filling has fallen out of a tooth on the lower right side and has left a sharp edge that irritates his tongue. He is otherwise asymptomatic.

History of complaint

The filling was placed about a year ago at a casual visit to the dentist precipitated by acute toothache triggered by hot and cold food and drink. He did not return to complete a course of treatment. He lost contact when he moved house and is not registered with a dental practitioner.

Medical history

The patient is otherwise fit and well.

Examination

Extraoral examination

He is a fit and healthy-looking adolescent. No submental, submandibular or other cervical lymph nodes are palpable and the temporomandibular joints appear normal.

Intraoral examination

The lower right quadrant is shown in Figure 1.1. The oral mucosa is healthy and the oral hygiene is reasonable. There is gingivitis in areas but no calculus is visible and probing depths are 3 mm or less. The mandibular right first molar is grossly carious and a sinus is discharging buccally. There are no other restorations in any teeth. No teeth have been extracted and the third molars are not visible. A small cavity is present on the occlusal surface of the mandibular right second molar.

■ ***What further examination would you carry out?***

Test of tooth vitality of the teeth in the region of the sinus. Even though the first molar is the most likely cause, the adjacent teeth should be tested because more than one tooth might be nonvital. The results should be compared with those of the teeth on the opposite side. Both hot/cold methods and electric pulp testing could be used because extensive reactionary dentine may moderate the response.

The first molar fails to respond to any test. All other teeth appear vital.

Investigations

■ ***What radiographs would you take? Explain why each view is required.***

Radiograph	Reason taken
Bitewing radiographs	Primarily to detect approximal surface caries, and in this case also required to detect occlusal caries.
Periapical radiograph of the lower right first molar tooth, preferably taken with a paralleling technique	Preoperative assessment for endodontic treatment or for extraction should it be necessary.
Panoramic radiograph	Might be useful as a general survey view in a new patient and to determine the presence and position of third molars.

■ ***What problems are inherent in the diagnosis of caries in this patient?***

Occlusal lesions are now the predominant form of caries in adolescents following the reduction in caries incidence over the past decades. Occlusal caries may go undetected on visual examination for two reasons. First, it starts on the fissure walls and is obscured by sound superficial enamel, and secondly lesions cavitate late, if at all, probably because fluoride strengthens the overlying enamel. Superimposition of sound enamel also masks small and medium-sized lesions on bitewing radiographs. The small occlusal cavity in the second molar arouses suspicion that other pits and fissures in the molars will be carious. Unless lesions are very large, extending

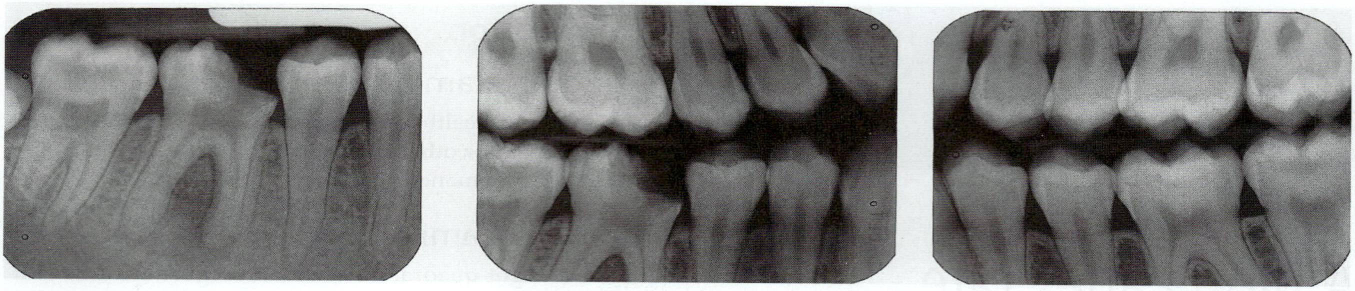

Fig. 1.2 Periapical and bitewing films.

into the middle third of dentine, they may not be detected on bitewing radiographs.

■ ***The radiographs are shown in Figure 1.2. What do you see?***

The periapical radiograph shows the carious lesion in the crown of the lower right first molar to be extensive, involving the pulp cavity. The mesial contact has been completely destroyed and the molar has drifted mesially and tilted. There are periapical radiolucencies at the apices of both roots, that on the mesial root being larger. The radiolucencies are in continuity with the periodontal ligament and there is loss of most of the lamina dura in the bifurcation and around the apices.

The bitewing radiographs confirm the carious exposure and in addition reveal occlusal caries in all the maxillary and mandibular molars with the exception of the upper right first molar. No approximal caries is present.

■ ***If two or more teeth were possible causes of the sinus, how might you decide which was the cause?***

A gutta percha point could be inserted into the sinus prior to taking the radiograph, as shown in Figure 1.1. A medium- or fine-sized point is flexible but resilient enough to pass along the sinus tract if twisted slightly on insertion. Points are radiopaque and can be seen on a radiograph extending to the source of the infection, as shown in another case in Figure 1.3.

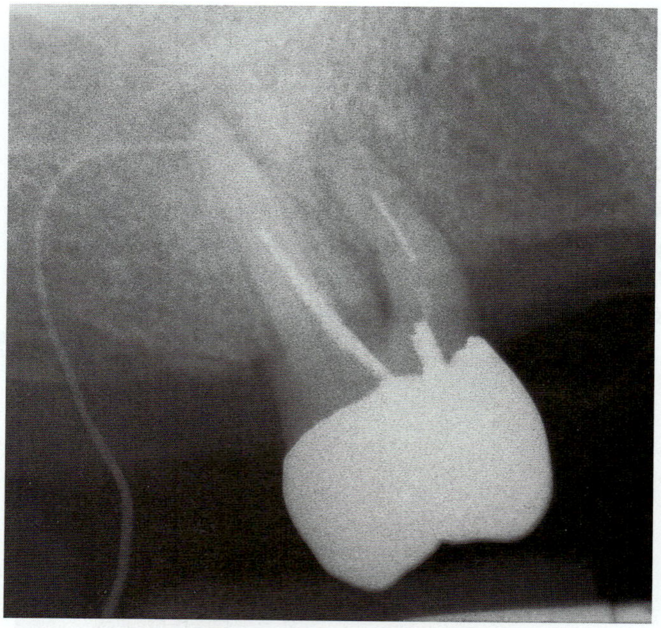

Fig. 1.3 Another case, showing gutta percha point tracing the path of a sinus.

Diagnosis

■ ***What is your diagnosis?***

The patient has a nonvital lower first molar with a periapical abscess. In addition he has a very high caries rate in a previously almost caries-free dentition.

Treatment

The patient is horrified to discover that his dentition is in such a poor state, having experienced only one episode of toothache in the past. He is keen to do all that can be done to save all teeth and a decision is made to try to restore the lower molar.

■ ***How will you prioritize treatment for this patient? Why should treatment be provided in this sequence?***

See Table 1.1.

■ ***What temporary restoration materials are available? What are their properties and in what situations are they useful?***

See Table 1.2.

■ ***Why is one molar so much more broken down than the others?***

It is difficult to be certain but the extensive caries is probably, in part, a result of the previous restoration. In view of the pattern of caries in the other molars, it seems likely that this was a large occlusal restoration and the history suggests it was placed in a vital tooth. It probably undermined the mesial cusps or marginal ridge. Three factors could have contributed to the extensive caries present only 1 year later: marginal leakage, undermining of the marginal ridge or mesial cusps leading to collapse, or failure to remove all the carious tissue from the tooth. Failure to remove all carious enamel and dentine is a common cause of failure in amalgam restorations.

Table 1.1 Sequence of treatment

Phase of treatment	Items of treatment	Reasons
Immediate phase	Caries removal from the lower right first molar, access cavity preparation for endodontics, drainage, irrigation with sodium hypochlorite and placement of a temporary restoration	Essential if the tooth is to be saved and to remove the source of the apical infection. There is also an urgent need to minimize further destruction of this tooth, which may soon be unrestorable. The temporary restoration is necessary to facilitate rubber dam isolation during future endodontic treatment, and it will also stabilize the occlusion and stop mesial drift.
Stabilization of caries	Removal of caries and placement of temporary restorations in all carious teeth in visits by quadrants/two quadrants	To prevent further tooth destruction and progression to carious exposure while other phases of treatment are being carried out.
Preventive treatment	Dietary analysis, oral hygiene instruction, fluoride advice	Should start immediately and extend throughout the treatment plan, to reduce the high caries rate and ensure the long-term future of the dentition.
Permanent restoration	Will depend on what is found while placing temporary restorations	Permanent restorations may be left until last; stabilization takes priority.

Table 1.2 Temporary restoration materials

Material	Examples	Properties	Situations
Zinc oxide and eugenol pastes	Kalzinol	Bactericidal, easy to mix and place, cheap but not very strong. Easily removed.	Suitable for temporary restoration of most cavities provided there is no significant occlusal load. Endodontic access cavities.
Self-setting zinc oxide cements	Cavit Coltosol	Harden in contact with saliva. Reasonable strength and easily removed.	Endodontic access cavities. No occlusal load.
Polycarboxylate cements	Poly-F	Adhesive to enamel and dentine, hard and durable.	Used when mechanical retention is poor. Strong enough to enable rubber dam placement when used in a badly broken down tooth.
Glass ionomer including silver reinforced preparations	Chem-fil Shofu Hi-Fi Ketac Silver	Adhesive to enamel and dentine, hard and durable. Good appearance.	As polycarboxylate cements and also useful in anterior teeth.

■ How would you ensure removal of all carious tissue when restoring the vital molars?

Removal of all softened carious tissue at the amelodentinal junction is essential and only stained but hard dentine can be left in place.

Removal of carious dentine over the pulp is treated differently. In a young patient with large pulp chambers there is always a tendency for the operator to be conservative but this might be counterproductive if softened or infected dentine were left below the restoration. Very soft or flaky dentine must always be removed. Slightly soft dentine can be left in situ provided a good well-sealed restoration is placed over it. Deciding whether to leave the last layers of softened dentine can be difficult and the decision rests to a degree on clinical experience. Pain associated with pulpitis indicates a need to remove more dentine or, if severe, a need for elective endodontics. Interpreting softened dentine in rapidly advancing lesions is difficult. The deepest layers are soft through demineralization but are not necessarily infected and may sometimes be left over the pulp. Also, bacterial penetration of the dentine is not reliably indicated by staining in rapidly advancing lesions. Removal of the last layers of carious dentine may require some courage in deep lesions.

More detailed information on caries removal is included in problem 9, 'A large carious lesion'.

■ What is the most important preventive procedure for this patient? Explain why.

Diet analysis. Caries requires dietary sugars, in particular sucrose, glucose and fructose, an acidogenic plaque flora and a susceptible tooth surface. Denying the plaque flora its substrate sugar is the most effective measure to halt the progression of existing lesions and prevent new ones forming. No preventive measure affecting the flora or tooth is as effective. A further advantage of emphasis on diet is that it forces the patient to acknowledge that they must take responsibility for preventing their own disease.

■ How would you evaluate a patient's diet?

Dietary analysis consists of two elements: enquiry into lifestyle and into the dietary components themselves. Information about the diet itself is of little value unless it is taken in context with the patient's lifestyle. Only dietary recommendations tailored to the patient's lifestyle are likely to be adopted.

The diet record should include all the foods and drinks consumed, the amount (in readily estimated units) and the time of eating or drinking.

In this case it should be noted that the patient is a 17-year-old student. Lifestyle often changes dramatically between the ages of 16 and 20. He may no longer be living at home and may be enjoying physical, financial and dietary independence from his parents. He may be poor and be eating a cheap carbohydrate-rich diet of snacks instead of regular meals. Long hours of studying may be accompanied by the frequent consumption of sweetened drinks.

Analysis of the diet itself may be performed in a variety of ways. The patient can be asked to recall all foods consumed over the previous 24 hours. This is not very effective, relying as it does on a good memory and honesty, and is unlikely to give a representative account. Relying on memory for more than 24 hours is too inaccurate.

The most effective method is for the patient to keep a written record of their diet for 4 consecutive days, including 2 working and 2 leisure days. The need for the patient to comply fully and assess their diet honestly must be stressed and, of course, the diet should not be changed because it is being recorded. Ideally the analysis should be performed before any dietary advice is given. Even the patient who does not keep an honest account has been made more aware of their diet. If they know what foods to omit from the sheet to make their dentist happy, at least the first step in an educative process has been made.

■ ***How will you analyse this patient's 4-day diet sheet shown in Figure 1.4? What is the cause of his caries susceptibility?***

Highlight sugar-rich foods and drinks as in Figure 1.4. Note whether they are confined to meal times or whether they are **eaten frequently** and spaced throughout the day as snacks. The number of **sugar attacks should be counted** and discussed with the patient. Also note the **consistency** of the food because dry and sticky foods take longer to be cleared from the mouth. Sugared drinks taken immediately before bed are highly significant because salivary flow is reduced during sleep and clearance time is greater. Identify foods with a high **hidden sugar** content because patients often do not realize that such foods are significant; examples are baked beans, breakfast cereals, tomato ketchup and 'plain' biscuits.

The diet sheet shows that the main problem for this patient is too many sugar-containing drinks, and frequent snacks of cake and biscuits. Most meals or snacks contain a high sugar item and some more than one. The other typical cause of a high caries rate in this age group is sweets, especially mints.

■ ***What advice will you give the patient?***

The principles of a safer diet are shown in Table 1.3 (p. 6).

Dietary advice is almost always provided using the health-belief model of health education. However, it is well-known that education about the risks and consequences of lifestyle, habits and diet is often ineffective. It is important to judge the patient's likely compliance and provide dietary advice that can be used to make small but significant changes rather than attempting to eradicate all sugar from the diet. As the diet improves, the advice can be adapted and extended.

Advice must be acceptable, practical and affordable. In this case the patient has already suffered serious consequences from his poor diet and this may help change behaviour.

The patient must be made aware that damage to teeth continues for up to 1 hour after a sugar intake. The explanation given to some patients may be no more than this simple statement. Many other patients can comprehend the concept (if not the detail) of a Stephan curve without difficulty.

The patient should be advised to use a fluoride-containing toothpaste. During the period of dietary change it would also be beneficial to use a weekly fluoride rinse as well. This could be continued for as long as the diet is felt to be unsafe.

Oral hygiene instruction is also important, but may be emphasized in a later phase of treatment. It will not stop caries progression, which is critical for this patient, and there is only a mild gingivitis.

■ ***Assuming good compliance and motivation, how will you restore the teeth permanently?***

The mandibular right first molar requires orthograde endodontic treatment and replacement of the temporary restoration with a core. Retention for the core can be provided by residual tooth tissue, provided carious destruction is not gross. The restorative material may be packed into the pulp chamber and the first 2–3 mm of the root canal. If insufficient natural crown remains, it may be supplemented with a preformed post in the distal canals. The distal canal is not ideal, being further from the most extensively destroyed area, but it is larger.

The other molar teeth will need to have their temporary restorations replaced by definitive restorations. Caries involved only the occlusal surface but removal of these large lesions has probably left little more than an enamel shell. Restoration of such teeth with amalgam would require removal of all the unsupported, undermined enamel leaving little more than a root stump and a few spurs of tooth tissue. Restoration could be better achieved with a radiopaque glass ionomer and composite hybrid restoration. The glass ionomer used to replace the missing dentine must be radiopaque so that it is not confused with residual or secondary caries on radiographs. A composite linked to dentine with a bonding agent would be an alternative to the glass ionomer.

■ ***Figure 1.5 shows the restored lower first molar 2 months after endodontic treatment. What do you see and what long-term problem is evident?***

There is good bone healing around the apices and in the bifurcation. Complete healing would be expected after 6 months to 1 year at which time the success of root treatment can be judged.

As noted in the initial radiographs, the lower right first molar has lost its mesial contact, drifted and tilted. This makes it impossible to restore the normal contour of the mesial surface and contact point. The mesial surface is flat and there is no defined contact point. In the long term there is a risk of caries of the distal surface of the second premolar, and the caries is likely to affect a wider area of tooth and extend further gingivally than caries below a normal contact. The area will also be difficult to clean and there is a risk of localized periodontitis. Tilting of the occlusal surface may also favour food packing into the contact unless the contour of the restoration includes an artificially enhanced marginal ridge.

This tooth may require a crown in the long term. Much of the enamel is undermined and the tooth is weakened by endodontic treatment. A crown would allow the contact to have a better contour but the problem is insoluble while the tooth remains in its present position. Orthodontic uprighting could be considered.

4 day diet analysis sheet for John Smith

	Thursday		Friday		Saturday		Sunday	
	Time	Item	Time	Item	Time	Item	Time	Item
Before breakfast			7.00	2 cups of tea with 2 sugars	7.30	4 chocolate biscuits tea with 2 sugars		
Breakfast	8.30	sausages pitta bread ketchup tea with 2 sugars	8.30	banana			8.00	chocolate puffed rice breakfast cereal 1 glass cola drink
Morning	9.20 11.15	1 glass cola drink hot chocolate chocolate bar	9.30	mug hot chocolate packet crisps can of diet cola drink	11.00	1 slice cherry cake	10.30	4 slices toast and peanut butter 1 piece cake
Mid-day meal	12.30	turkey salad sandwich 1 glass cola drink tea with 2 sugars	1.00 pm	2 pieces cheese on toast, garlic sausage 1 slice cake 1 glass cola drink	12.30	1 slice cake tea with 2 sugars	1.00 pm	fish pie 1 glass cola drink
Afternoon	4.00 pm	fizzy drink chocolate bar 1 slice cake	4.30 pm 5.00 pm	ham 1 piece cake tea with 2 sugars 1 glass cola drink	3.00 pm	sausages, beans, toast. an orange 1 can cola drink	2.00 pm 4.30 pm 6.00 pm	tea with 2 sugars 1 biscuit 1 piece cake tea with 2 sugars bar of chocolate
Evening meal	6.00 pm	salad, garlic sausage, ham, coleslaw	7.30 pm	burger and chips 1 can of cola drink	8.00 pm	spaghetti bolognaise ice cream	9.00 pm	fish and chips, peas 1 cola drink
Evening	10.30 pm	sausages crisps 1 glass fizzy drink			9.30 pm	tea with 2 sugars		

Fig. 1.4 The patient's diet sheet.

Table 1.3 Dietary advice

Aims	Methods
Reduce the amount of sugar	Check manufacturers' labels and avoid foods with sugars such as sucrose, glucose and fructose listed early in the ingredients. Natural sugars (e.g. honey, brown sugar) are as cariogenic as purified or added sugars. When sweet foods are required, choose those containing sweetening agents such as saccharin, acesulfame-K and aspartame. Diet formulations contain less sugar than their standard counterparts. Reduce the sweetness of drinks and foods. Become accustomed to a less sweet diet overall.
Restrict frequency of sugar intakes to meal times as far as possible	Try to reduce snacking. When snacks are required select 'safe snacks' such as cheese, crisps, fruit or sugar-free sweets, such as mints or chewing gum (which not only has no sugar but also stimulates salivary flow and increases plaque pH). Use artificial sweeteners in drinks taken between meals.
Speed clearance of sugars from the mouth	Never finish meals with a sugary food or drink. Follow sugary foods with a sugar-free drink, chewing gum or a protective food such as cheese.

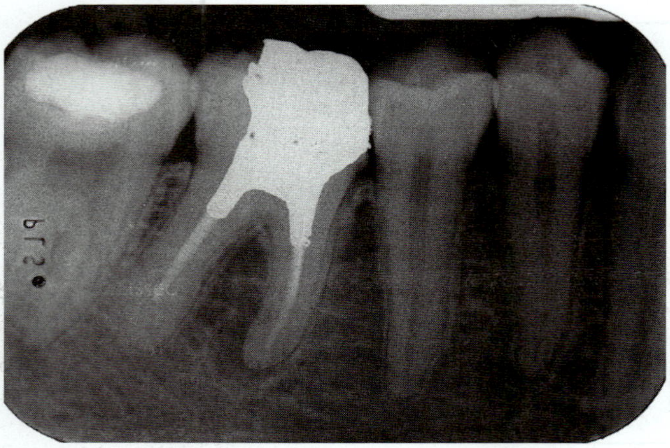

Fig. 1.5 Periapical radiograph of the restored lower first molar.

Why not simply extract the lower molar?

Extraction of the lower right first molar may well be the preferred treatment. The caries is extensive, restoration of the tooth will be complex and expensive and problems will probably ensue in the long term. The missing tooth might not be readily visible.

To a large degree the decision will depend on the patient's wishes. If he would be happy with an edentulous space, the extraction appears an attractive proposition. However, if a restoration is required, a bridge will require preparation of two further teeth. A denture-based replacement is probably not indicated but an implant might be considered at a later date. Any hesitancy or uncertainty on the patient's part might well influence you to propose extraction.

Another factor affecting the decision is the condition and long-term prognosis of the other molars. If further molars are likely to be lost in the short or medium term it makes sense to conserve whichever teeth can be successfully restored.

Case 2

A multilocular radiolucency

SUMMARY

A 45-year-old African man presents in the accident and emergency department with an enlarged jaw. You must make a diagnosis and decide on treatment.

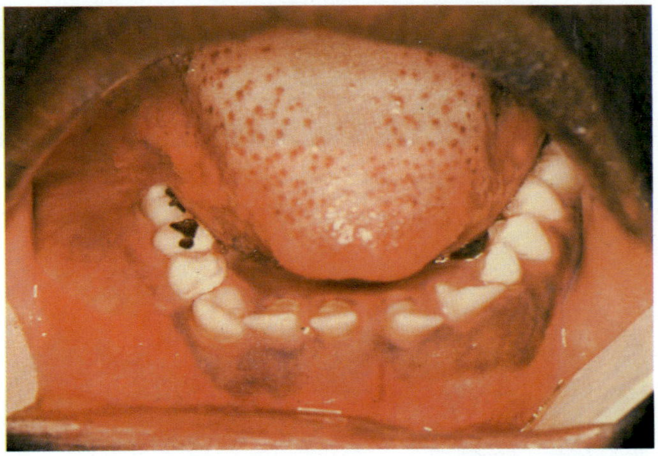

Fig. 2.1 The patient on presentation.

History

Complaint

The patient's main complaint is that his lower back teeth on the right side are loose and that his jaw on the right feels enlarged.

History of complaint

The patient has been aware of the teeth slowly becoming looser over the previous 6 months. They seem to be 'moving' and are now at a different height from his front teeth, making eating difficult. He is also concerned that his jaw is enlarged and there seems to be reduced space for his tongue. He has recently had the lower second molar on the right extracted. It was also loose but extraction does not seem to have cured the swelling. Although not in pain, he has finally decided to seek treatment.

Medical history

He is otherwise fit and healthy.

Examination

Extraoral examination

He is a fit-looking man with no obvious facial asymmetry but a slight fullness of the mandible on the right. Palpation reveals a smooth rounded bony hard enlargement on the buccal and lingual aspects. Deep cervical lymph nodes are palpable on the right side. They are only slightly enlarged, soft, not tender and freely mobile.

Intraoral examination

■ ***What do you see in Figure 2.1?***

There is a large swelling of the right posterior mandible visible in the buccal sulcus, its anterior margin relatively well defined and level with the first premolar. The lingual aspect is not visible but the tongue appears displaced upwards and medially suggesting significant lingual expansion. The mucosa over the swelling is of normal colour, without evidence of inflammation or infection. There are two relatively small amalgams in the lower right molar and second premolar

If you could examine the patient you would find that all his upper right posterior teeth are extracted and that the lower molar and premolars are 2–3 mm above the height of the occlusal plane. Both teeth are grade 3 mobile but both are vital.

■ ***What are the red spots on the patient's tongue?***

Fungiform papillae. They appear more prominent when the tongue is furred, as here, for instance when the diet is not very abrasive.

■ ***On the basis of what you know so far, what types of condition would you consider to be present?***

The history suggests a relatively slow-growing lesion, which is therefore likely to be benign. While this is not a definitive relationship, there are no specific features suggesting malignancy, such as perforation of the cortex, soft tissue mass, ulceration of the mucosa, numbness of the lip or devitalization of teeth. The character of the lymph node enlargement does not suggest malignancy.

The commonest jaw lesions that cause expansion are the odontogenic cysts. The commonest odontogenic cysts are the radicular (apical inflammatory) cyst, dentigerous cyst and odontogenic keratocyst. If this is a radicular cyst it could have arisen from the first molar, though the occlusal amalgam is relatively small and there seems no reason to suspect that the tooth is nonvital. A residual radicular cyst arising on the extracted second or third molar would be a possibility. A dentigerous cyst could be the cause if the third molar is unerupted. The possibility of an odontogenic keratocyst seems unlikely, because these cysts do not normally cause

Radiographic view	Reason
Panoramic radiograph or an oblique lateral	To show the lesion from the lateral aspect. The oblique lateral would provide the better resolution but might not cover the anterior extent of this large lesion. The panoramic radiograph would provide a useful survey of the rest of the jaws but only that part of this expansile lesion in the line of the arch will be in focus. An oblique lateral view was taken.
A posterior-anterior (PA) of the jaws	To show the extent of mediolateral expansion of the posterior body, angle or ramus.
A lower true (90°) occlusal	To show the lingual expansion which will not be visible in the PA jaws view because of superimposition of the anterior body of the mandible.
A periapical of the lower right second premolar and the first molar	To assess bone support and possible root resorption.

much expansion. An odontogenic tumour is a possible cause and an ameloblastoma would be the most likely one, because it is the commonest, and arises most frequently at this site and in this age group. There is a higher prevalence in Africans than other racial groups. An ameloblastoma is much more likely than an odontogenic cyst to displace the teeth and make them grossly mobile. A giant cell granuloma and numerous other lesions are possibilities but are all less likely.

Investigations

■ ***Radiographs are obviously indicated. Which views would you choose? Why?***

Several different views are necessary to show the full extent of the lesion. These are listed in the 'Radiographic view' table above.

■ ***These four different views are shown in Figures 2.2–2.5. Describe the radiographic features of the lesion (shown in 'Feature of lesion' table on p. 9).***

■ ***Why do the roots of the first molar and second premolar appear to be so resorbed in the periapical view when the oblique lateral view shows minimal root resorption?***

The teeth are foreshortened in the periapical view because they lie at an angle to the film. This film has been taken using the bisected angle technique and several factors contribute to the distortion:

- the teeth have been displaced by the lesion, so their crowns lie more lingually, and the roots more buccally;
- the lingual expansion of the jaw makes film packet placement difficult, so it has had to be severely tilted away from the root apices;
- failure to take account of these two factors when positioning and angling the X-ray tubehead.

Radiological differential diagnosis

■ ***What is your principal differential diagnosis?***

1. Ameloblastoma
2. Giant cell lesion.

■ ***Justify this differential diagnosis.***

Ameloblastoma classically produces an expanding multilocular radiolucency at the angle of the mandible.

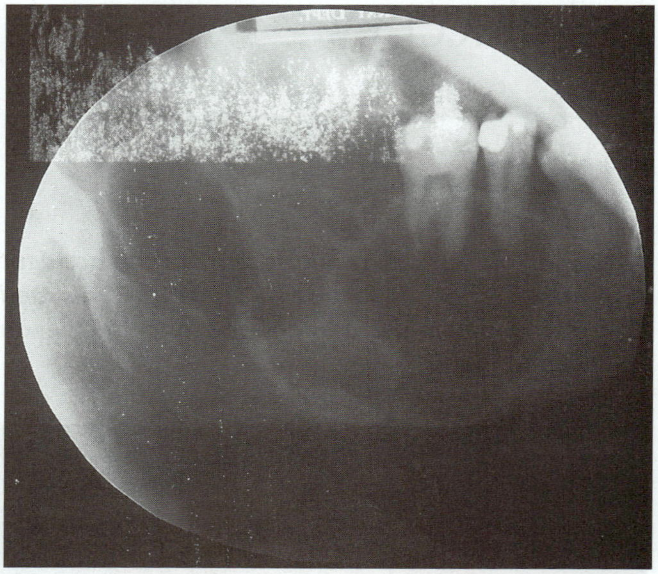

Fig. 2.2 Oblique lateral view.

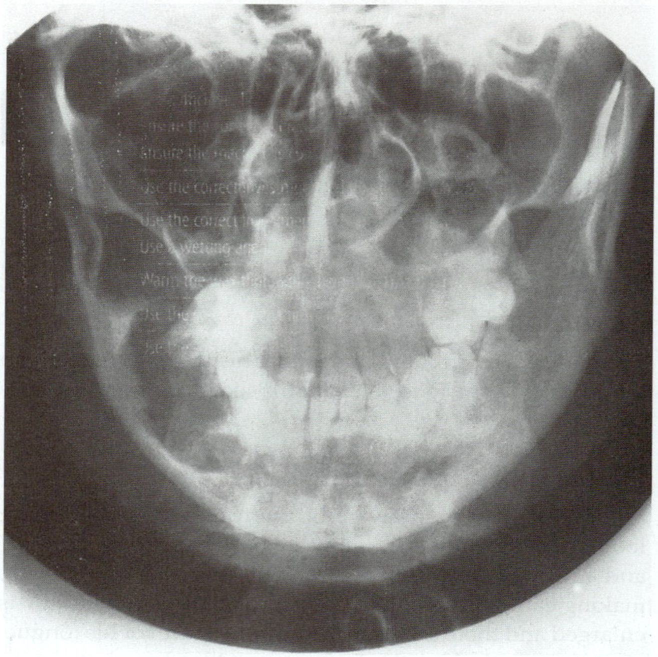

Fig. 2.3 Posterior-anterior view of the jaws.

Feature of lesion	Radiographic finding
Site	Posterior body, angle and ramus of the right mandible.
Size	Large, about 10 × 8 cm, extending from the second premolar, back to the angle and involving all of the ramus up to the sigmoid notch, and from the expanded upper border of the alveolar bone down to the inferior dental canal.
Shape	Multilocular, producing the *soap bubble* appearance.
Outline/edge	Smooth, well defined and mostly well corticated.
Relative radiodensity	Radiolucent with distinct radiopaque septa producing the multilocular appearance. There is no evidence of separate areas of calcification within the lesion.
Effects on adjacent structures	Gross lingual expansion of mandible, expansion buccally is only seen well in the occlusal films. Marked expansion of the superior margin of the alveolar bone and the anterior margin of the ascending ramus. The involved teeth have also been displaced superiorly. The roots of the involved teeth are slightly resorbed, but not as markedly as suggested by the periapical view. The cortex does not appear to be perforated.

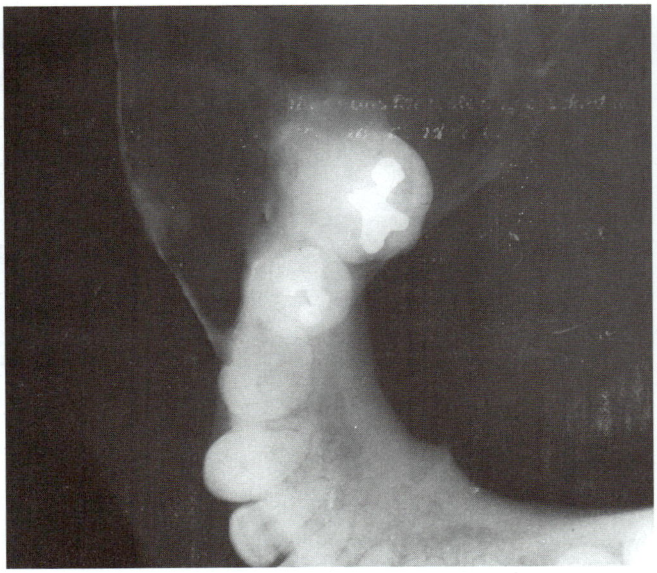

Fig. 2.4 Lower true occlusal view.

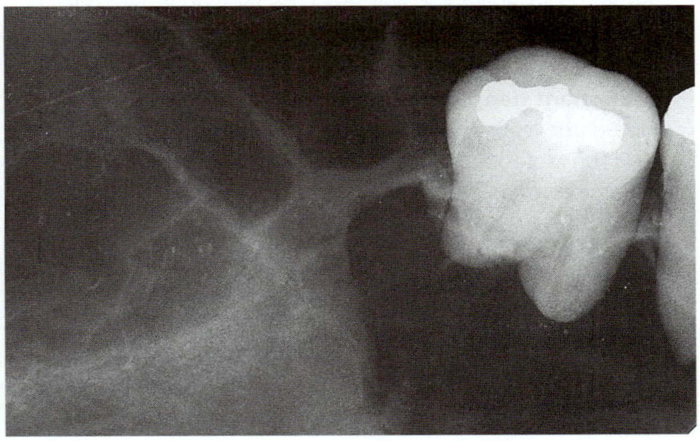

Fig. 2.5 Periapical view of the lower right first permanent molar.

As noted above, it most commonly presents at the age of this patient and is commoner in his racial group. The radiographs show the typical multilocular radiolucency, containing several large cystic spaces separated by bony septa, and the root resorption, tooth displacement and marked expansion are all consistent with an ameloblastoma of this size.

A giant cell lesion. A central giant cell granuloma is possible. Lesions can arise at almost any age but the radiological features and site are slightly different, making ameloblastoma the preferred diagnosis. Central giant cell granuloma produces expansion and a honeycomb or multilocular radiolucency, but there would be no root resorption and the lesion would be less radiolucent (because it consists of solid tissue rather than cystic neoplasm), often containing wispy osteoid or fine bone septa subdividing the lesion into a honeycomb-like pattern. However, these typical features are not always seen. The spectrum of radiological apearances ranges from lesions which mimic odontogenic and solitary bone cysts to those which appear identical to ameloblastoma or other odontogenic tumours. The aneurysmal bone cyst is another giant cell lesion which could produce this radiographic appearance with prominent expansion. Adjacent teeth are usually displaced but rarely resorbed. However, aneurysmal bone cyst is much rarer than central giant cell granuloma in the jaws.

What types of lesion are less likely and why?

Several lesions remain possible but are less likely either on the basis of their features or relative rarity.

Rarer odontogenic tumours including particularly odontogenic fibroma and myxoma. These similar benign connective tissue odontogenic tumours are often indistinguishable from one another radiographically. Odontogenic myxoma is commoner than fibroma but both are relegated to the position of unlikely diagnoses on the basis of their relative rarity and the younger age group affected. Both usually cause unilocular or apparently multilocular expansion radiolucency at the angle of the mandible that displace adjacent teeth or sometimes loosen or resorb them. A characteristic, though inconsistent feature is that the internal dividing septa are usually fine and arranged at right angles to one another, in a pattern sometimes said to resemble the letters 'X' and 'Y' or the strings of a tennis racket. In myxoma, septa can also show the bubbly *honeycomb* pattern described in giant cell granuloma.

Odontogenic keratocyst. This is unlikely to be the cause of this lesion but in view of its relative frequency it might still be included at the end of the differential diagnosis. It should be included because it can cause a large multilocular radiolucency at the angle of the mandible in adults, usually slightly younger than this patient. However, the growth pattern of an odontogenic keratocyst is quite different from the present lesion. Odontogenic keratocysts usually extend a considerable distance into the body and/or ramus before causing significant expansion. Even when expansion is evident, it is usually a broad-based enlargement rather than a localized expansion. Adjacent teeth are rarely resorbed or displaced.

What lesions have you discounted and why?

Dentigerous cyst is a common cause of large radiolucent lesions at the angle of the mandible. However, the present lesion is not unilocular and does not contain an unerupted tooth. Similarly, the **radicular cyst** is unilocular but associated with a nonvital tooth.

Malignant neoplasms, either primary or metastatic. As noted above, the clinical features do not suggest malignancy and the radiographs show an apparently benign, slowly enlarging lesion.

Further investigations

Is a biopsy required?

Yes. If the lesion is an ameloblastoma the treatment will be excision, whereas if it is a giant cell granuloma, curettage will be sufficient. A definitive diagnosis based on biopsy is required to plan treatment.

Would aspiration biopsy be helpful?

No. If odontogenic keratocyst were suspected, this diagnosis might be confirmed by aspirating keratin. It would also be helpful in trying to decide whether the lesion were solid or cystic. It would not be particularly helpful in the diagnosis of ameloblastoma.

What precautions would you take at biopsy?

An attempt should be made to obtain a sample of solid lesion. If this is an ameloblastoma and an expanded area of jaw is selected for biopsy it will almost certainly overlie a cyst in the neoplasm. A large part of many ameloblastomas is cyst space and the stretched cyst lining is not always sufficiently characteristic histologically to make the diagnosis. If the lesion proves to be cystic on biopsy, the surgeon should open up the cavity and explore it to identify solid tumour for sampling.

The surgical access must be carefully closed on bone to ensure that healing is uneventful and infection does not develop in the cyst spaces. The expanded areas may be covered by only a thin layer of *eggshell* periosteal bone. Once this is opened it may be difficult to replace the margin of a mucoperiosteal flap back onto solid bone.

The histological appearances of the biopsy are shown in Figures 2.6 and 2.7. What do you see?

The specimen is stained with haematoxylin and eosin. At low power the lesion is seen to consist of islands of epithelium separated by thin pink collagenous bands. Each island has a prominent outer layer of basal cells, a paler staining zone within that, and sometimes a pink keratinized zone of cells centrally. One of the islands shows early cyst formation (*c* shown in Figure 2.6). At higher power, the outer basal cell layer is seen to comprise elongate palisaded cells with reversed nuclear polarity (nuclei placed away from the basement membrane). Towards the basement membrane many of the cells have a clear cytoplasmic zone and the overall appearance looks like piano keys. Above the basal cell layer is a zone of very loosely packed stellate cells with large spaces between them. There is no inflammation.

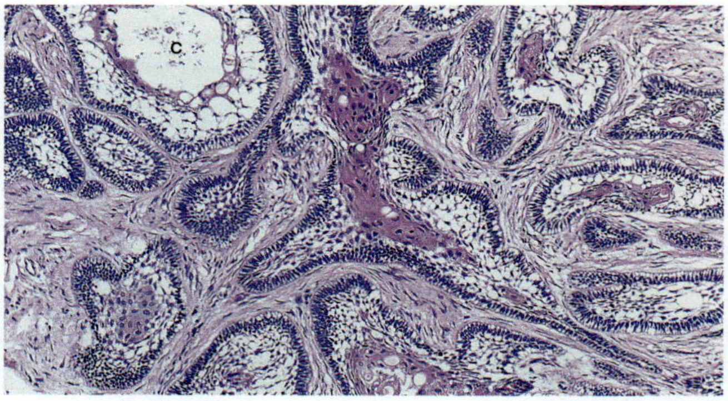

Fig. 2.6 Histological appearance of biopsy at low power.

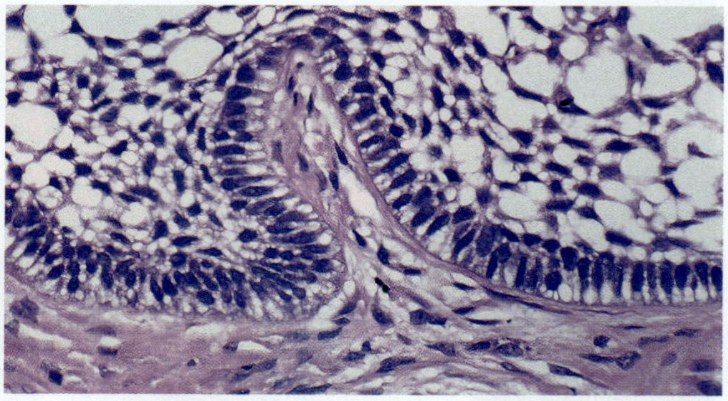

Fig. 2.7 Histological appearance of biopsy at high power.

How do you interpret these appearances?

The appearances are typical and diagnostic of ameloblastoma. The elongate basal cells bear a superficial resemblance to preameloblasts and the looser cells to stellate reticulum. The arrangement of the epithelium in islands with the stellate reticulum in their centres constitutes the follicular pattern of ameloblastoma.

Diagnosis

The final diagnosis is ameloblastoma, of the solid/multicystic type.

Does the type of ameloblastoma matter?

Yes, it is important for treatment. There are several different types of ameloblastoma and not all exhibit spread into the

Table 2.1 Types of ameloblastoma

Type	Features	Invades surrounding bone?
Solid/multicystic	The conventional and commonest type. Usually contains multiple cysts and has a multilocular radiographic appearance. Plexiform, follicular and mixed histological variants exist but have no bearing on behaviour or treatment.	Yes, in a quarter or less of cases
Unicystic	An ameloblastoma with only one cyst cavity and no separate islands of tumour, or just a few limited to the inner part of the fibrous wall. Presents radiographically as a cyst, sometimes in a dentigerous relationship. Can only be diagnosed definitively as a unicystic ameloblastoma by complete histological examination after treatment.	No
Desmoplastic	A rare variant with sparse islands of ameloblastoma dispersed in dense fibrous tissue. Radiographically forms a fine honeycomb radiolucency that may resemble a fibro-osseous lesion with a margin that is difficult to define. No large cysts are present. As frequent in the maxilla as in the mandible.	Yes, in most cases
Peripheral	A solid/multicystic ameloblastoma that develops as a soft tissue nodule outside bone, usually on the gingiva. Usually detected when small and readily excised. This variant is very rare.	No (the lesion is outside bone)

surrounding medullary cavity. Their characteristics are shown in table 2.1.

Treatment

What treatment will be required?

The ameloblastoma is classified as a benign neoplasm. However, it is locally infiltrative and in some cases permeates the medullary cavity around the main tumour margin. Ameloblastoma should be excised with a 1 cm margin of normal bone and around any suspected perforations in the cortex. If ameloblastoma has escaped from the medullary cavity, it may spread extensively in the soft tissues and requires excision with an even larger margin. The lower border of the mandible may be intact and is sometimes left in place to avoid the need for full thickness resection of the mandible and a bone graft. This causes a low risk of recurrence, but such recurrences are slow growing and may be dealt with conservatively after the main portion of the mandible has healed. The fact that the ameloblastoma is of the follicular pattern is of no significance for treatment.

What other imaging investigations would be appropriate for this patient?

In order to plan the resection accurately, the extent of the tumour and any cortical perforations must be identified. Cone beam computed tomography (CBCT, computed tomography (CT) and/or magnetic resonance imaging (MRI) would show the full extent of the lesion in bone and surrounding soft tissue respectively.

Case • 3

An unpleasant surprise

SUMMARY

A 30-year-old lady develops acute shortness of breath following administration of amoxicillin. What would you do?

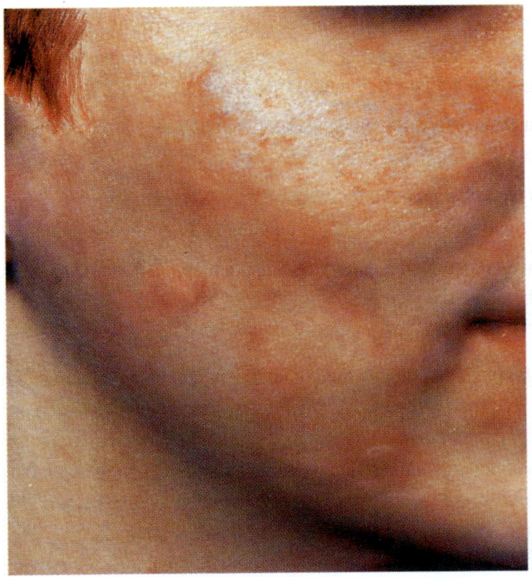

Fig. 3.1 The patient's face as she starts to feel unwell.

History

Complaint

The patient complains that she feels unwell, hot and breathless.

History of complaint

The patient has an appointment for routine dental treatment involving scaling and a restoration under local anaesthesia and antibiotic prophylaxis. She took a 3 g oral dose of amoxicillin 45 minutes ago.

Medical history

You checked the medical history before administering the amoxicillin and so you know that the patient is a well-controlled asthmatic taking salbutamol on occasions. She also suffers from eczema, as do her mother and her two children, and uses a topical steroid cream as required. The patient has had antibiotic cover before and refuses treatment without. See Case 44 for further discussion.

Dental history

The patient has been a regular attender for a number of years. She has had previous courses of penicillin from her general medical practitioner for chest infections.

■ ***What is the likely diagnosis?***

Anaphylaxis, arising from hypersensitivity to the amoxicillin.

Examination

■ ***The patient's face is shown in Figure 3.1. What do you see?***

There is patchy erythema. In the most inflamed areas there are well-defined raised oedematous weals, for instance at the corner of the mouth and on the side of the chin. This is a typical urticarial rash and indicates a type 1 hypersensitivity reaction.

■ ***What would you do immediately?***

- Reassure the patient.
- Assess the vital signs including blood pressure, pulse and respiratory rate.
- Lie the patient flat (as there is no difficulty breathing).
- Call for help.
- Obtain oxygen and your practice emergency drug box.

■ ***What are the signs and symptoms of anaphylaxis?***

The signs and symptoms vary with severity. The classical picture is of:

- a red urticarial rash
- oedema that may obstruct the airway
- hypotension due to reduced peripheral resistance
- hypovolaemia due to the movement of fluid out of the circulation into the tissues
- small airways obstruction caused by oedema and bronchospasm.

Involvement of nasal and ocular tissue may cause rhinitis and conjunctivitis. There may also be nausea and vomiting.

■ ***What does urticarial mean?***

The word urticarial comes from the Latin for nettle rash. An urticarial rash has superficial oedema that may form separate flat raised blister-like patches (as in Fig. 3.1) or be diffuse. In the head and neck it is often diffuse because the tissues are lax. Markedly oedematous areas may become pale by compression of their blood supply but the background is erythematous. Patients often know an urticarial rash by the lay term *hives*.

■ ***What is the pathogenesis of anaphylaxis?***

Anaphylaxis is an acute type 1 hypersensitivity reaction triggered in a sensitized individual by an allergen. The allergen enters the tissues and binds to immunoglobulin E (IgE) that is already bound to the surface of mast cells, present in almost all tissues. Binding of allergen to IgE induces degranulation and the release of large amounts of inflammatory mediators, particularly histamine. This causes the vasodilatation, increased capillary permeability and bronchospasm.

■ ***Type 1 hypersensitivity is also known as immediate hypersensitivity but onset was delayed for 45 minutes. Why?***

Acute anaphylactic reactions may occur within seconds or may be delayed for up to an hour depending on the nature of the allergen and the route of exposure. It takes time for an oral dose of antibiotic to be absorbed and pass through the circulation to the tissues, in this case 45 minutes. The reaction would be expected about 30 minutes after intramuscular administration of an allergen but almost instantaneously after intravascular administration. The time of onset is unpredictable. Some allergens such as peanuts and latex can cause rapid reactions despite being applied topically. The variability in onset of reactions explains why patients should be observed for an hour after administration of antibiotic cover.

On examining for the signs noted above you discover that the patient is breathless and a wheeze can be heard during both inspiration and expiration indicating small airways obstruction. She feels hot and has a pulse rate of 120 beats per minute and blood pressure of 120/80 mmHg. She is conscious but the effects are becoming more severe and the rash now affects all the face and neck region and has spread onto the upper aspect of the thorax. The appearance of one arm is shown in Figure 3.2.

Treatment

■ ***What treatment would you perform?***

Before the breathing problems were noted you correctly laid the patient flat. However, their lungs must now be raised above the rest of their body to prevent oedema fluid collecting in the lungs.

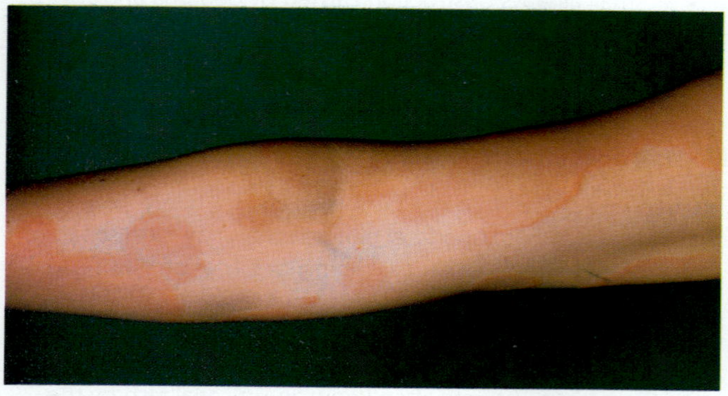

Fig. 3.2 The patient's arm 5 minutes later.

Allow the patient to adopt the most comfortable position for breathing and give oxygen (5 litres per minute) by facemask.

Because there is bronchospasm, give the following drugs in order:

Adrenaline (epinephrine) 1 : 1000, 500 micrograms intramuscularly. The easiest form to administer is a preloaded 'EpiPen' or 'Anapen', which are available for both adults (300 micrograms/dose) and children (150 micrograms/dose). Alternatively, a Min-I-Jet prepacked syringe and needle assembly or a standard vial of adrenaline solution, both containing 1 milligram in 1 millilitre (1 : 1000), may be used. However, both of these latter methods require a delay in administration to prepare the injection. You need to be familiar with whichever form is held in your practice as delay in calculating doses and volumes is clearly undesirable. Adrenaline (epinephrine) may also be given subcutaneously but the absorption is slower and this route is no longer recommended. Note that autoinjectors are designed for self-administration and so provide a slightly lower dose than is recommended. The recommended site for the intramuscular injection is the anterolateral aspect of the middle of the thigh, where there is most muscle bulk. If clothing prevents access, the upper lateral arm, into the deltoid muscle, is an alternative site. In an emergency it may be necessary to inject through clothing but this is not recommended. In the past the tongue has been proposed a potential site because it is familiar to dentists, but it is highly vascular allowing rapid uptake of drug and unlikely to be acceptable to the conscious patient.

Chlorphenamine (chlorpheniramine) 10 mg intravenously will counteract the effects of histamine.

Hydrocortisone 100–200 mg intravenously or intramuscularly.

Intravenous fluid. Only required if hypotension develops. A suitable regime would be 1 litre of normal saline infused over 5 minutes with continuous monitoring of the vital signs.

The last three actions require intravenous access and this may be difficult to achieve in an individual with reduced circulatory volume and hypotension. Finding and entering a collapsed vein is difficult even for the experienced and is best attempted as soon as adrenaline has taken effect. If necessary massage the arm towards the hand to try to inflate the vein. The importance of gaining venous access depends on circumstances. If medical or paramedical help is likely to arrive quickly, no more than adrenaline may be required. If not, these extra drugs may be important. Though the circulation may be maintained effectively by adrenaline, its action is short lived and you will only have a limited number of doses available. It is probably worthwhile inserting a Venflon-type intravenous cannula or at least a butterfly needle for any patient that develops difficulty breathing. If the reaction becomes more severe, it may be more difficult to insert later.

The presentation of drugs useful for anaphylaxis is shown in Figure 3.3.

■ ***Why must the drugs be given in this order?***

Adrenaline is the life-saving drug and must be given straight away, before circulatory collapse. It is rapidly acting.

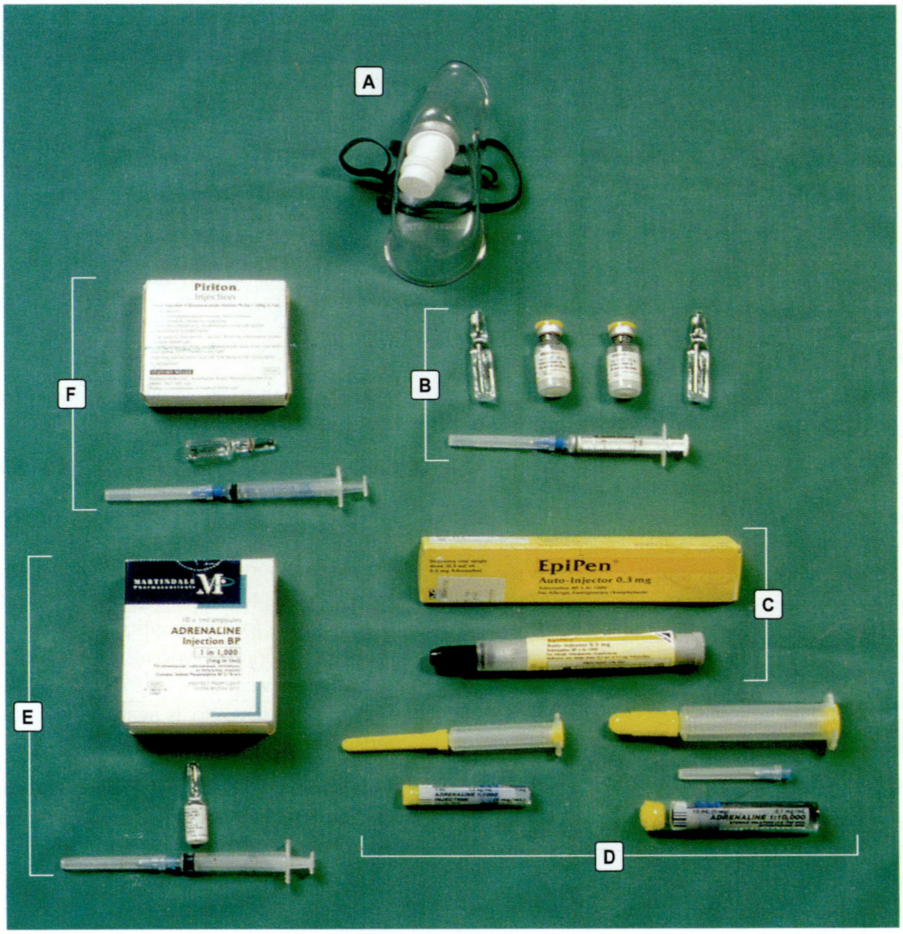

Fig. 3.3 Typical presentations of drugs used to treat anaphylaxis.

A. Oxygen mask.

B. Hydrocortisone. Vials of lyophilised powder for reconstitution in water for injection, NOT saline. Administer with a conventional syringe and needle.

C. Adrenaline* in an Epipen disposable autoinjector spring-loaded syringe, boxed, and below with the plastic covers removed from each end. Press directly onto the skin and the spring-loaded needle is unsheathed and the drug is injected automatically. A similar device, the Anapen, has a spring-loaded needle that springs out when a button at the opposite end is pressed. Both deliver 300 micrograms of adrenaline.

D. Adrenaline in Min-I-Jet format. The yellow plastic cover is removed from the back (right hand end) of the syringe barrel and front of the glass cartridge and the cartridge is screwed into the syringe barrel. Available in two types, with needle fitted (left, recommended) and with luer lock fitting for a conventional needle (slower to use). After removing front cover and fitting needle, if required, use as a conventional syringe. Versions with finer needles for subcutaneous administration are available but the intramuscular route is preferred and the version with the larger 21 gauge needle should be used.

E. Adrenaline as traditional ampoule, ready to inject with a conventional syringe.

F. Chlorpheniramine as traditional ampoule, ready to inject with a conventional syringe.

**Note that epinephrine is now the recommended name for adrenaline internationally but that adrenaline is still the most widely used name in the UK.*

Chlorphenamine (chlorpheniramine) is less potent and slower acting and cannot alone counteract pulmonary oedema or bronchospasm, which indicate a severe reaction. Hydrocortisone is the lowest priority; it takes up to 6 hours to act and is not immediately life saving.

■ *After giving all three drugs, the patient recovers. What would you do next?*

- Abandon dental treatment.
- Continue to monitor the vital signs.
- Continue to administer oxygen.
- Arrange transfer of the patient to an appropriate secondary care facility.
- Advise the patient of the need for formal investigation of their probable allergy.

■ *Can you relax now the immediate crisis is over?*

No, definitely not. The response of the patient needs to be closely observed. Adrenaline (epinephrine) is highly effective but has a very short half-life. Recurrence of bronchospasm, a drop in blood pressure or worsening oedema indicates a need for further adrenaline (epinephrine). This is likely to be needed about 5 minutes after the previous administration and it can be repeated again as often as necessary. However, the chlorphenamine (chlorpheniramine) will start to become effective and no more than two doses of adrenaline (epinephrine) should be necessary.

Late relapse, hours later, is also possible. Mast cells also release other potent inflammatory mediators and some have long half-lives. The hydrocortisone prevents this late relapse.

■ ***Can an anaphylactic reaction be controlled without adrenaline (epinephrine)?***

If the only features are a rash and mild swelling not involving the airway it may be appropriate to give chlorphenamine (chlorpheniramine) and hydrocortisone in the first instance and observe the response. However, if bronchospasm, hypotension or oedema around the airway develops, adrenaline (epinephrine) will be needed. Adrenaline (epinephrine) should be administered as early as possible to be effective and it is better not to delay unless the signs and symptoms are very mild.

Further points

■ ***Why is adrenaline (epinephrine) effective?***

Adrenaline (epinephrine) is the prototypical adrenergic agonist and has both alpha and beta receptor activity. Alpha receptor-mediated action on arterioles causes vasoconstriction and thus reverses oedema. Beta receptor-mediated actions include increasing the cardiac output by increasing the force of contraction and heart rate (beta 1) and bronchodilatation (beta 2). Mast cell degranulation is also suppressed.

■ ***Why was this patient at high risk of anaphylaxis?***

She has a history of asthma and a family history of eczema. This indicates atopy and an increased risk of developing hypersensitivity to a wide range of substances. It is important to take a thorough allergy history, particularly regarding drugs, rubber and other dental materials in all patients. No patient should be exposed to a possible allergen until you have sought advice.

■ ***Why had this patient no history of allergy to penicillin?***

The patient may have been sensitized by the previous courses of penicillins. This underlines the unpredictability of allergic reactions. Patients who have been administered any medication should be monitored for an appropriate time in case of acute adverse effects, the period depending on the route of administration (see above).

■ ***How can penicillin allergy develop in patients who have never taken penicillins?***

It is thought that sensitization may also develop in response to very small quantities of penicillins in the environment. Veterinary uses of penicillins leave residues in meat and milk, and these may pass to babies via their mother's milk. Penicillins are ubiquitous and there is probably a genetic predisposition to explain why only a few individuals develop hypersensitivity.

Table 3.1 Emergency drugs

Drug	Dose
Glyceryl trinitrate spray	400 micrograms/dose
Salbutamol aerosol inhaler	100 micrograms/puff
Adrenaline injection	1 : 1000 1 mg/ml
Aspirin dispersible	300 mg
Glucagon injection	1 mg
Oral glucose solution	Gel, tablets or powder
Midazolam	5 mg/ml or 10 mg/ml
Oxygen	

■ ***Can patients be tested for penicillin allergy?***

Yes, but it carries a risk of anaphylaxis and must be performed with care in a specialized centre. Only 10–20% of patients who report penicillin allergy are actually hypersensitive but not all can be tested. It is recommended that testing be reserved only for those who give a convincing history of a type 1 reaction and who also have a definite requirement for penicillin. In most cases a safe alternative antibiotic, for example clindamycin, is available and so testing is not performed.

■ ***Why is there no corticosteroid or antihistamine in my dental emergency drugs box; it is claimed to contain the recommended drugs?***

The Resuscitation Council UK has published guidance on medical emergencies and resuscitation, revised in May 2008. Their recommendations have been endorsed by the General Dental Council. They state that the emergency drugs listed in Table 3.1 should be available in all dental surgeries in the UK:

Of the drugs recommended for this case, only oxygen and adrenaline are included. The guidance specifically notes that antihistamines and corticosteroids are not first line drugs for treatment of anaphylaxis. As noted above, this is true, but this drug box is a minimum specification for general practice only. Much more diverse emergency drug boxes are used by those working in hospitals, health clinics and some specialist practices, where dentists may be trained in advanced trauma life support (ATLS) or have other specialist skills through their involvement with conscious sedation or special care dentistry.

The list must also be modified to circumstances. In remote areas where medical help may be delayed, it will be essential to have these additional drugs for longer term treatment and also for the dentist to be able to gain venous access. These drugs and skills should be within the remit and capabilities of any dental practitioner.

Dentists must be familiar with the actions and effects of drugs they may need to use, so it is the dentist's responsibility to ensure that they are properly informed about any additional drugs they elect to hold. The General Dental Council also provides guidance that every practice should have two people available and trained in medical emergencies whenever treatment is being carried out. All the dental team must practice simulated emergencies together on a regular basis.

Other possibilities

■ ***If you discovered that you had just administered a penicillin orally to a patient known to be allergic to penicillins, what would you do?***

Absorption of only a very small amount of the penicillin is needed to trigger an allergic response so there is no point in thinking that inducing vomiting would be helpful. The best thing to do would be to administer the chlorphenamine (chlorpheniramine) and steroid immediately, prepare the adrenaline (epinephrine) and oxygen and administer the adrenaline (epinephrine) immediately any signs begin to develop. The patient would still have to seek medical care as soon as possible because the late phases of the reaction might still develop even if the immediate phases were prevented.

■ ***Suppose the patient had been a child?***

Allergy in children is usually triggered by dietary allergens rather than drugs but latex allergy is possible and children with frequent medical exposure to latex, as in catheters, are at risk. Doses of adrenaline are reduced to 250 micrograms for ages 6–12 years and 120 micrograms for ages 6 months to 6 years. Giving these doses might prove difficult if you do not have specific paediatric formulations in your emergency drug kit. Autoinjectors provide 300 or 150 micrograms and Min-I-Jet devices are designed to give a full adult dose. Children with severe allergies may carry autoinjection devices with the correct paediatric dose and should be asked to bring them when they attend for dental treatment.

Case • 4

Gingival recession

SUMMARY

A 30-year-old woman has gingival recession. Assess her condition and discuss treatment options.

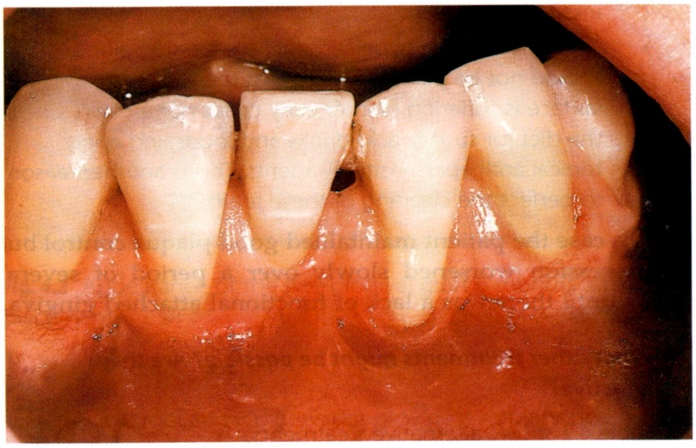

Fig. 4.1 The appearance of the lower incisors.

History

Complaint

The patient is worried about the gingival recession around her lower front teeth, which she feels is worsening.

History of complaint

She remembers noticing the recession for at least the previous 5 years. She thinks it has worsened over the last 12 months. There has recently been some sensitivity to hot and cold and gingival soreness, most noticeably on toothbrushing or eating ice cream.

Dental history

The patient has been a patient of your practice for about 10 years and you have discussed her recession at previous visits and reassured her. She has a low caries rate and generally good oral hygiene.

Medical history

She is a fit and healthy individual and is not a smoker.

■ ***What further specific questions would you ask to help identify a possible cause?***

How often do you brush your teeth? Provided brushing is effective, cleaning once a day is sufficient to maintain gingival health. However, most patients clean two or three times each day and some brush excessively in terms of frequency, duration and force used. Trauma from brushing is considered a factor in some patients' recession, and recession may indicate a need to reduce the frequency and duration of cleaning while maintaining its effectiveness. In this instance the patient has a normal toothbrushing habit but should clean no more than twice each day and for a sensible period of time.

Have you had orthodontic treatment? A lower incisor is missing, suggesting that some intervention may have taken place. Fixed orthodontics in the lower labial segment is occasionally associated with gingival recession in patients with thin buccal gingiva, narrow alveolar processes and correction of severe crowding. Plaque control may be compromised during the wearing of an orthodontic appliance and, even over a relatively short period, this can contribute to the problem. In this instance the patient had undergone extraction of the incisor but had not worn an appliance.

Examination

Intraoral examination

■ ***The appearance of the lower incisors is shown in Figure 4.1. What do you see?***

- Missing lower left central incisor.
- Unrestored teeth.
- No plaque is visible except for a small amount at the cervical margin of the lower left lateral incisor.
- Gingival recession affecting all lower incisors and, to a lesser extent, the lower canines.
- Apart from the abnormal contour, the buccal gingivae are pink and healthy and the interdental papillae are normal.
- Reduction in width of keratinized (cornified) attached gingival epithelium. In places, attached gingiva appears absent.

■ ***What clinical assessments would you make, how would you make them and why are they important?***

See Table 4.1.

On performing these clinical examinations you find that all probing depths are 1–2 mm with no bleeding. The width of keratinized gingiva varies with the degree of recession. The lower left lateral incisor has no attached gingiva and tension on the lip displaces the gingival margin. No teeth have increased mobility and no possible occlusal factors are present. There is no reason to suspect loss of vitality and all teeth respond to testing.

Case • 5

A missing incisor

SUMMARY

A 9-year-old boy is referred to you in the orthodontic department with an unerupted upper left central incisor. What is the cause and how may it be treated?

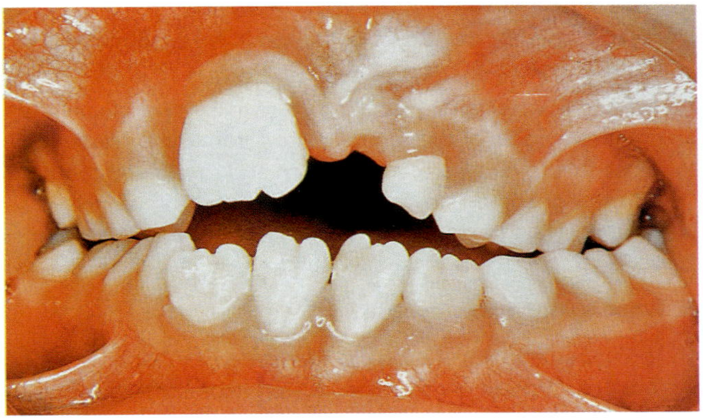

Fig. 5.1 The appearance of the patient on presentation.

History

Complaint

The patient's upper left central incisor has not erupted although he is 9 years old. The mother is very concerned about her son's appearance and is anxious for him to be treated.

History of complaint

The upper left deciduous predecessor had been present until about 4 months ago. It was extracted by the patient's general dental practitioner in an attempt to speed up the eruption of the permanent successor. Despite this, there has been no change in appearance. The upper permanent central incisor on the opposite side erupted normally at 7 years of age.

Medical history

The patient has suffered from asthma since he was 4 years old. This is controlled using salbutamol (Ventolin).

Examination

Extraoral examination

There are no extraoral signs or symptoms and the patient is an active, happy boy.

Intraoral examination

■ ***The appearance of the mouth is shown in Figure 5.1. What do you see?***

The patient is in the early mixed dentition stage and the teeth present are:

6EDCB1	BCDE6
6EDC21	12DE6

No upper left central incisor is present, but there is a pale swelling high in the upper labial sulcus above the edentulous space and the upper left B. There has been some loss of space in the region of the absent upper central incisor.

There is a tendency to an anterior open bite which is slightly more pronounced on the right.

There is mild upper and lower arch crowding and a unilateral crossbite on the left. If you were able to examine the patient you would discover that this is associated with a lateral displacement of the mandibular position. The lower centre line is shifted to the left.

There are no restorations but the mouth is not very clean.

■ ***What are the possible causes of an apparently absent upper central incisor?***

The incisor may be missing or have failed to erupt. Possible causes include the following:

Missing	Developmentally absent Extracted Avulsed
Failure to erupt	Dilaceration and/or displacement as a result of trauma Scar tissue preventing eruption Supernumerary tooth preventing eruption Insufficient space as a result of crowding Pathological lesion (e.g. cyst or odontogenic tumour)

■ ***What specific questions would you ask the parents?***

The most important questions are related to trauma. Avulsion or dilaceration would follow significant trauma which is likely to be recalled by the parent. The parent should be asked whether the deciduous predecessor was discoloured. If it was this would provide evidence of loss of vitality, perhaps related to trauma.

Extraction would be unusual and a cause should be readily obtained in the history.

In response to your questioning the parent reports that the patient fell on his face when he was much younger. At the time of the accident there was considerable injury to his lips and teeth, but no tooth loss was noticed and no dental opinion was sought.

■ *What are the likely causes of the anterior open bite and shift in the lower centre line?*

The anterior open bite is probably associated with a thumb-sucking or similar habit. The shift in the centre line is probably caused by the combination of crowding and early exfoliation of the lower left C.

■ *Give a differential diagnosis for the cause of the missing incisor. Explain each possibility.*

Dilaceration of the central incisor as a result of the injury appears the most likely cause. However, it is unclear whether the injury was severe enough to cause dilaceration. Dilaceration usually follows intrusion and the intruded tooth might well have re-erupted into its normal position. The swelling in the sulcus does not lie on the normal eruption path of the central incisor, and dilaceration could explain the abnormal position.

A supernumerary tooth or an odontome would be the next most likely possibility if trauma is not the cause. Supernumerary teeth are not uncommon in the premaxilla (1–3% of the population), and the late-forming (tuberculate) type which often lies adjacent to the crown of the permanent incisor frequently causes delay or failure of eruption.

A pathological lesion appears unlikely but cannot be excluded. There is no evidence of alveolar expansion to suggest a cyst, which would be the most likely cause and could arise from the tooth itself, a supernumerary or an odontome. An unexpected lesion remains a remote possibility.

■ *What causes have you excluded and why?*

Crowding appears to be an unlikely cause. It would have to be very severe to cause a delay of up to 2 years and this patient's teeth are only mildly crowded. Crowding is a very unusual cause for failure of eruption of a central incisor because resorption and loss of the B would provide enough space for eruption.

Scarring of the alveolus delays eruption because it slows resorption of bone over the tooth and because fibrosis and thickening of the mucoperiosteum resists tooth movement. This is an unlikely cause because there is no reason to suspect scarring, the deciduous predecessor having been extracted only 4 months ago.

Avulsion can be excluded because it seems that the tooth has never erupted and there is no recent history of trauma.

Developmental causes of absence appear most unlikely. The swelling in the upper sulcus would seem to indicate that the tooth is present but has failed to erupt. A missing central incisor without other missing teeth would be an extremely rare finding.

Investigations

Radiographs are required to determine whether or not the unerupted tooth is present, to establish whether it is the cause of the swelling in the sulcus and detect possible supernumerary teeth.

■ *What radiographic views would you request and why?*

See Table 5.1.

The radiographs of the patient are shown in Figures 5.2–5.4.

■ *What do the radiographs show?*

The panoramic radiograph confirms the presence of a full complement of developing permanent successors, excluding the third molars, which would not be expected to have formed. However, a crypt should be present between the ages of $8^1/_2$ and 10 years of age and there is a suggestion of early crypt formation in the lower left quadrant. The unerupted permanent upper left central incisor is clearly visible on this radiograph; its shape is not normal but the root shape cannot be seen in this view. It is not possible to establish the labiopalatal position of the tooth in this film nor to detect an adjacent supernumerary tooth which may lie outside the tomographic focal trough.

The periapical view gives considerably more detail. The upper left central incisor has an intact but distorted root. Its apical development appears normal and similar to that of the right central incisor but the foreshortened appearance suggests dilaceration. Using this film in conjunction with the panoramic view and applying the principle of vertical parallax you can see that the crown of the central incisor is labially positioned. This is consistent with the swelling in the sulcus being caused by the crown of the tooth. No supernumerary tooth is present.

The lateral view completes the picture and shows clearly the displaced crown of the central incisor. From the three films it is possible to deduce that the crown and root of the tooth are misaligned, the crown deflected labially with its incisal edge pointing forwards into the labial sulcus and the root developing in the normal direction.

■ *What is your final diagnosis?*

The upper left central incisor is dilacerated, probably as a result of intrusion of the deciduous predecessor in the injury sustained in infancy.

Treatment

■ *What are the options for treatment?*

If the dilaceration were severe, the tooth would require extraction. Then either of the following options could be selected:

1. Align the adjacent teeth, ideally with fixed appliances, using the central incisor space. The lateral incisor would replace the central incisor and could be masked to simulate it. In the short term this could be accomplished by an adhesive restoration but in the longer term a permanent restoration would be necessary. The canine might also need restoration or masking so that it would not appear incongruous, especially in a patient with slender lateral incisors. This option is not ideal because the final appearance is often poor.

Table 5.1 Radiographic views and their purposes

View	Reason
Dental panoramic radiograph	To provide a general view of the developing dentition and establish the presence or absence of the permanent teeth and any supernumeraries.
Upper standard occlusal or periapicals of the edentulous area, taken with a paralleling technique	To provide a more detailed view of the region, in particular the root morphology and any adjacent structures such as supernumerary teeth or pathological lesions. These may lie outside the focal trough of the radiograph or be obscured by superimposition of other structures in the panoramic view. If periapical views are taken they should include the adjacent teeth in case these were damaged in the original accident. In addition the standard occlusal and panoramic view can be used together to establish the relationship of unerupted structures relative to the dental arch, using the principle of (vertical) parallax. Objects lying nearer to the X-ray tube (labially positioned) appear to move in the opposite direction to the tube relative to a fixed point. Those further away (palatally positioned) appear to move in the same direction as the tube.
Lateral view	Confirms the presence of any distortion of the tooth, if dilacerated, and confirms the relationship of the tooth to the labial swelling in a third dimension.

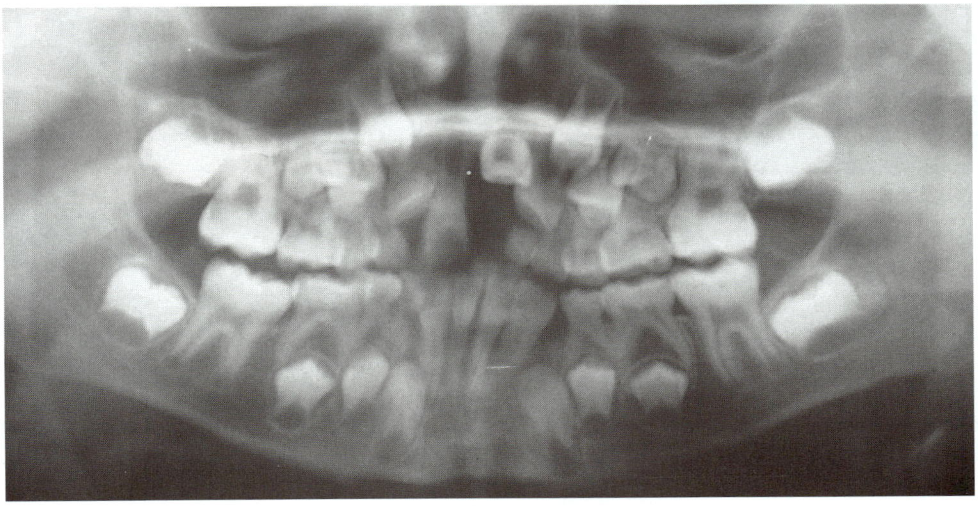

Fig. 5.2 Dental panoramic radiograph.

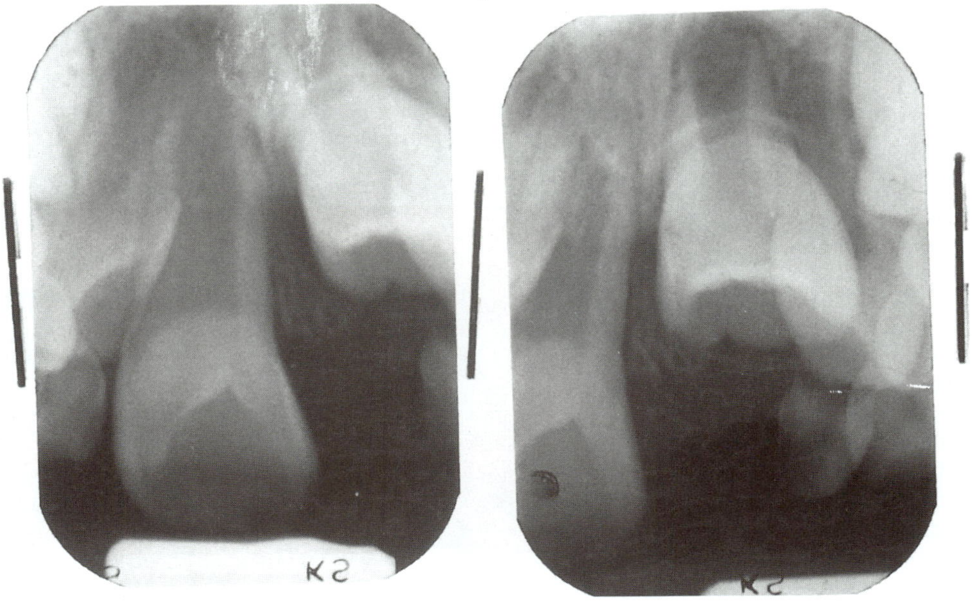

Fig. 5.3 Periapical views.

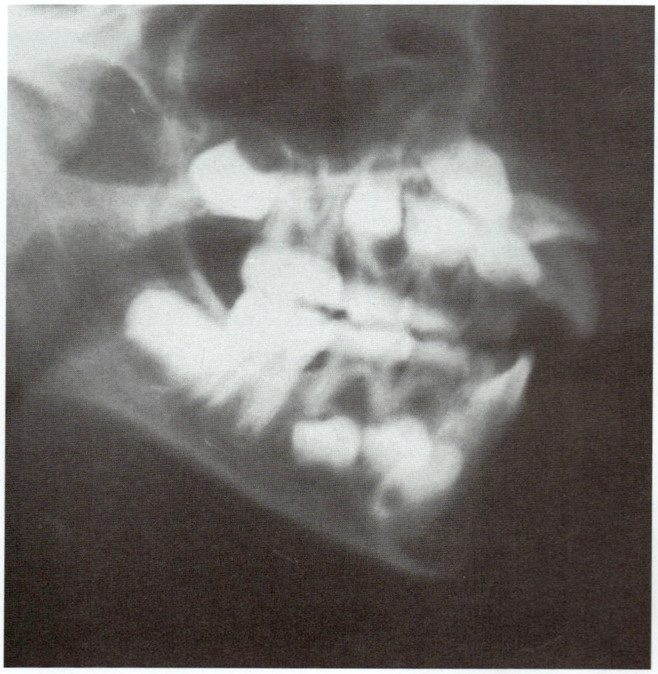

Fig. 5.4 Lateral view.

2. Immediate replacement of the extracted central incisor by a denture or adhesive bridge with a permanent restoration or possibly a single tooth implant in adulthood (see Case 35).

If, on the radiographs, the dilaceration does not appear to be too severe or lies in the apical portion of the root, consideration could be given to aligning the tooth orthodontically. This would involve regaining any lost space followed by localized surgical exposure of the crown of the tooth and applying extrusive traction with an orthodontic appliance.

■ *What factors affect the selection of a particular treatment?*

- Position and severity of the dilaceration (see above)
- The size of overjet
- Degree of crowding
- Position and condition of the other permanent teeth
- The general condition of the mouth
- The attitude of the child and parent

■ *Assuming none of these factors prevents the ideal treatment, what would you recommend for this case?*

In this case the ideal treatment is to extrude and align the dilacerated tooth into the arch.

The dilaceration appears to be in the root and relatively mild. Therefore, an attempt should first be made to regain the lost space to accommodate the central incisor crown. This would be best achieved by extraction of both upper Cs and the upper left B to encourage eruption of permanent lateral incisors. Some months later the dilacerated tooth should be surgically exposed and an orthodontic attachment with a length of gold chain placed on its palatal surface for extrusion.

■ *Should a fixed or removable appliance be used?*

As the tooth movements are relatively simple an upper removable appliance can be used at this stage. More control and more accurate tooth positioning would be achieved with a fixed appliance. However, the patient will probably require further fixed appliance treatment at a later age and the fine adjustment of tooth position could be performed then.

■ *Design a suitable removable appliance.*

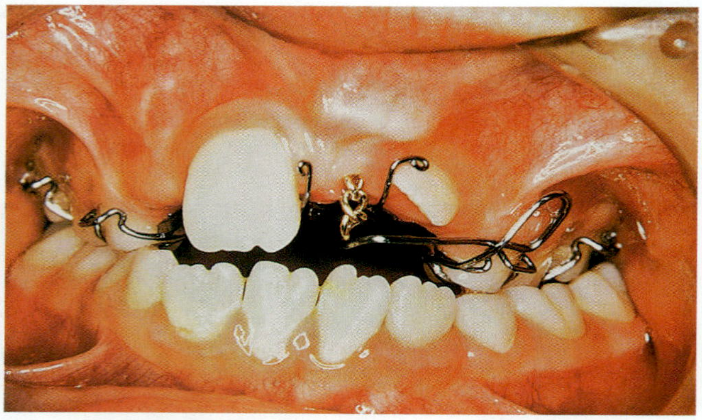

Fig. 5.5 The fitted extrusion appliance.

The appliance consists of:

- — cribs on D | D (0.6-mm wire)
- — cribs on 6 | 6 (0.7-mm wire)
- — finger springs on 1| and |2 (0.5-mm wire) to retract and regain the space for the |1
- — a buccal arm to extrude |1 (0.7-mm wire) attached to the gold chain bonded to |1

■ *Figure 5.6 shows the position of the dilacerated tooth after approximately 18 months of active treatment. What further treatment may be necessary at a later stage of dental development?*

Ideally it would be appropriate to relieve the crowding in the permanent dentition and align the teeth, correcting the unilateral posterior crossbite and eliminating the mandibular displacement. Details of appropriate treatment cannot be finalized until the patient passes from mixed dentition to permanent dentition at about 10–12 years of age.

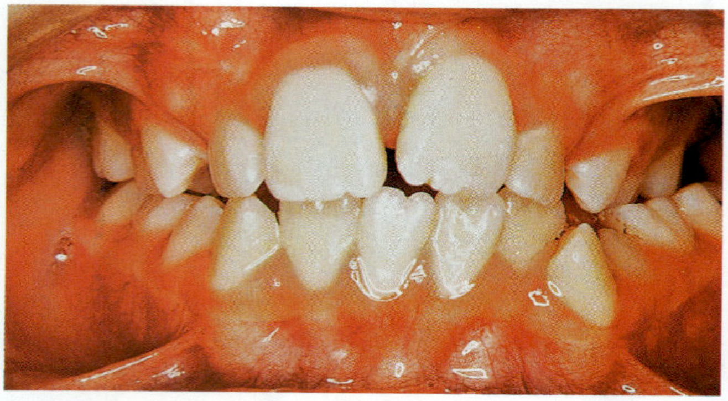

Fig. 5.6 After 18 months of treatment.

Case 6

Down's syndrome

SUMMARY

A 40-year-old male patient presents to you in your dental surgery with a loose tooth. What is the cause and what will you do?

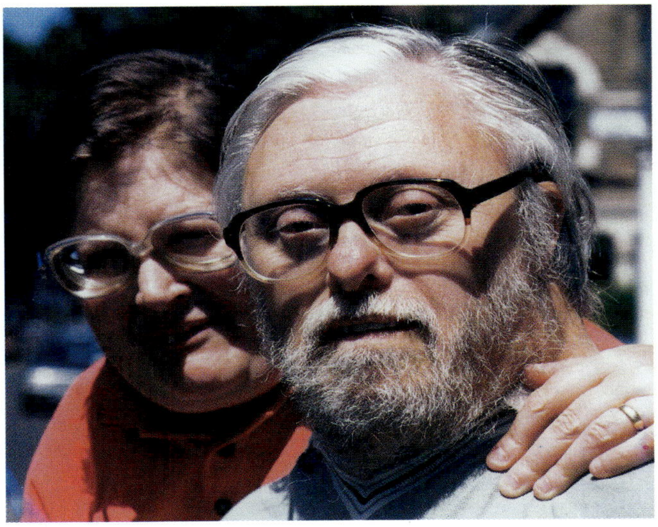

Fig. 6.1 The patient on presentation.

History

Complaint

The patient has been complaining of a sore, loose lower back tooth for 1 week. It is particularly sore when eating and the patient often flinches whilst chewing.

History of complaint

There were no recent symptoms from this tooth until 1 week ago. When the pain started, the patient's mother noticed that he stopped bruxing.

Dental history

He has been seen in your practice for several years and attends with his mother on most occasions (Figure 6.1).

You have been monitoring his periodontitis for many years. The patient achieves a moderate degree of oral hygiene but cleaning posteriorly is always suboptimal. He has had a series of episodes of acute symptoms from this tooth but has always refused to let you extract it.

Medical history

The patient has Down's syndrome. He has a patent ventriculoseptal defect that is unrepaired and a mild to moderate learning disability. He reports recurrent upper respiratory tract infections.

Social history

The patient lives at home with his parents and works part-time in a supermarket. He does not smoke or drink any alcohol.

■ ***What are the causes of Down's syndrome?***

Down's syndrome is caused by complete or partial trisomy of chromosome 21. The majority of patients have a complete third copy of the chromosome, but there are several different ways in which cells can acquire additional chromosome 21 DNA. This is important because not all individuals with Down's syndrome have a similar phenotype. The types of trisomy 21 are explained in Table 6.1.

■ ***How does this cause the condition?***

The long arm of chromosome 21 includes a region called the Down syndrome critical region. Genes at this site encode transcription factors that control development, including that of the brain. An increase in copy number of genes in this region is thought to account for most of the neurological and facial, and possibly other, features of Down's syndrome. Other genes have been identified for leukaemia and other complications.

■ ***What is the risk of having a child with Down's syndrome?***

Because most cases are caused by chromosomal non-disjunction during egg formation, the risk is linked to *maternal* age. The risk rises markedly after 40 years. The risk in a mother aged 30 is approximately 1 in 1000 but this rises to almost 1 in 100 at age 40 years and higher after that.

Prenatal screening relies on a variety of tests, including ultrasound screening. The most accurate tests require amniocentesis and are reserved for those at the highest risk. The newest tests promise accurate diagnosis on the basis of a blood test. The combination of prenatal testing and termination of pregnancy has resulted in falling incidence in many parts of the world. This is somewhat compensated for by a generalized increase in maternal age and greater life expectancy for those affected.

Two-thirds of affected fetuses die during normal development and the frequency of trisomy 21 in the population is 1 in 650–1000 live births.

Table 6.1 Types and causes of Down's syndrome

Type of trisomy	% of patients	Cause	Significance
Free trisomy Down's syndrome	95%	A 'free' third copy of chromosome 21 in every cell. Meiotic non-disjunction (failure of chromosomes or chromatids to separate during cell division) in development of the egg (95%) or sperm (5%) results in gametes with an extra copy of chromosome 21. After fertilization and embryogenesis, every cell carries a copy of the third chromosome	Commonest type. Not inherited
Translocation Down's syndrome	2%	One copy is translocated to another chromosome, most often chromosome 14 or 21, in a cell division during development of the egg, or occasionally sperm. Sometimes the translocation affects only the child. Occasionally the translocation is stable and can be passed from generation to generation	About half of cases have a familial pattern of inheritance
Mosaic Down's syndrome	2%	Patients are a mosaic of normal cells and cells with trisomy 21. The gametes are normal but non-disjunction during a somatic division in embryogenesis gives some cells trisomy. If the trisomy arises early a large proportion of the patient's cells are affected; if late, fewer are affected	The features vary depending on which cells are affected. Some patients may be of Down's appearance but normal intelligence or vice versa, and the features are often mild. Not inherited
Other types	1%	Caused by a variety of different chromosomal rearrangements involving chromosome 21	

■ ***The patient has 'mild to moderate learning difficulty'. What does this mean?***

A wide range of terms may be used to describe intellectual ability. Terms such as mental retardation, intellectual impairment and mental subnormality are no longer used in the UK, though they are considered acceptable in other cultures. Learning difficulty and learning disability are considered synonymous in the UK. Mental incapacity is a legal term used to describe ability to make informed decisions. It relates to intellectual ability but is not the same as learning difficulty.

Learning difficulty is defined as a significant impairment of intelligence and social functioning acquired before adulthood. The definitions are from the Education Act 1996 and the Special Educational Needs and Disability Act 2001 that define the educational needs and aid the individual in gaining access to legal protections and rights.

Learning difficulty is usually divided into mild, moderate and severe, but these definitions are not always helpful in health care because they are based on analysis of social functioning as well as psychometric testing. The categories do not correlate directly with intelligence, though they are often equated, as shown in Table 6.2.

The majority of individuals with Down's syndrome have mild to moderate learning difficulty. Regardless of learning difficulty, all those with Down's syndrome will require lifelong help with accommodation and supportive working. Some can lead largely independent lives with support whereas, for others, daily supervision will be necessary.

■ ***Before you examine the patient, are there significant medical features of Down's syndrome that you need to consider immediately?***

Yes, there are several, but the one of immediate importance is general joint laxity that involves the atlantoaxial joint. Care must be taken positioning the head and neck to avoid dislocation, which would have severe consequences. In practice this is most likely to affect patients under general anaesthesia or sedation. However, individuals with Down's syndrome also have poor muscle tone so that the joint is not fully stable even when conscious. Simply ensuring head support, including lateral support, is sufficient. About 15% of patients are affected in this way, though only 1–2% are at high risk of spinal cord compression. Examination of a conscious patient poses minimal risk.

Table 6.2 Categories of learning difficulty

Learning difficulty/ disability	Indicative IQ	Effects
Mild	50–70	Most can lead normal lives but may need assistance in handling difficult situations
Moderate	35–49	Need to use simple language when talking. Can generally attend to the basic tasks of life after training but more complex activities such as using money usually require support within a special residential environment
Severe	20–34	Many able to look after themselves but with careful and close supervision

■ ***Is the patient able to give consent for the examination?***

Capacity to give consent must be assessed in line with the Mental Capacity Act 2005. You need to assess capacity to consent at each visit in relation to the treatment to be carried out. As this individual works part-time in a supermarket and has presented for treatment independently, it is very likely that his consent would be valid for examination but not necessarily for any treatment.

In the meantime, you can proceed with examination and diagnosis.

Examination

Extraoral examination

■ ***How can you recognize Down's syndrome?***

Down's syndrome has a readily recognized physical appearance, characteristic facies and signs affecting the hands that are readily recognized in the dental setting. These include:

- Short stature
- Short neck
- Obesity

- Short limbs
- Broad head and sloping forehead
- Round face
- Large lips
- Flat nasal bridge
- Oblique slanting eye fissures
- Epicanthic skin folds on the inner corner of the eyes
- White spots on the iris (Brushfield spots)
- Short stubby hands and fingers
- Inward-curving fifth finger
- However the individual features and their prominence vary considerably between individuals. The patient's appearance is shown in Figure 6.1.

There are multiple slightly tender mobile cervical lymph nodes.

Intraoral examination

The tongue appears large and makes examination of the lower teeth a little difficult. The oral hygiene is generally good anteriorly but there is fairly thick plaque around the gingival margins of the molar teeth. There are a few small restorations and no dental caries. The lower right second molar is grade II mobile and tender on pressure.

■ ***Interpret these findings in the light of Down's syndrome.***

Recurrent upper respiratory tract infections are common in individuals with Down's syndrome and noted by the patient. This is likely to account for the lymphadenopathy but you need to consider alternative explanations.

The tongue is not enlarged, but appears so. It has a forward posture, associated with mouth breathing, and poor muscle tone. This is more prominent in children with Down's syndrome and becomes less prominent in late childhood. Poor tongue control can lead to problems with speech and swallowing.

Individuals with Down's syndrome have a lower prevalence of dental caries than the normal population, though this can be overcome by high levels of dietary sugar. Caries resistance has been claimed to be due to high titres of secretory IgA against *Streptococcus mutans* in saliva and a high salivary pH. However, late eruption, spacing of the teeth and shallow fissures also contribute and may be as important.

There is predisposition to plaque-induced gingivitis and periodontitis that might account for the mobile lower molar. Immune function, particularly neutrophil function, is impaired and thought to be the cause, though the exact causes are not defined. There are also changes in complement and antibody levels, required for optimum neutrophil function. Mouth-breathing contributes to gingivitis. Once periodontitis develops, the teeth have short conical roots and are more quickly compromised.

Bruxism is a feature of Down's syndrome. The patient stopped bruxing when symptoms started, suggesting pain of periodontal ligament origin, and this is consistent with the tooth mobility and pain on eating.

These and other oral features of Down's syndrome are listed in Table 6.3.

Table 6.3 Oral features of Down's syndrome

Fissured lips
Open-mouth posture and mouth-breathing
Tongue protrusion
Lack of muscle tone
Fissuring of the dorsal surface of the tongue
Drooling
Bruxism
Developmental absence of some teeth
Teeth with short conical roots
Interdental spacing
Delayed eruption
Small teeth, including conical crown forms
Shallow fissures
Hypoplastic/hypocalcified enamel
Class 3 skeletal pattern and malocclusion
Taurodontism (0.54–5.6%)
Prone to periodontal disease
Prone to intraoral candidal infection and angular cheilitis
Resistant to dental caries

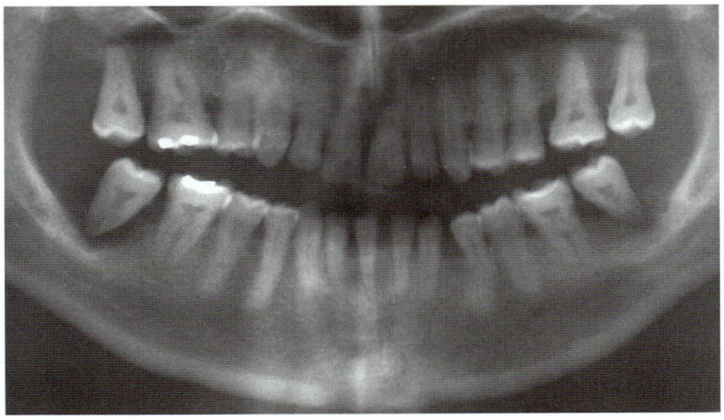

Fig. 6.2 Panoramic radiograph.

Investigations

■ ***What investigations should be carried out and why?***

As periodontitis is the most likely cause for the tooth mobility, the patient's periodontal assessment should be updated with pocket depths around as many teeth as possible and a radiographic survey, unless recent films are available. Periapical radiographs are the view of choice but may not be possible because of the combination of the tongue and lack of cooperation. A panoramic radiograph is a suitable second choice provided the patient can sit still for the required period. Alternatively, an oblique lateral is a good choice; the exposure is very short and the film is held against the patient's face, so that the effects of movement during exposure are minimized.

In this case, you already have a panoramic radiograph that was taken a year ago and shows the cause of the problems.

■ ***The panoramic radiograph is shown in Figure 6.2. What do you see?***

Consistent with Down's syndrome, there are missing third molars and small teeth with short conical roots and spacing anteriorly. There are only a few shallow restorations but there is marked periodontitis.

There is generalized horizontal bone loss posteriorly with almost complete bone loss around the lower right third molar. Calculus is present in all posterior interdental spaces.

Diagnosis

■ ***What is your diagnosis?***

Extensive bone loss due to advanced periodontal disease with apical involvement and, almost certainly, a perioendodontic lesion.

Treatment

■ ***Will the patient need antibiotic cover for whatever treatment you prescribe?***

No. The unrepaired ventriculoseptal defect is not currently considered to require antibiotic cover for dental treatment. However, the patient remains at risk of bacterial endocarditis and infections such as this need to be treated vigorously and without delay. As the patient must understand the risk, signs and symptoms of endocarditis, most of the responsibility will rest with carers, whose involvement will be essential.

More detailed information on endocarditis is given in Case 44.

■ ***What treatment would you recommend?***

In principle, individuals with Down's syndrome must be offered the same standard of care as other patients. In this case the prognosis for this tooth in any individual would be poor. When the predisposition to periodontitis, endocarditis and infection is taken into account, the only treatment that can be recommended is extraction. This had been recommended before but was refused.

In the longer term, there is a need for continuing periodontal treatment and monitoring. Removal of subgingival calculus is a priority.

If sedation or general anaesthesia is required, then extraction of the lower left second molar and scaling and root planing could all be carried out in one episode.

■ ***Does the level of learning difficulty help in planning treatment?***

Only slightly. Knowing that the cause of the learning disability is Down's syndrome is probably more useful than the level of disability itself. Individuals with Down's syndrome are generally considered to be friendly, tolerant, cheerful, gentle and patient but somewhat stubborn. This stereotype often holds true, but all are individuals and vary considerably. They all have their own range of abilities that you will need to assess. Some will be anxious about dentistry.

A third of patients will suffer additional psychiatric disorders that may include Alzheimer's disease, attention deficit hyperactivity disorder, autism, depression, bipolar disorder or psychosis. These have more profound effects on dental treatment. The most severely affected will not be amenable to dentistry without general anaesthetic.

It is important to evaluate how treatment has been provided in the past. This patient has been treated in the practice for several years and has had some restorative work carried out, which indicates good cooperation for treatment under local anaesthetic. On the basis of what is known about this patient, he may require only standard types of support such as behaviour management or inhalation sedation, possibly with oral sedation. Intravenous sedation or general anaesthesia might be considered for more demanding treatments.

■ ***Can the patient refuse to accept the extraction? He has before.***

All patients over the age of 16 take responsibility for their own treatment. The degree of capacity required for consent to be valid increases with the complexity of the procedure. If the patient understands the risks of endocarditis and the advantages and disadvantages of extracting the tooth, his opinion is final.

If you believe that the patient does not understand the issues, then he does not have capacity to consent because he cannot make an informed decision. It is still possible to provide treatment within the framework set by the Mental Capacity Act 2005, which governs consent. This states that:

i. A patient is assumed to have capacity to consent unless proven otherwise. Such a loss of capacity may be permanent or temporary.

ii. Capacity has to be assessed at each visit, in relation to the treatment and recorded.

iii. A person must be able to understand, retain, and weigh the information given and communicate their decision to have capacity.

iv. When a person lacks capacity to consent, treatment must be provided within 'best interest' of the patient and consideration given to all the relevant circumstances. The person should be encouraged to participate in the decision-making process. Consideration must be given to past and present wishes, feelings, values and beliefs that would influence the decision. Consult with family, next of kin, carer, lasting power of attorney, or deputy of court as appropriate.

v. Individuals can nominate a lasting power of attorney who can give or withhold consent on their behalf for health care decisions in the event that they lack capacity.

vi. 'Advance directives' can be made to advise of treatment that the person does not wish to undergo in the event that that person lacks capacity. These can only rule out specific items and cannot require specific treatment to be carried out. In order to be binding the directive must show capacity and validity applicable to the specific situation.

If the patient cannot make an informed decision, it will be necessary to ensure that any proposed treatment is reasonable and in the patient's best interests, and the least restrictive option in terms of the individual's basic rights, based upon section 5 of the Mental Capacity Act 2005. This states:

> For those who lack capacity the following conditions must be met:
>
> - The treatment is undertaken in connection with another person's care or treatment;
> - The person doing it takes reasonable steps to establish whether the recipient has capacity;
> - There is reasonable belief that the recipient lacks capacity;
> - There is reasonable belief that the treatment is in the best interests of the patient;
> - If restraint is to be used to carry out the treatment, there is reasonable belief both that it is necessary to undertake treatment in order to prevent harm to the person and that the treatment is a proportionate response to the likelihood of the person suffering harm and the seriousness of that harm.

In the event that the patient does not have capacity, the proposed treatment must be discussed with parents, legal guardians or carers and may also be agreed by two dentists or doctors. The NHS consent form for those who lack capacity (consent form 4) should be used.

Delay is not an appropriate response. There is a need for urgent treatment and failure to follow through and deliver it would be negligent.

Long-term management

Are there any long-term issues to consider in planning dental treatment?

Yes, the reduced life expectancy must be taken into account when planning treatment. The mean lifespan for people with Down's syndrome has increased significantly in the last decades and currently stands at about 50 years, with some individuals reaching 60 years or more.

Congenital heart disease carries significant mortality in the long term. It is also possible for patients to acquire cardiac defects in later life, either de novo or as developmental defects reveal themselves in later life.

There is also a predisposition to atherosclerosis as part of generalized premature ageing. Mitral valve prolapse affects about half of adults *without* congenital heart defects. It is now recommended to have a second cardiac assessment in early adulthood as most deaths result from cardiac causes.

Eyesight is often impaired and may worsen with age as a result of opacification of the lens, making oral care more difficult.

In later life, three-quarters will develop Alzheimer's disease. The pathogenesis of the neurological degeneration is the same as that in normal individuals, but accelerated because of an extra copy of the amyloid precursor protein carried on the extra chromosome 21. Microscopic evidence of senile plaques and amyloid deposition in the brain is present in all those reaching 40 years of age. Dementia is an increasing problem as the lifespan increases.

Table 6.4 General features of Down's syndrome.

Cardiovascular	Cardiovascular defect 40–50% Ventriculoseptal defect 33% Atrioseptal defect 10% Tetralogy of Fallot 6% Isolated patent ductus arteriosus 4%
Musculoskeletal	Short broad hands Short stature Obesity from adolescence Inwardly curved fifth finger Single palmar flexion crease Hypoplasia of maxillary sinuses Absence of frontal/sphenoidal sinuses Joint, including atlantoaxial, instability Large fontanelles with late closure Persistent frontal suture (metopic suture) Muscular hypotonia
Skin	Early skin ageing Early greying of hair
Endocrine	Hypothyroidism Diabetes Reduced fertility
Haematological	Acute leukaemia (in childhood)
Immunological	Impaired cellular immunity Impaired neutrophil function Susceptibility to infection, especially fungal and including angular cheilitis
Neurological	Learning disability Epilepsy Autism Attention deficit hyperactivity disorder Obsessive compulsive disorder Tourette's syndrome Hearing loss, usually conductive in type Depression Alzheimer's disease Dementia Poor eyesight
Gastrointestinal tract	Duodenal atresia Imperforate anus Tracheo-oesophageal fistula Hirschsprung's disease Coeliac disease Reduced peristalsis/constipation

With all this patient's problems, perhaps he should be referred for specialist care?

There is no reason why the majority of individuals with Down's syndrome should not be treated in general dental practice. Despite this, they and their carers often report difficulty gaining access to dental care. Dentists may be reluctant to take on care for a variety of reasons, often of spurious validity. It is important that all such patients are able to obtain care in an appropriate local setting, ideally with other family members. Specialized services are available, but often stretched. They may be able to provide advice and backup when medical support or treatment under sedation or anaesthetic is required. This would be prudent because the airway may be compromised by the tongue, poor nasal patency and short neck. However, most individuals with Down's syndrome need only routine dental care from a caring, patient and well-informed dentist.

■ ***What other features of Down's syndrome may be present?***

There are many features associated with Down's syndrome that will only be seen in a minority of patients, as shown in Table 6.4. Many have implications for dental diagnosis or treatment.,

Acknowledgements

Figure 6.1 by kind permission of the Down's Syndrome Association (**www.downs-syndrome.org.uk**).

Case 7

A dry mouth

SUMMARY

A 50-year-old lady presents to you in your hospital dental department complaining of dry mouth. Identify the cause and plan treatment.

History

Complaint

She complains of dryness which makes many aspects of her life a misery. The dryness is both uncomfortable and renders eating and speech difficult. She is forced to keep a bottle of water by her side at all times.

History of complaint

She first noticed the dry mouth about 4 or 5 years ago though it may have been present for longer. At first it was only an intermittent problem but over the last 3 years or so the dryness has become constant. Recently the mouth has become sore as well as dry.

Medical history

The patient describes herself as generally fit and well but has had to attend her medical practitioner for poor circulation in her fingers. They blanch rapidly in the cold and are painful on rewarming. She has also used artificial tears for dry eyes for the last 2 years but takes no other medication.

Examination

Extraoral examination

She is a well-looking lady without detectable cervical lymphadenopathy. There is no facial asymmetry or enlargement of the parotid glands and the submandibular glands appear normal on bimanual palpation. Her eyes and fingers appear normal.

Intraoral examination

■ ***The appearance of the patient's mouth is shown in Figures 7.1 and 7.2. What do you see? How do you interpret the findings?***

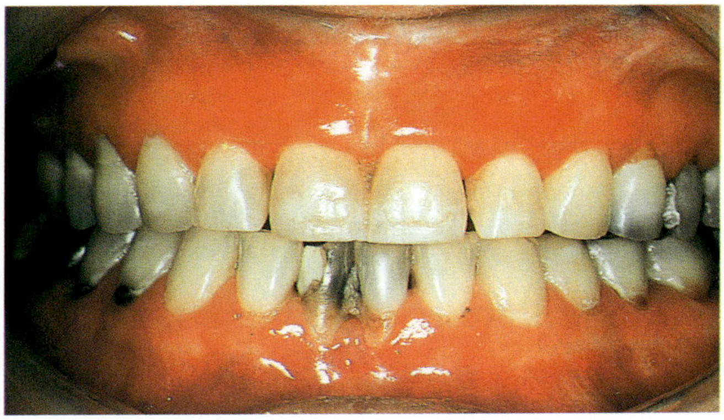

Fig. 7.1 Appearance of the patient's anterior teeth.

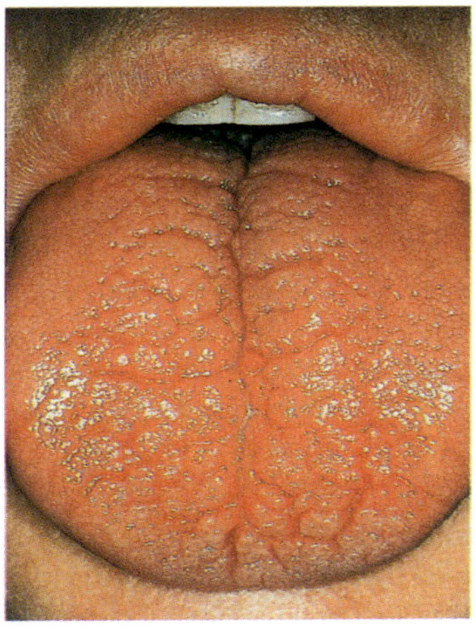

Fig. 7.2 Appearance of the patient's tongue.

The alveolar mucosa appears 'glazed' and translucent or thin (atrophic) suggesting long-standing xerostomia. Some oral debris adheres between the teeth, again suggesting dryness, which causes plaque to be thicker and more tenacious. There are carious lesions and restorations at the cervical margins of the lower anterior teeth, indicating a high caries rate. The tongue is lobulated and fissured. Both features suggest a lack of saliva.

If you were able to examine the patient you would find that her mouth does feel dry. Gloved fingers and mirror adhere to the mucosa making examination uncomfortable. Parts of the mucosa, especially the palate and dorsal tongue appear redder than normal. No saliva is pooling in the floor of the mouth and what saliva can be identified is frothy and thick. Small amounts of clear but viscid saliva can be expressed from all four main salivary ducts.

■ ***What are the common and important causes of xerostomia and how are they subdivided?***

In true xerostomia the salivary flow is reduced. The term 'false xerostomia' describes the sensation of dryness despite normal salivary output.

■ ***On the basis of the history and examination which cause is the most likely? Why?***

Sjögren's syndrome is the most likely cause. It is the commonest single medical disorder causing xerostomia. It also

Type of xerostomia	Common causes
False	Mouth breathing Mucosal disease Psychological
True	Drugs Dehydration Sjögren's syndrome Irradiation Neurological Developmental anomaly

causes dry eyes and predominantly affects female patients of middle age. Sjögren's syndrome is sometimes defined by the presence of dry eyes and mouth, with or without an autoimmune/connective tissue disorder. This patient meets these criteria though they are rather imprecise and further investigations would be required to confirm the diagnosis.

■ ***Which causes have you excluded and why?***

Drugs are by far the commonest cause of true xerostomia but this patient is not taking any medication.

Dehydration is a common cause in elderly people who may have a habitual low fluid intake, especially when institutionalized. It also accompanies cardiac or renal failure or diuretic drugs. (The combination of drugs and disease probably explains the apparent association of xerostomia with age). These are not factors in this case.

False xerostomia is very common. Those who sleep with an open mouth will have xerostomia on waking, compounded by the normal reduction in salivary secretion at night. Diseases causing oral mucosal roughness such as lichen planus or candidosis may cause a sensation of dryness but no such condition is present. False xerostomia may be a feature, sometimes a central one, in psychiatric disorders. However, this patient's mouth is genuinely dry. The history of prolonged and unremitting dryness over a period of years almost always indicates a salivary disorder and the appearance of the mucosa and the high caries rate indicate true xerostomia.

Neurological and developmental causes, such as aplasia of gland or atresia of ducts, are very rare and need not be considered further until common causes have been investigated. There is no history of irradiation of the head and neck.

■ ***What is Sjögren's syndrome and how may the condition be subclassified?***

Sjögren's syndrome is a poorly understood autoimmune disorder in which exocrine glands are destroyed. In primary Sjögren's syndrome the salivary and lacrimal glands are those most affected (though there are often nonspecific systemic signs of autoimmune disease such as Raynaud's phenomenon) and there is sometimes salivary gland swelling. Other exocrine glands and organs are also affected. In secondary Sjögren's syndrome there is an accompanying connective tissue disorder such as rheumatoid arthritis, systemic lupus erythematosus or mixed connective tissue disease. Other exocrine glands are less severely affected in the secondary form, the mouth is usually less dry and salivary glands are very rarely enlarged.

Investigations

■ ***What simple test differentiates false and true xerostomia?***

Measuring the whole salivary flow rate. This may be done by asking the patient to tilt their head forward to allow all saliva to flow into a graduated specimen container for 10 minutes. Although this patient is strongly suspected to have true xerostomia it would still be a useful test because it provides a baseline reading against which disease severity and progression may be judged.

When you measure the flow, the patient has a whole salivary flow rate of 0.1 ml/minute.

■ ***What salivary flow rate would you consider to indicate xerostomia?***

Approximately 500 ml of saliva are secreted daily, mostly during eating and drinking, and very little at night. Rates vary greatly between individuals but less than 2 ml in 10 minutes (0.2 ml/minute) unstimulated whole saliva flow is generally considered to indicate xerostomia.

This patient has true xerostomia.

■ ***What further investigations are required and why is each performed?***

Although a number of investigations will be required to confirm the diagnosis, the immediate problem is one of soreness. A dry mouth is not usually sore unless there is superimposed candidal infection. Smears, a saliva sample or a therapeutic trial of antifungal agent are required to exclude this possibility.

The diagnosis of Sjögren's syndrome is straightforward when the clinical presentation is florid, and may then be based on history and examination alone. However, numerous investigations are required in most patients with suspected Sjögren's syndrome in whom there are just a few early signs (Table 7.1). Many investigations are possible but only the minimum required to make the diagnosis need be performed. A selection is usually necessary because every test will be negative in a small proportion of patients and none is completely specific.

The results of this patient's investigations are:

Salivary culture	10 000 cfu *Candida* sp./ml
Smear for candida	Hyphae present
Red cell indices	Normal
White cell count/differential count	Normal
Platelets	Normal
ESR	20 mm/hour
Ig levels	Normal
Autoantibodies	
RA latex	Negative
Antinuclear	Weak positive
Antithyroid	Negative
ssA	Positive
ssB	Positive
Urine glucose	Normal

Table 7.1 Investigations for patients with Sjögren's syndrome

Sample	Test	Relevance
Saliva	Whole salivary flow rate	See above; differentiates false from true xerostomia.
	Culture for candidal count	To exclude superimposed candidosis.
	Stimulated parotid flow	Accurate estimation of maximum possible parotid salivary flow.
Blood tests	Full blood picture	Mild anaemia is common in all autoimmune conditions and may require treatment.
	Erythrocyte sedimentation rate (ESR)	Relatively nonspecific but raised in inflammatory conditions, useful for monitoring their activity after treatment.
	Immunoglobulin levels	Often raised in autoimmune disorders and may be markedly raised in primary Sjögren's syndrome.
	Autoantibody screen	Autoantibodies are a frequent finding in autoimmune disease. This appears to be a partly nonspecific effect and many different autoantibodies may be seen. The exact combination in the routine screen varies between centres but usually includes rheumatoid factor, antinuclear, antithyroid, antiparietal cell and antimitochondrial antibody. Additional autoantibodies which may be seen in Sjögren's syndrome are antisalivary gland duct antibody and ssA and ssB autoantibodies (anti-Ro and anti-La) directed against extractable nuclear antigens. None of these antibodies is individually helpful in diagnosis but the presence of more than one is typical. They may help diagnosis of connective tissue disease in secondary Sjögren's syndrome and ssA and ssB may indicate patients at risk of specific complications. Antisalivary gland duct antibody is not related to either the periductal infiltrates seen on biopsy or the pathogenesis of the disease.
Urine	Glucose	Occasionally useful to exclude unsuspected diabetes as a cause of dehydration.
Salivary gland	Sialogram	In established disease a sialogram almost always shows characteristic changes.
	Other imaging techniques	Pertechnetate scintigraphy is a complex but useful test of secretion from individual glands. It is useful if sialography is not possible but involves a significant radiation dose. Magnetic resonance imaging is useful to delineate the extent of salivary gland swelling if present.
	Minor salivary gland biopsy	The histological appearances of salivary glands are characteristic in established disease. Biopsy of major glands is difficult but the same changes may be seen in the minor glands of the lips and cheeks provided a sufficient sample is removed (6–8 glands).
	Parotid gland biopsy	Biopsy of the tail of the parotid is possible without significant risk to branches of the facial nerve. It provides an excellent sample and may be useful when other techniques have failed or when other conditions need to be excluded. It may also be helpful in the diagnosis of lymphoma in swollen parotid glands. However, it is rarely performed.
Eye	Schirmer test	This measures lacrimal secretion. Narrow filter paper strips are placed with one end under the lower eyelid and the length wetted after 5 minutes is recorded. In practice the test is not very reproducible. (It is also uncomfortable and may cause corneal abrasions when the eye is very dry and for this reason is no longer recommended). Ophthalmological examination is preferable but the Schirmer test remains widely used.
	Ophthalmological examination	Examination by an ophthalmologist using a slit lamp will detect conjunctival splits and Rose Bengal staining identifies dried tear secretion on the front of the eye. Though these changes are rarely helpful in diagnosis, examination and follow up are required to prevent long-term complications of dry eyes.

■ ***The parotid sialogram is shown in Figure 7.3. What do you see? What is your interpretation?***

The sialogram shows punctate sialectasis. The major duct is seen but almost no major or minor duct branches are visible. Small round spots of contrast medium are scattered throughout the gland, apparently unconnected with the duct tree. These features have some similarities to those in chronic nonspecific sialadenitis but are much more even and affect the whole gland equally. These features are characteristic of Sjögren's syndrome.

■ ***The minor salivary gland biopsy is shown in Figures 7.4 and 7.5. What do you see?***

The low power view shows several minor salivary glands. A minimum of 6–8 glands is required for reliable diagnosis and this sample is sufficient. Even at this low magnification, dark foci of inflammatory cells are visible (though they cannot be identified as such) and it can be seen that the lobular structure of the glands is largely intact.

The high power view shows one gland lobule. Centrally there are three small ducts surrounded by a dense lymphocytic infiltrate. The infiltrate is sharply defined and within the lymphocytic focus there is complete loss of acinar cells (acinar atrophy). Around the lymphocytes there is a zone of essentially normal uninflamed mucous salivary gland.

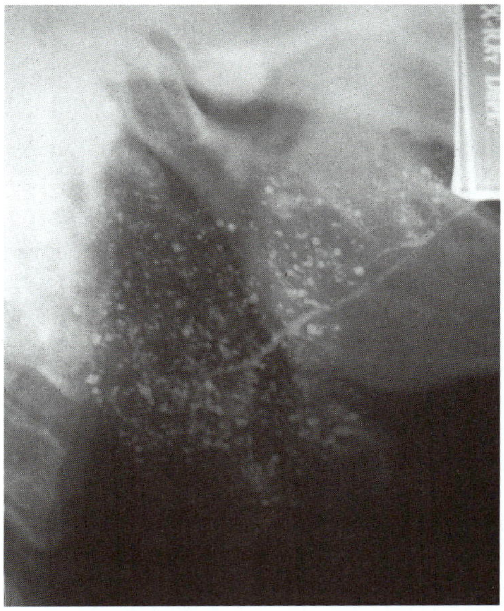

Fig. 7.3 Parotid sialogram.

■ ***How do you interpret these histological appearances?***

The focal lymphocytic sialadenitis centred on ducts and concentric sharply defined zones of acinar atrophy

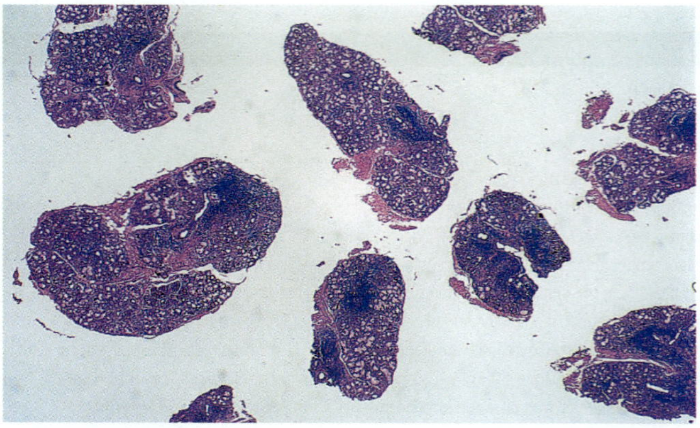

Fig. 7.4 Minor salivary gland biopsy; low power.

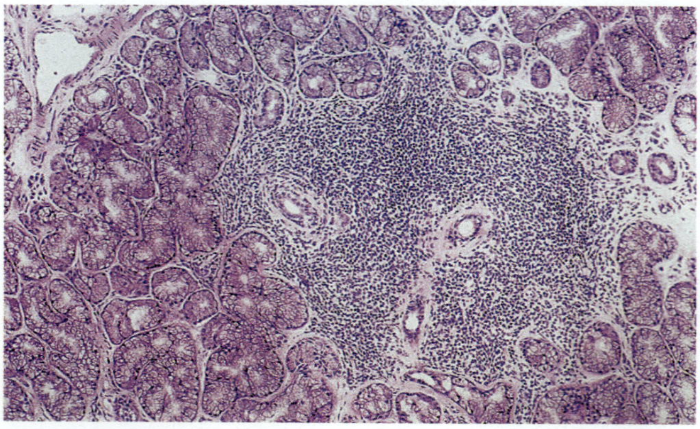

Fig. 7.5 Minor salivary gland biopsy; high power.

surrounded by normal acini are characteristic of Sjögren's syndrome.

Diagnosis

What is your final diagnosis?

The patient has primary Sjögren's syndrome. The diagnosis was suspected on the basis of history and examination, and is confirmed by the characteristic sialogram and biopsy findings. The primary form of Sjögren's syndrome is indicated by the lack of autoimmune/connective tissue disease and the positivity for ssA and ssB autoantibodies. The presence of Raynaud's phenomenon, the severity of the xerostomia and dryness of the eyes are also more consistent with the primary form. In addition the patient has candidosis which is the probable cause of the soreness.

Treatment

How could you contribute to the management of this patient?

Control of the underlying disease is not possible but the patient requires treatment for complications and continued follow up:

- Treat candidosis and follow up regularly for recurrence.
- Preserve what salivary secretion remains; saliva is more effective than saliva substitutes.
  - Sip water rather than drinking it, so as to expand remaining saliva and not wash it from the mouth.
  - Whenever possible avoid drugs which cause xerostomia.
  - Maintain fluid intake.
  - Stimulate residual salivary flow using chewing gum (sugar-free).
  - Consider using pilocarpine in severe cases (though side-effects and an appropriate dosing regimen can be problematic).
- Prevent and treat dental caries
  - Avoid sweets or overuse of citrus fruit to stimulate salivary flow.
  - Appropriate dietary analysis, preventive advice and fluoride treatment.
  - Treat caries.
- Consider using saliva substitutes though these are generally unsatisfactory and not liked by patients.
  - Carboxymethyl-cellulose and similar starch-based liquids.
  - Mucin-based preparations are more effective and generally better tolerated.
- Warn patient about, and follow up for, attacks of acute bacterial ascending sialadenitis in the major glands, which destroys residual gland function. Treat aggressively if it develops.
- Ensure continued ophthalmological follow up.
- Inform patient's general medical practitioner to ensure follow up for other complications. Involvement of other exocrine glands can lead to dry skin, dry vagina, pancreatic dysfunction and lung disease.
- Warn patient and follow up for development of persistent salivary gland swelling.
- Provide continued reassurance and care for patients with this distressing condition.

What is the significance of the development of salivary gland swelling?

This is usually the first sign of lymphoma development; 10% or more of patients with primary Sjögren's syndrome eventually develop lymphoma and in some cases gland swelling is the presenting sign. The lymphoma is usually a form of low grade B-cell lymphoma (MALT type) which has a slow indolent growth pattern, remains localized to the salivary glands for a long period and initially responds well to treatment. However, high grade lymphoma may also develop. Persistent gland swelling would be an indication for biopsy.

Case 8

Painful trismus

SUMMARY

A 27-year-old woman is unable to open her mouth normally. What is the diagnosis and how should she be managed?

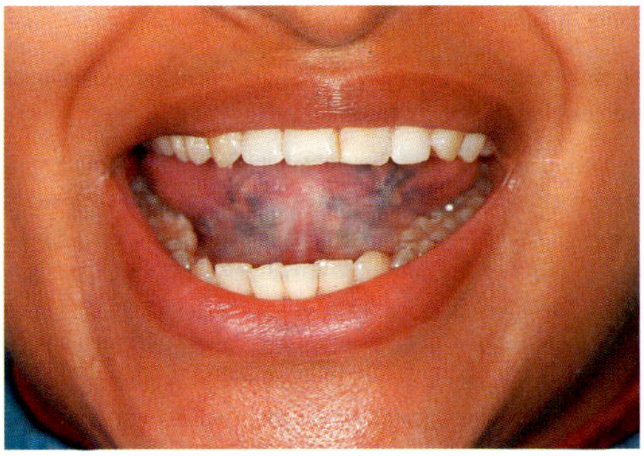

Fig. 8.1 The patient on presentation showing maximal opening.

History

Complaint

The patient is unable to open her mouth more than half the normal distance.

History of complaint

She has had sporadic painless clicks from her right jaw joint for many years. Recently the click has become louder and painful. On occasions there has been some hesitancy of opening just at the position where the click would normally be felt. Three days ago, while eating a particularly chewy piece of meat, she felt a sudden pain in front of the right ear and since that time she has been unable to open her mouth more than about half way.

Medical history

The patient is otherwise well but she has suffered from previous episodes of knee pain and was seen by a rheumatologist who diagnosed generalized hypermobility of her joints.

Social history

The patient used to be a keen and successful gymnast as a teenager.

Examination

Extraoral examination

The patient is apyrexial and appears well. There is no facial swelling and the skin colour over the preauricular regions is normal. There is tenderness on palpation over the right condyle but no tenderness on the left side. There is generalized muscular tenderness, particularly of the right masseter and the right lateral pterygoid muscles. Examination of the fingers, wrists and elbows shows an increased range of joint movement.

Intraoral examination

■ ***The patient's appearance is shown in Figure 8.1. She is trying to open her mouth to the maximum extent. What do you see?***

There is limited mouth opening and a deviation towards the right side. If you were able to examine the patient you would find that the opening, measured between the tips of the incisor teeth, is 23 mm. Lateral excursions of the mandible were measured at 8 mm to the right and 1 mm to the left. The patient readily achieved a normal position of maximum intercuspation between upper and lower teeth.

Differential diagnosis

■ ***The patient has trismus. What is trismus?***

The definition of trismus is reduced opening caused by spasm of the muscles of mastication but the term is used loosely for all causes of limited opening. True trismus is usually temporary.

■ ***What are the causes of trismus?***

Causes of limitation of opening include:

Intra-articular causes	Internal derangement of the joint
	Fractured condyle
	Traumatic synovitis
	Septic arthritis
	Osteoarthrosis
	Inflammatory arthritis, (e.g. rheumatoid or psoriatic)
	Ankylosis (secondary to trauma or infection)
	Lesions of the condylar head (e.g. osteochondroma)
Extra-articular causes	Trauma (e.g. fractured mandible not involving the condyle)
	Postsurgical removal of impacted lower third molar or recent prolonged dental treatment
	Acute infections of the oral tissues especially involving the cheeks or the muscles of mastication, usually dental in origin

	Muscle spasm of masticatory muscles (e.g. myofascial pain)
	Disease of masticatory muscles (e.g. myositis ossificans)
	Scarring of muscles, skin or mucosa (e.g. submucous fibrosis, scleroderma or after radiotherapy)
	Inflammatory conditions of the oral mucosa (e.g. painful ulcerative conditions or other forms of stomatitis)
	Tetanus

■ *What are the common causes of pain in the temporomandibular joint?*

There are three conditions that are common and they are usually classified according to the 'Research Diagnostic Criteria' or RDC system.

Myofascial pain dysfunction syndrome, also known as arthromyalgia or, inappropriately, temporomandibular joint pain-dysfunction. In this condition the masticatory muscles, which move the joint, are the source of the pain and the condition has little or nothing to do with the joint itself. The pain is described as a diffuse ache over the side of the face and has a tight, heavy or dragging quality. The pain can be mild or severe and usually fluctuates in intensity, with bouts of exacerbation lasting hours or sometimes days. Two presentations are seen, one with pain that is worst in the early morning and one in which it builds up through the day and is worst in the early evening. Movements of the jaw are sometimes painful, but not always, and mouth opening is sometimes restricted. Tight bands within tense muscles are thought to be the cause. The condition also affects other parts of the musculoskeletal system, where it may be termed fibromyalgia.

Internal derangement of the temporomandibular joint (TMJ) is the term used to describe instability or abnormal position of the articular disc, usually anterior displacement. This gives rise to clicking and locking of the TMJ.

Osteoarthrosis or degenerative joint disease is also commonly seen in the TMJ and the condyle in particular. Although commonly ascribed to wear and tear, the cause is probably a failure of cartilage repair with a genetic predisposition. Fibrillation (cracking and fraying) of the articular cartilage and loss of proteoglycans lead to break up of the articular surface. This causes pain on movement, especially when the joint is loaded, for instance during chewing. There is restriction of movement in all directions. Crepitus (a grating or crunching noise and sensation) is also evident.

■ *Why do temporomandibular joints click?*

Laxity of the posterior distal ligaments allows the disc to move forward into an abnormal position and it may momentarily obstruct forward condylar translation during jaw movements. The disc may be trapped and stretched forwards but further movement releases it suddenly and it snaps back into its normal position, giving rise to the audible and palpable click that the patient appreciates. This is an opening click.

A closing click arises during closing and is caused by the condyle rapidly repositioning posteriorly, displacing the disc anteriorly or medially.

Both are associated with a disc that fails to move in a coordinated manner. When a patient has both an opening and a closing click they are said to suffer from reciprocal clicks. The mechanisms of clicks are shown in Figure 8.2.

■ *Why do joints lock in internal derangement?*

Sudden locking of the jaw (inability to open) implies total obstruction of forward condylar movement (translation). There are two types of lock: a closed lock and an open lock. Locking and clicking are presentations of the same process – internal derangement of the joint.

If the discal ligaments become very stretched or even ruptured, the disc may move anteriorly into a very displaced position and become fixed in the anterior fornix of the joint space. This completely obstructs forward translation of the condyle. Locking of this type can be acute in onset but usually follows many years of reciprocal clicking. In this case the condyle is stuck behind the disc, the patient cannot open their mouth and so the condition is known as closed lock.

In an open lock the mouth is locked open and the condyle is in a forward position. This happens in subluxation or dislocation of the joint.

Movements of the temporomandibular joint and mechanisms of clicks and open lock are shown in Figure 8.2.

■ *Does this patient have an intra-articular or extra-articular cause for the locking? Explain why.*

In trismus of extra-articular origin the joint and its capacity to move are unaffected. This condition can be imagined by thinking of the patient as having a piece of string tied between the tip of their nose and the point of the chin. The mouth is unable to open in a vertical direction but lateral and protrusive movements are not restricted. Therefore translation of the condyles permits normal protrusive and lateral excursions despite the fact that the mouth cannot be opened. In this case there is both deviation on opening and restricted lateral excursion, suggesting that the cause is not extra-articular.

When the cause is intra-articular, forward translation of the condyle is normally the first movement to be lost. This component of joint movement occurs in the upper joint space and is required for opening and lateral excursion. Thus, in intra-articular causes of trismus there is usually limitation of movement *in all directions*, as in the present case.

Movements possible in intra- and extra-articular trismus and locking are shown in Figure 8.3.

■ *What is the most likely cause?*

There is no history of surgery or trauma, no suggestion of fracture, no inflammation visible over the joint to suggest arthritis and no systemic cause for arthritis. Traumatic synovitis is a possibility but does not usually cause selective impairment of movement; all joint movements are painful. This leaves internal derangement involving the intra-articular disc as the most likely cause. The progression of clicking to locking with pain and intra-articular trismus of rapid onset is typical of closed lock and fits with the pattern of symptoms and signs seen in this case.

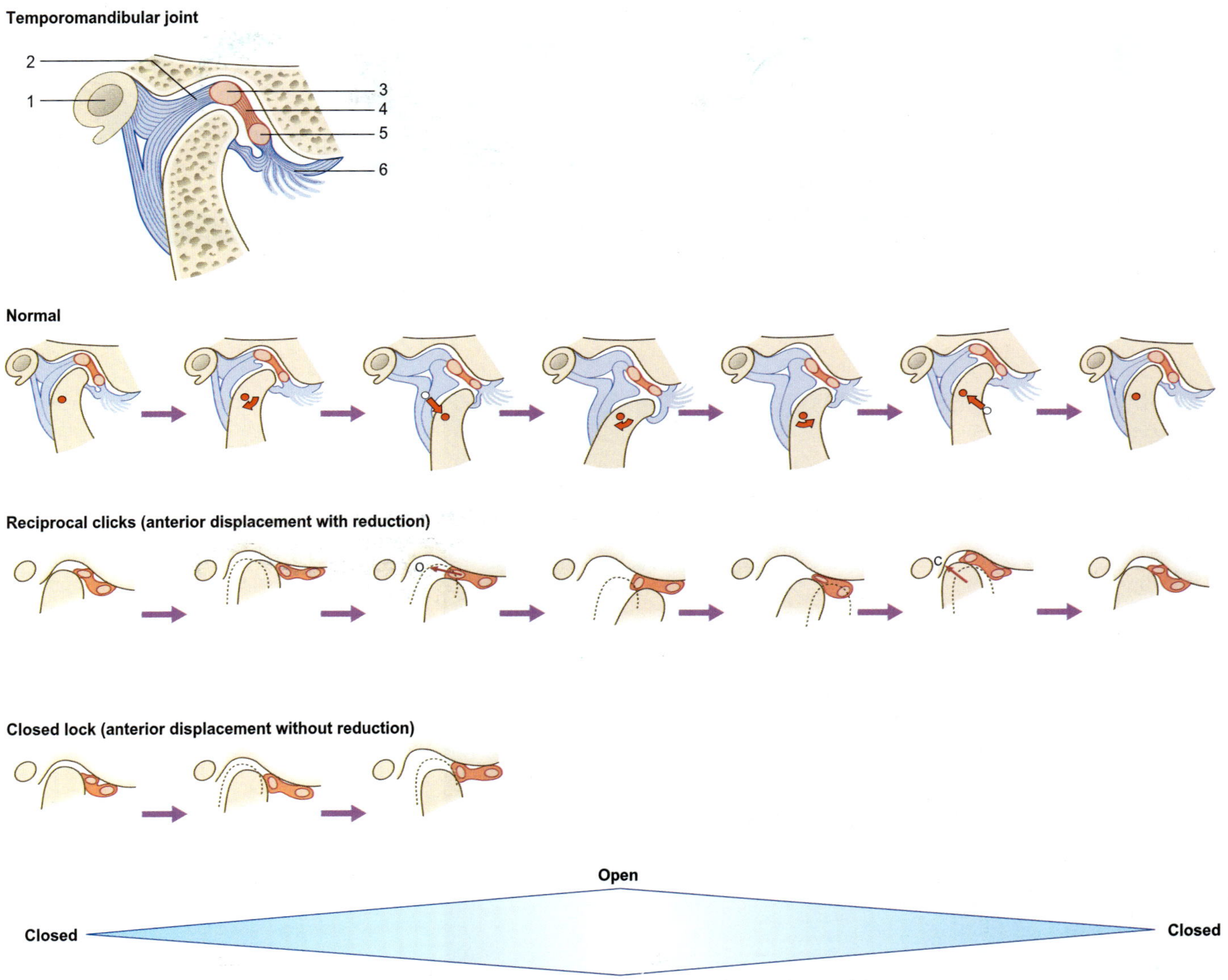

Fig. 8.2 Movements of the temporomandibular joint during the normal opening and closing cycle, with reciprocal clicking and in closed lock. The structure of the normal temporomandibuar joint is shown in the upper panel, with the components of the articular disc and joint capsule. The top row shows the normal opening and closing cycle. Rotation occurs in the lower joint compartment and translation in the upper. The mechanism of reciprocal clicking is shown in the middle row with arrows indicating the sudden movements of disc and condyle that cause opening (O) and closing (C) clicks respectively. The bottom row shows partial opening in a patient with closed lock as a result of anterior displacement of the disc with reduced translation and opening. 1, External auditory meatus; 2, bilaminar region of disc; 3, posterior band of disc; 4, intermediate zone of disc; 5, anterior band of disc; 6, insertion of lateral pterygoid.

In this case the patient is still able to translate the left condyle forward, causing deviation to the right on opening. Lateral excursion to the right was normal at 8 mm. Therefore the cause of the restricted opening is internal derangement of the right joint.

Investigations

■ *What investigations may help?*

Plain radiographs will probably show no abnormality because there is no change in the bony structures of the joint. If a pathological process other than internal derangement is suspected then radiography may be helpful. A dental panoramic tomogram is usually the first view of choice with other tomographic projections including spiral tomography cone beam CT or CT giving additional information. Alternatively transpharyngeal or transcranial projections give clearer views but with a higher radiation dose.

Magnetic resonance imaging (MRI) would show the malpositioned disc and this may sometimes be helpful in diagnosis. Images from this patient's magnetic resonance scan are shown in Figure 8.4.

Arthrography – radiography with a contrast medium injected into the joint – is possible. Lower joint space

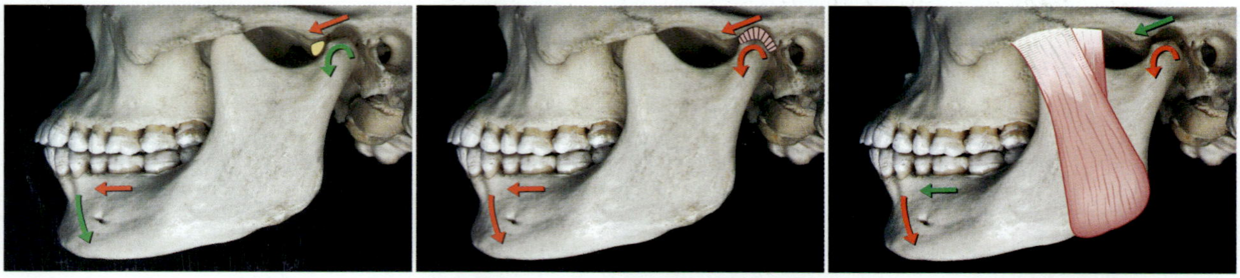

Fig. 8.3 Movements possible in intra- and extra-articular trismus. Green arrows indicate movements that are possible and red arrows those which are impossible. Left, intra-articular trismus: closed lock caused by an anteriorly displaced disc (yellow). Middle, intra-articular trismus: ankylosis (red). Right, extra-articular trismus: spasm or fibrosis of masseter muscle (red).

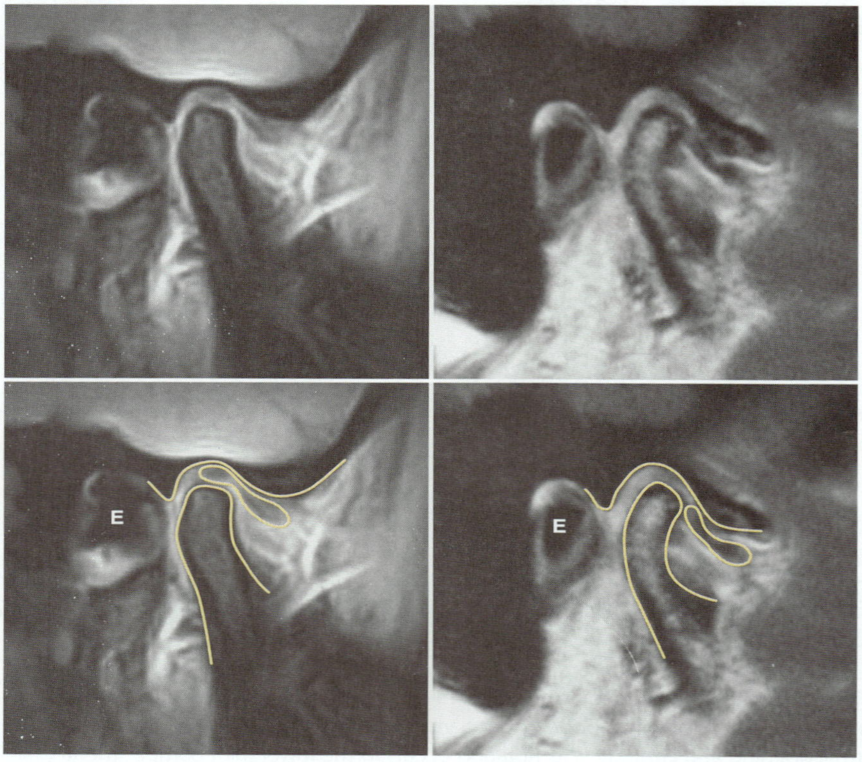

Fig. 8.4 T1 weighted magnetic resonance imaging of the right temporomandibular joint. A normal joint is shown on the left and the patient's joint on the right with the external auditory meatus labeled E. In this technique air, dense cortical bone and the disc all appear dark. In the lower panels the condyle, temporal bone and disc are outlined.

arthrograms are more helpful but it is more difficult to inject medium into the lower joint space.

Serology for rheumatoid factor and an autoantibody profile may be indicated if a polyarthropathy is suspected. However, some causes of arthritis are seronegative, for instance psoriasis and ankylosing spondylitis.

In this, and most other cases, the clinical picture is sufficiently clear to make the diagnosis and these investigations are not normally required.

Treatment

How should this condition be managed?

Most cases of closed lock resolve spontaneously. A consensus view supports conservative management for a period of at least 3–6 months with prescription of analgesics if required. The joint should be mobilized gently as the condition permits.

Forced manipulation of the joint, especially in the early phase, is generally not helpful. It used to be thought that dislocated discs should be surgically repositioned during an open joint operation. This produces about a 90% cure but the same result is obtained spontaneously without surgical intervention.

Proponents of open joint surgery argue that the disc needs to be pulled back into its normal anatomical position and the posterior attachments shortened to keep it there. However, MRI studies have shown that the disc often relapses following surgery and also that an anterior position of the disc is often perfectly compatible with normal joint function. It seems likely that the condyle may adapt to the altered disc position by a process of remodelling.

■ ***Suppose there is no improvement after 6 months?***

In a few cases limitation persists longer than 6 months and then may respond to arthrocentesis – injection of sterile saline or Hartmann's salt solution into the joint to break down adhesions between the disc and the bony joint components. This procedure can be performed either blind or under arthroscopic guidance and is sometimes referred to as *lysis and lavage*. In the event that this procedure is not successful, surgical meniscectomy and disc replacement may be indicated but is required in only a very small number of patients.

Another possibility

■ ***Is there any significance in the history of joint hypermobility?***

Yes. Those with hypermobile joints are at higher risk of temporomandibular joint derangement, as well as damage to other joints. However, only a small proportion of patients with temporomandibular joint derangement will have this particular predisposing factor. Joint hypermobility would not be a result of the patient's childhood gymnastics but those with mobile joints are likely to perform well in such sports.

Case • 9

A large carious lesion

SUMMARY

How will you deal with a large carious lesion in a maxillary molar tooth?

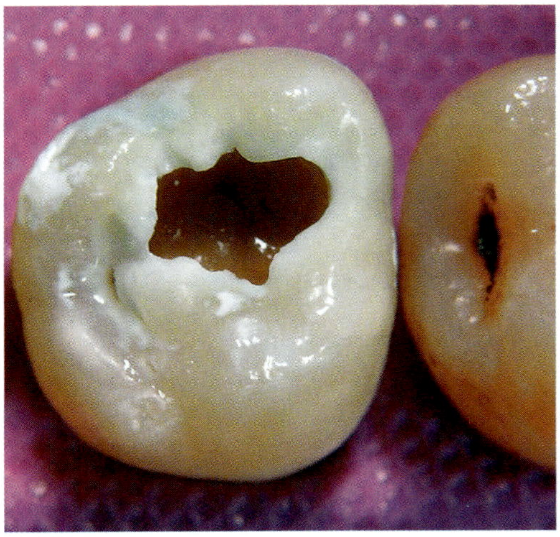

Fig. 9.1 The patient's upper second molar on presentation.

History

Complaint

A 30-year-old patient complains of severe attacks of pain, each of a few seconds duration and fading slowly, but she cannot identify which tooth is responsible. Hot, cold or sweet foods or cold air on the upper right jaw make the pain worse.

History of complaint

The pain has been present intermittently for several months but has only recently become severe. There is no pain on biting.

Dental history

The patient attends on a casual basis for dental treatment. Despite the fact that this carious lesion is very large, it is the only lesion in an otherwise intact arch and there have been no other lesions noted in the last 3 years. The patient is therefore classified as a low risk for dental caries.

Medical history

The patient is fit and well.

Examination

Extraoral examination

The extraoral examination reveals no significant abnormality.

Intraoral examination

There is no tenderness or swelling over the buccal or palatal roots.

■ ***The maxillary right second molar is shown in Figure 9.1. What do you see and how do you assess the problem so far?***

The history is classical of acute pulpitis and repeated attacks of pain – as opposed to continuous severe pain – probably indicate that the pulp can be preserved if the caries is treated. The fact that there is no pain on biting and no tenderness over the roots also suggests a reversible pulpitis and excludes periapical periodontitis.

There is a deep, cavitated lesion on the occlusal surface with extensive exposed carious dentine. Opaque white demineralization of the marginal, unsupported enamel indicates that it is also carious, despite not having fractured off. The dark colour of the tooth distally suggests that caries undermines enamel to the distal marginal ridge and it certainly involves the dentine supporting the enamel of the mesial approximal surface.

This is a relatively small upper second molar. Females have slightly smaller teeth, and when second molars are this small, the third molar may not have developed. This may influence the decision to restore or extract the tooth.

Investigations

■ ***What investigations would you carry out?***

A test of tooth vitality (sensitivity) is required even though the symptoms suggest a vital pulp. This is a large cavity in a molar and partial pulp vitality is a possibility.

A radiograph is required for a variety of reasons. The proximity of the lesion to the pulp and its lateral extent, undermining cusps and the approximal enamel, will affect restorability. Pulp size reduction by reactionary dentine will also be visible. It may also be possible to see evidence of periapical periodontitis, widening of the periodontal ligament and loss of the lamina dura. The ideal views would be a bitewing or periapical depending on your suspicions about pulp vitality or caries in other teeth.

When you perform these investigations, the tooth responds quickly and strongly to ethyl chloride (cold), indicating a hypersensitive pulp, though the proximity of the pulp to the cavity may also contribute to this strong response.

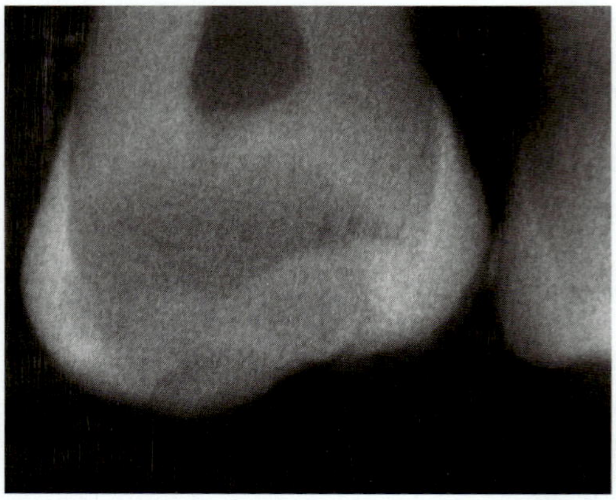

Fig. 9.2 Radiograph of the tooth.

■ ***The radiograph is shown in Figure 9.2. What do you see?***

The coronal radiolucency indicating caries is extensive. It reaches the inner third of the dentine close to the pulp. There appears to be a bridge of intact dentine between the lesion and the pulp chamber. Caries has undermined most of the occlusal enamel and also the distal enamel, but there are no separate approximal lesions or cavitation present. The coronal pulp chamber is rounded and much reduced in size, with the pulp horns obliterated by reactionary ('tertiary') dentine.

There is slight radicular 'burn-out' of the dentine immediately above and below the mesial and distal amelodentinal junction. This could be mistaken for caries extending from the crown into the distal root, but the shape and site of the relative radiolucency do not suggest caries.

Diagnosis

■ ***What is your diagnosis?***

Acute pulpitis in the maxillary second molar caused by extensive occlusal caries. The pulp appears vital and there is no evidence of periapical periodontitis. The pulp does not appear exposed radiographically.

Treatment

■ ***Is this tooth restorable?***

Yes. The prognosis must be guarded as the pulp may still lose vitality, as a result of either the caries or restoration. There is no indication for immediate endodontic treatment.

■ ***What will you do first?***

The patient is in pain and the immediate response must be to relieve it. Pulpitis does not respond to analgesic drugs and the appropriate treatment is restoration.

If a permanent restoration cannot be placed immediately, a temporary dressing could be placed following partial excavation of caries. This would relieve pain by removing the stimulus (bacterial products and acid penetrating the dentine) and by insulating the inflamed pulp from the triggering stimuli. Eugenol-containing temporary filling materials have an obtundent effect on the pulp, reducing pain. However, it must be noted that eugenol-containing materials must not be used if the final restoration to be placed is an adhesive composite as the eugenol adversely affects the bond/polymerization process. A second alternative might be to place a longer-term provisional restoration with a calcium hydroxide lining, in an attempt to induce further reactionary dentine formation in the pulp. However, the carious lesion does not appear to be in imminent danger of breaching the pulp.

Removal of caries will leave a weakened crown, more susceptible to fracture under normal occlusal loading. An immediate definitive restoration is the best course of action.

Subsequently, the patient needs a full caries risk assessment and an intensive preventive regime that may include topical fluorides if other lesions are found. Further details are given in problem 1.

■ ***Why not extract this tooth?***

Such a large lesion in a casual dental patient might well lead to extraction if that were the patient's wish. However, this is a young patient and she may not have a third molar or, if it is present, it may not erupt spontaneously after extraction of the second molar. Even though the prognosis may be guarded there is a good chance that this tooth could be retained for many years. This would be the better immediate option because the condition of the rest of the dentition has not yet been fully assessed.

Operative treatment

■ ***How will you provide analgesia?***

A buccal infiltration of local anaesthetic including a vasoconstrictor should be sufficient. There is no continuous pulpal pain to suggest that obtaining analgesia will be a problem. If this fails, palatal infiltration would be an appropriate next step, or intraligamentary injection.

■ ***Is rubber dam essential for this restoration?***

Yes, it is required. There is a risk of pulp exposure. Though this is small, contamination of the cavity by oral bacteria could reduce the chances of success of subsequent endodontic treatment.

The lesion is extensive and it may be that some carious tissue will have to be retained. The marginal seal of the restoration will be critical to its final success. An adhesive restoration will require a controllable, dry field to achieve the best seal. Rubber dam will also help by controlling the soft tissues, improving visibility and access. The final quality of restorations placed under rubber dam is considered to be higher than those placed without.

■ ***What materials could you use to restore the cavity?***

The choice of restorative material will be a compromise between physicochemical properties, the skill of the dentist placing the restoration and the ability of the patient to maintain it. Choices for this cavity are shown in Table 9.1.

Table 9.1 Potential direct restorative materials for this tooth

Material	Advantages	Disadvantages
Resin composite	Good appearance, favourable wear characteristics and mechanical properties, intact enamel margins	Technique sensitivity (moisture control, multiple increments), high polymerization shrinkage and shrinkage stress
Glass ionomer cement	Less technique-sensitive (more moisture-tolerant than resins), bulk fill possible, fluoride released, dynamic chemical exchange, bonds to both enamel and dentine	Good initial, but poorer long-term, appearance and mechanical properties than composite (brittle fracture and abrasion resistance lower after initial set)
Adhesive layered restoration ('sandwich' or laminate) of resin composite and glass ionomer cement (GIC)	Most useful for very deep cavities with margins primarily in dentine. Good mechanical properties with GIC as dentine replacement, composite replacing enamel. Good appearance and long-lasting. No base or lining required	Technique sensitivity as for composite, choice between using GIC or resin-modified GIC as the dentine replacement, and their poor resistance to acid-etch, bulk GIC required for strength and durability
Amalgam	Least technique-sensitive, good mechanical properties, longevity	Poor appearance, risk of overpreparation to provide macroretention (possibly may be partly overcome with bonded amalgams)

■ *Which is the most appropriate choice for this cavity?*

There is no absolutely correct answer, for the reasons given in the previous paragraph. In this case the decision was made to use resin composite. Composite would adhere well to the extensive supragingival enamel margins and the depth of the cavity might not have been sufficient to accommodate a layered restoration. The material will help support the surrounding tooth structure due to its adhesive and mechanical properties. One disadvantage of composite alone is the need to place the restoration in small increments to reduce shrinkage stress on the cavity margin. This is especially important in this case where there is considerable poorly supported enamel, but can be overcome by using the latest low-shrink composite materials (for which less than 0.9% shrinkage by volume is claimed).

■ *How do you gain access to the lesion? How much enamel will you remove?*

The lesion is already open, making access to the dentine straightforward, but much of the occlusal enamel is unsupported and weakened. Ideally, enamel at the margins should be completely sound to ensure etching and adhesion are effective. Unfortunately, this is not always easy to assess clinically. All frosted, demineralized, unsupported and friable enamel must be removed. Pressure with a hand instrument will fracture off unsupported enamel if unsure. Compromises might have to be made to conserve the cusp enamel. Once the enamel joining the cusps and forming the thick outer ring of the occlusal surface is lost, much of the strength of the crown is lost. A tungsten carbide or diamond bur in an air-turbine handpiece or hand instruments may be used to remove the enamel and introduce a slight bevel if required. (Figure 9.3.)

■ *How should you remove the carious dentine?*

Conventionally, carious dentine is removed with large slowly revolving rose-head, carbon-steel burs and hand excavators. Possible alternative techniques are shown in Table 9.2.

No method is completely guaranteed to remove only the necessary amount of caries. The best methods are those that give the most tactile feedback to the operator because assessment of softening and texture is critical to remove the optimum amount of dentine. These include the mechanical and chemomechanical methods.

Table 9.2 Techniques for excavation of carious dentine

Technique	Mechanism/advantages
Burs	Mechanical, rotary
Hand excavators	Mechanical, non-rotary
Air-abrasion (alumina/bioglass), ultrasonics, sono-abrasion, air polishing	Mechanical, non-rotary
Caridex, Carisolv gel, enzyme-based gels	Chemo-mechanical
Lasers	Ablative
Photoactive disinfection (PAD), ozone	Oxidative destruction and bacterial killing

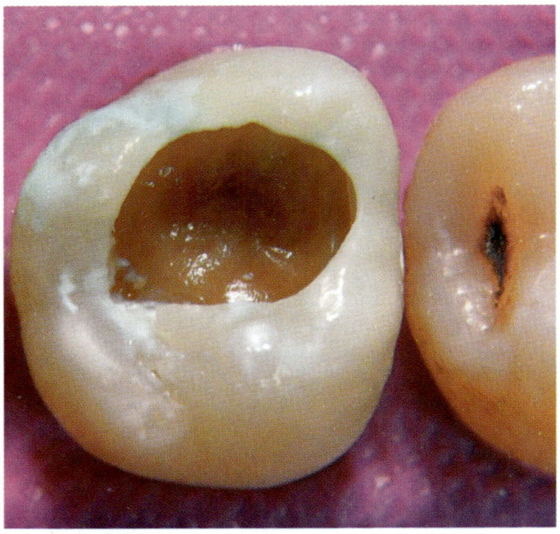

Fig. 9.3 The lesion after unsupported enamel removal.

■ *How much carious dentine needs to be removed?*

The 'correct' amount to remove is the minimum required to restore the tooth successfully and prevent disease progression. In order to achieve this, it is necessary to understand the structure of different parts of a carious lesion.

There is a continuous spectrum of degrees of dentine destruction in caries. At the advancing front (at the depth of the lesion closest to the pulp) there is demineralization (and remineralization during reversal). Behind that, the tubules are widened by demineralization and can be more easily penetrated by bacteria. Between this layer and the surface is progressive destruction of the dentine by both demineralization and proteolysis induced by bacteria. The dentine structure is destroyed and numerous bacteria live within it.

This continuous spectrum of destruction is conventionally divided into zones to aid understanding, but it must be appreciated that this is an artificial concept and that the boundaries of the zones are based on histological examination, not clinical appearance.

Dentine caries can be divided into zones of destruction, bacterial penetration and demineralization, or caries-infected and affected zones. The features of the zones are shown in Table 9.3.

In addition there are changes in the dentine caused by reactions of the pulp–dentine complex. These are not part of the caries process (they may be induced by trauma, attrition or age, for example) but they are present to some degree in carious but vital teeth and form an integral part of the overall picture. The pulp–dentine defence reactions are shown in Table 9.4.

During caries removal, the aim should be to remove all dentine that contains bacteria. Dentine that is only softened by acid can partially remineralize and repair, and may be retained under certain circumstances. Thus it will be necessary to identify the layer or zone of the lesion that clinically corresponds to the level of the red line in Table 9.3 and in Figure 9.4.

How can you recognize this level clinically?

This is difficult to do with any accuracy. The relatively smooth lines marking the edges of the zones in Figure 9.4 do not reflect the irregularly shaped advancing front and the small

Table 9.3 Histological layers of dentine caries

Location	Dentine caries zones		Features
Superficial (closest to enamel)	Destruction	Infected	Irreversibly denatured and demineralized, highly infected, 'necrotic' dentine with little residual tubular structure and lateral clefts. Loss of odontoblast processes
Middle	Bacterial penetration	Infected	Bacteria penetrate along tubules widened by demineralization. But there is less damage to the tubular structure. Loss of odontoblast processes, less loss of mineral and collagen breakdown
Deepest (closest to pulp)	Demineralization	Affected	Tubules widened by acid diffusing ahead of the advancing bacteria, dentine softened but structurally intact. Loss of odontoblast processes

Table 9.4 Pulp–dentine complex responses to dentine caries

Reaction/change	Effect
Peritubular reactionary dentine	Forms on the inner wall of tubules where odontoblast processes remain alive. Gradually obliterates tubules around the sides of the carious lesion and between it and the pulp. Occlusion of the tubules makes the dentine translucent and more radiodense. This is known as the translucent zone (not to be confused with the translucent zone in enamel caries, which is quite different) The circumpulpal dentine has the largest tubule diameter and is softer and more porous than dentine further from the pulp. Peritubular sclerosis is therefore a very useful reaction in the deepest layers
Regular reactionary dentine ('tertiary' dentine)	Forms in the pulp below the lesion, obliterating pulp horns and increasing the amount of dentine between caries and the pulp. Only slowly formed reactionary dentine is regular and it forms a good barrier to caries, even though it does not always form at the most useful sites
Irregular reactionary dentine ('tertiary' dentine)	A rapidly formed reactionary dentine in the pulp below caries. As regular reactionary dentine, but forms a less well-organized, more permeable and less effective barrier

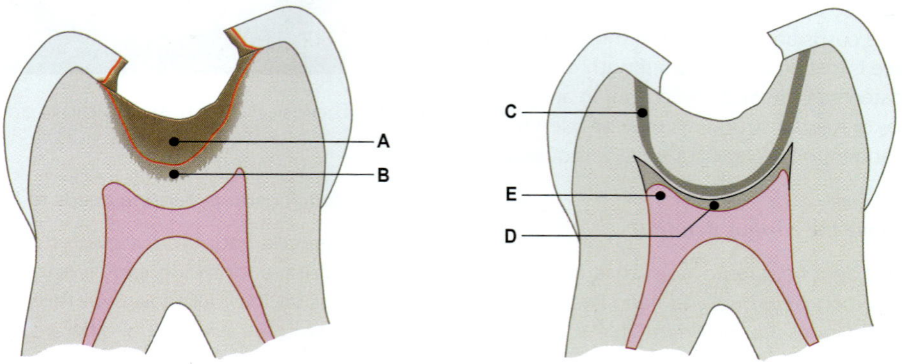

Fig. 9.4 The zones of dentine caries and pulp–dentine defence reactions. Left panel, zones of caries: **A** Infected dentine (including the zones of dentine destruction and bacterial penetration along intact tubules); **B** affected, demineralized dentine. Right panel, pulp defence reactions: **C** translucent zone formed by peritubular sclerosis surrounds the lesion; **D** regular and/or irregular reactionary ('tertiary') dentine that has reduced the size of the pulp; **E** pulpitis, an immunological and inflammatory reaction triggered by odontoblast damage, but not helpful in resisting the advance of caries.

tongues of bacteria that penetrate tubules in advance of the main lesion.

It is universally accepted that not *all* bacteria have to be removed during excavation. Those that are sealed from the oral environment, the primary source of their substrate, will either die or become dormant. Provided the restoration provides a good seal, small numbers of retained bacteria will not be sufficient to allow caries to progress below the restoration. Removal of grossly infected dentine is relatively straightforward. All superficial, very soft, wet, often more darkly stained dentine is highly infected and is readily excavated.

Whether the underlying caries-affected dentine, which can potentially be repaired by the dentine–pulp complex, may be spared is a decision that must be made on a case-by-case basis. It is usually preserved in the cavity depths to protect the pulp but cleared from around the enamel–dentine junction to ensure that the peripheral seal is effective.

Caries-affected dentine is often stained and is softer than the surrounding healthy dentine. A possible clinical indicator that the boundary zone between infected and affected dentine has been reached is that the cavity surface is both scratchy and sticky to a sharp dental probe. Unfortunately this sensation cannot be appreciated in the words from a textbook and requires experience of the sensation!

■ *Can caries detector dyes help identify the zones in carious dentine?*

The original caries detector dyes, developed in the 1970s and based on propylene glycol solutions, were claimed to stain collagen that had become denatured by the carious process. However, they tended to penetrate too far into dentine and stain acid-denatured collagen, thus staining both infected and affected zones, and even sound dentine. Removing all dye-stained dentine therefore risked excessive and unnecessary dentine removal.

New caries indicators under development detect bacterial metabolism and have the potential to identify the infected zone more accurately in future.

■ *The appearance after initial caries removal is shown in Figure 9.5. What do you see?*

The dentine surface is still friable and flakes parallel with the surface, along clefts that are the result of bacteria breaking out of the tubules. The base of the cavity must still be in the infected zone. It is *just* starting to feel scratchy with a probe. Further caries should be removed.

■ *The final extent of excavation is shown in Figure 9.6. What do you see?*

Further dentine has been removed around the periphery. Affected dentine over the pulp has been retained. It does not show the gross flaking seen in Figure 9.5, but is still stained but dry, appearing matt. It is still noticeably soft but distinctly scratchy with a sharp probe. Consideration must be given of the relative hardness of the dentine retained at the base of the final cavity. If it is too soft, there is a risk that cohesive failure could occur within the dentine itself on shrinkage of an adhesive restorative material.

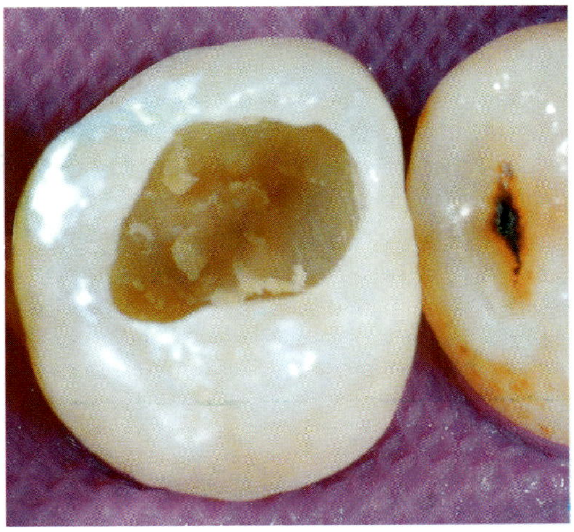

Fig. 9.5 Initial removal of grossly infected dentine.

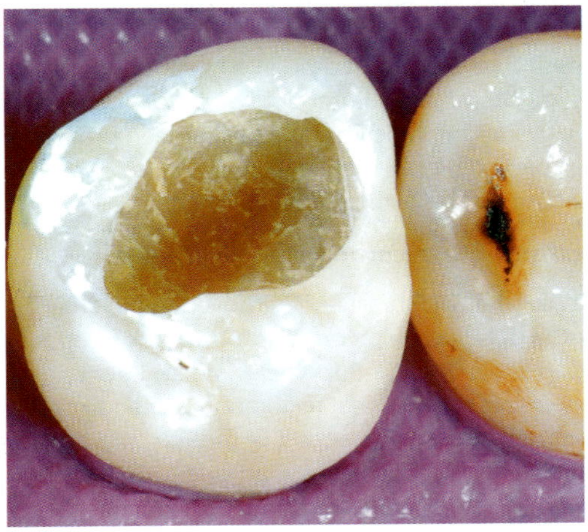

Fig. 9.6 Final caries excavation.

■ *Should this restoration have a mesial box?*

The amelodentinal junction is clearly visible in Figure 9.6 and both mesial and distal enamel have lost all, or most, of their support. There is an argument that the unsupported enamel will fracture, leading to failure of the restoration. If amalgam were being used, then both mesial and distal boxes would definitely be required.

Conversely, removing the mesial or distal enamel would seriously compromise the strength of the remaining crown and predispose to cuspal fracture, particularly buccally. Modern adhesive materials have good compressive strength and adhesion to the whole of the dentine and enamel inner surface of the cavity and will provide support for the enamel. It must be accepted that leaving this enamel does incur a small risk of failure, but the potential benefit of a more conservative approach outweighs the risk. Approximal caries, adverse occlusion or the possibility that the patient might not return immediately if the tooth fractured would influence this decision.

■ ***Surely caries has been left under this restoration and it will fail?***

In the recent past, this cavity would have been considered inadequate, with soft and stained dentine remaining on the cavity floor. There are almost certainly bacteria remaining in the dentine. If this cavity were to be prepared for amalgam, with its inherently poor marginal seal, the restoration would probably fail fairly quickly. However, the principles of caries removal have been revolutionized partly by the advent of adhesive restorations, which seal effectively, and partly by recognition that dentine caries may remineralize.

There is a risk that this more conservative approach will lead to failure if the quality of the overlying restoration is suboptimal. Leaving more caries than was accepted in the past does carry a risk, but the affected dentine has been left behind for specific reasons. This conservative approach will require continued monitoring for success.

Annual review will permit any visual changes to the restoration and its seal to be noticed. Early in its life, the restoration may develop some staining along sections of the margin and this does not constitute failure of the seal. However, if staining is accompanied by roughness to a sharp dental probe (not accounted for by fracture of composite 'flash'), this might indicate the seal has been breached and the restoration would require repair or possibly replacement, depending on the extent of the breakdown.

■ ***What is stepwise excavation?***

A technique in which caries is removed in increments to allow the dentine–pulp complex to heal the deeper layers of caries-affected dentine. Superficial infected dentine is removed and a provisional restoration placed to seal in the remaining tissue. Over a period of months, the deepest affected dentine remineralizes and develops an appearance similar to arrested carious dentine: darker, harder and drier than previously. Peritubular and reactionary dentine are also laid down around the lesion and at the pulp interface during this period.

If this technique were to be followed, the restoration would be removed after approximately 9 months, further carious dentine excavated and a permanent restoration placed. Current evidence suggests that this is clinically unnecessary. The peripheral seal of modern adhesive restorations is now so good that arrest and remineralization are predictable.

The notes might record that this tooth has been excavated conservatively and re-restoration can be delayed until either the restoration peripheral seal fails or, perhaps, some unsupported enamel fractures off. At that stage a decision can be made about further excavation. After removal of the failed restoration, if the cavity floor is hard and dry, no further dentine removal may be necessary.

■ ***Does the cavity require a lining for pulp protection?***

The purposes of cavity linings are:

1. to protect the pulp from the bacterial infection and diffusion of bacterial acid and toxins
2. to seal, impregnate and mechanically reinforce any layer of caries-affected dentine that may have been retained
3. to stimulate the dentine–pulp complex to lay down tertiary dentine as a defence response, usually when using calcium hydroxide-based linings
4. to protect the pulp from thermal, electrical and mechanical stimuli transmitted through the overlying restoration.

Many adhesive restorative materials and bonding agents carry out all these functions perfectly adequately and so the value of a separate lining is nowadays seriously debatable. However, it is still a common practice amongst some dentists to place a minimal lining at the base of a deep cavity close to the pulp, often using a calcium hydroxide or glass ionomer cement.

The final restoration is shown in Figure 9.7. It was finished using composite finishing burs and polishing discs and pastes to improve the final lustre of the restoration surface.

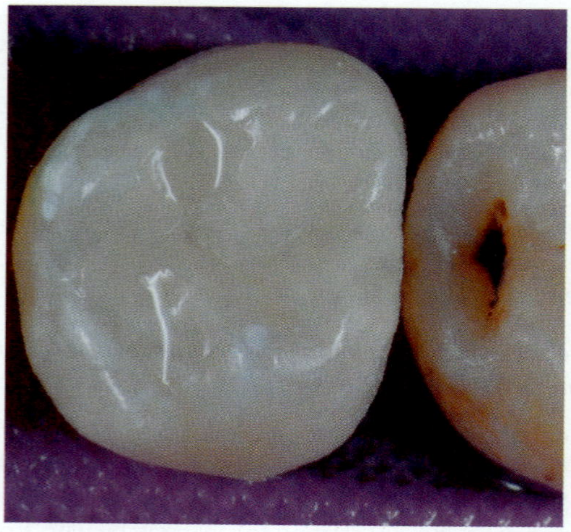

Fig. 9.7 The final restoration.

Case • 10

A lump on the gingiva

SUMMARY

A 48-year-old man presents to you in general dental practice with a gingival swelling. What is the cause and what would you do?

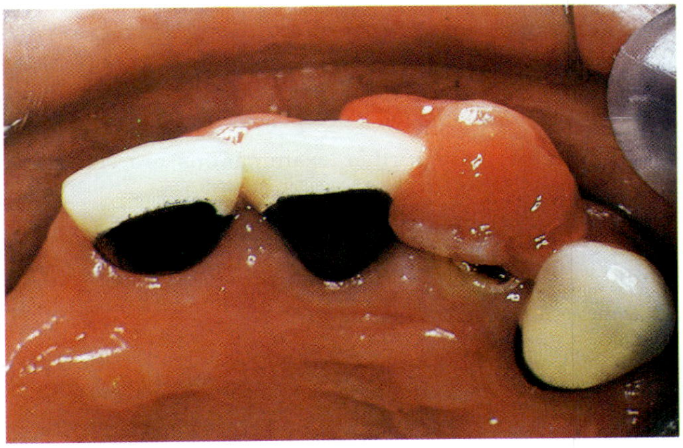

Fig. 10.1 Appearance of the swelling.

History

Complaint

The patient complains of a lump on the gum at the front of his mouth on the left side. It sometimes bleeds, usually after brushing or eating hard food but it is not painful.

History of complaint

The swelling has been present for 4 months and has grown slowly during this period. It was never painful but now looks unsightly. The patient gives no history of other mucosal or skin lesions.

Medical history

The patient has hypertension, controlled with atenolol 50 mg daily.

Examination

Extraoral examination

He is healthy looking but slightly overweight. There are no palpable cervical lymph nodes.

Intraoral examination

The patient is partially dentate and has relatively few and extensively restored teeth. He wears an upper partial denture. The root of the upper lateral incisor is present and its carious surface lies at the level of the alveolar ridge. The teeth on each side of the lesion are restored with metal–ceramic crowns.

There is a mild degree of marginal gingivitis. Most of the interdental papillae are rounded and marginal inflammation is present around crowns. Flecks of subgingival calculus are visible.

■ ***The appearance of the lesion is shown in Figure 10.1. Describe its features.***

Feature	Appearance
Site	Appears to arise from the gingival margin of the lateral incisor root or the interdental papilla mesially
Size	Approximately 10 × 7 mm
Shape and contour	Irregular rounded nodule. It is not possible to say whether it is pedunculated or sessile, though from its size and the fact that it overlies the lateral incisor root, it is probably pedunculated
Colour	Patchy red and pink with a thin grey translucent sheen. The surface is almost certainly ulcerated

If you were able to palpate the lesion you would find that it is fleshy and soft and attached by a thin base to the gingival margin. It bleeds readily from between the tooth and lesion when pressed with an instrument but it is not tender.

■ ***From the information in the history and examination so far, what is your differential diagnosis?***

Likely:

— Pyogenic granuloma (if the patient had been female, pregnancy epulis might have been considered)

— Fibrous epulis

Less likely:

— Peripheral giant cell granuloma

— Sinus papilla (parulis)

Unlikely:

— Papilloma

— Benign hamartoma or neoplasm

— Malignant neoplasm.

■ ***Justify your differential diagnosis.***

A very wide range of lesions may affect the gingiva and many possible causes cannot be excluded on the basis of the information given so far. However, the gingiva is the site of predilection for a number of inflammatory hyperplastic lesions comprising fibrous tissue and epithelium. All are associated with poor oral hygiene and the lesion is almost certainly one of this type on statistical grounds.

Pyogenic granuloma is a localized proliferation of granulation tissue or very vascular fibrous tissue. It arises in association with a local irritant such as poor oral hygiene, calculus or the margin of a restoration. The present lesion has many features of the pyogenic granuloma: it is asymptomatic, soft and vascular, bleeds readily, and has an ulcerated surface. If the patient had been female, a pregnancy epulis (a variant of pyogenic granuloma arising during pregnancy) would have been possible.

Fibrous epulis (gingival fibroepithelial polyp/nodule) is a nodule of more fibrous hyperplastic tissue. It is not usually ulcerated, is firmer on palpation and does not bleed so readily. Some fibrous epulides develop from pyogenic granulomas by maturation of the fibrous tissue and some arise de novo. They are usually associated with a local irritant in the same manner as pyogenic granulomas. The current lesion could well be a fibrous epulis, though its vascularity and red colour are more suggestive of pyogenic granuloma. These two names are really no more than convenient labels for lesions at opposite ends of a spectrum ranging from granulation tissue to dense fibrous tissue. All are hyperplastic.

Peripheral giant cell granuloma is another hyperplastic lesion which seems to develop in response to a local irritant. Clinically it may have a deep red maroon or blue colour, but is otherwise indistinguishable from pyogenic granuloma or fibrous epulis. However, histologically it is distinctive, containing numerous multinucleate osteoclast-like giant cells lying in a very cellular vascular stroma. The giant cell epulis is commoner in children, though it can arise in an adult. While it cannot be excluded, it is a less likely diagnosis for the present lesion.

Sinus papilla (parulis) is essentially a pyogenic granuloma developing at the opening of a sinus. Infection and inflammation are the stimuli inducing hyperplasia. If the sinus heals, the sinus papilla may disappear or it may mature and shrink into a small fibrous nodule. The usual site is on the alveolar mucosa and the lesion is usually no more than 4 or 5 mm across. This is an unlikely cause.

Papillomas are lesions of proliferating epithelium. Their exact cause is not always clear though it is generally considered that most are caused by human papilloma virus infection. Others do not appear to contain virus and may be benign neoplasms. Papillomas may arise at any site in the oral cavity but are often seen at the gingival margin and lips. Sometimes patients have warts on their fingers as well. Papillomas usually have a white spiky or frond-covered surface or a smoother cauliflower-like surface and neither is seen in the present lesion. Papillomas do not bleed easily and this seems an unlikely diagnosis.

It would not be useful to list the many other possible causes, but a few groups of lesions might also be considered.

Hamartomas and benign neoplasms can arise at all sites. If this were such a lesion a haemangioma would be likely in view of the vascularity. A haemangioma could appear very similar to a pyogenic granuloma.

Odontogenic tumours can occasionally arise extraosseously in the gingiva but usually form uninflamed sessile nodules.

Malignant neoplasms occasionally present in the gingiva. Metastatic deposits are commoner than primary lesions and leukaemia is the most likely cause. Kaposi's sarcoma might also be considered in an HIV-positive individual. Both these lesions are vascular, may bleed on pressure and ulcerate.

Further examination and investigations

■ ***What further examinations and investigations would you perform? Explain why.***

The definitive diagnosis will require a biopsy, and excision is indicated. However a number of other investigations (Table 10.1) need to be performed to identify possible causes. If the cause is left untreated the lesion may recur after excision.

The results of these further examinations are shown in Table 10.1.

Differential diagnosis

■ ***What is the most likely diagnosis?***

On the basis of the clinical appearance and the results of the tests in Table 10.1 the lesion is almost certainly a pyogenic granuloma or fibrous epulis.

Treatment

■ ***What treatment would you provide?***

- Excision biopsy
- Removal of causative factors, i.e. plaque and calculus
- Provide treatment for the generalized periodontitis
- Extract or restore the lateral incisor root.

Table 10.1 Investigations and findings

Test	Reason	Findings in this patient
Periodontal examination	To assess pocketing around the lesion and detect subgingival calculus, a common cause	There is generalized chronic adult periodontitis with loss of attachment of 3–4 mm. There is a 5-mm probing depth adjacent to the lesion, most of which is false pocket below the lesion. This pocket and others contain subgingival calculus
Tests of vitality of the adjacent incisor and canine	To determine whether the cause could be irritation from a periapical infection draining into the pocket	Both teeth are vital on electric pulp testing
Periapical view of the incisor and canine	Not useful for diagnosis but might be indicated on the basis of probing or vitality tests	Not indicated

Table 10.2 Obtaining a report on a biopsy specimen

Aim	Procedure
Avoid distortion or crushing of specimen	If a suture has been placed through the lesion to hold it and prevent it being lost in the vacuum, do not remove it. Cut the thread a centimetre or so from the lesion
Ensure rapid and efficient fixation	Place immediately in 10 times the tissue volume of 10% formol saline (available in biopsy containers from pharmacies, hospital suppliers and some pathology departments). In the absence of fixative, postpone the biopsy if possible. Spirits and other solutions used in dental surgeries are ineffective. An unfixed specimen will autolyse (rot) on the way to the laboratory
Provide the pathologist with sufficient clinical information to enable diagnosis	Fill in a request form or write a letter including the patient's name, age and sex, a complete clinical description of the lesion, the differential diagnosis and medical history. Include any details of previous lesions or lesions elsewhere in the mouth. Do not forget your own name and practice address and phone number
Protect those handling the specimen in transit	Package the specimen according to the Post Office regulations for sending hazardous materials through the post. Make sure the container is labelled with a hazard sticker identifying the contents as formalin. Place the specimen container in either an unbreakable second container or box with padding. Include enough absorbent material (e.g. tissue) to soak up all the formalin in the pack in the event of breakage. Label the package 'Pathology specimen – handle with care' and send by first-class post

■ ***Would you perform this biopsy in general dental practice? What complications might develop?***

Yes: this amounts to no more than the removal of a flap of gingiva, and ideally this would be performed in general practice. The only significant complication might be bleeding because this is a very vascular lesion. However, haemostasis should not prove a problem because pressure can be readily applied to the gingival margin.

■ ***How would you obtain a report on the biopsy specimen?***

Most histopathology departments, either specialized oral pathology departments associated with dental schools, or departments in district general or other hospitals, provide postal or courier pathology services for the dentists and/or medical practitioners in their area.

The steps to be taken after removal are shown in Table 10.2.

Diagnosis

■ ***The microscopic appearances of the biopsy specimen are shown in Figures 10.2 and 10.3. What do you see and how do you interpret them?***

The surface is ulcerated and covered by a slough of fibrin containing nuclei of inflammatory cells. At higher power you would be able to identify these as neutrophils. Below the surface is a pale-stained tissue in which the endothelial lining of numerous small blood vessels stands out. The vessels have a radiating pattern and point towards the surface reflecting a pattern of growth outwards from the centre. Between the vessels there is a little fibrin and the tissue is oedematous or myxoid or both. More deeply there is a cluster of inflammatory cells and collagen bundles are more prominent between the vessels.

The lesion is a nodule of ulcerated maturing granulation and fibrous tissue.

■ ***What is the diagnosis?***

Pyogenic granuloma.

Other possibilities

■ ***Is a more conservative approach to treatment ever justified?***

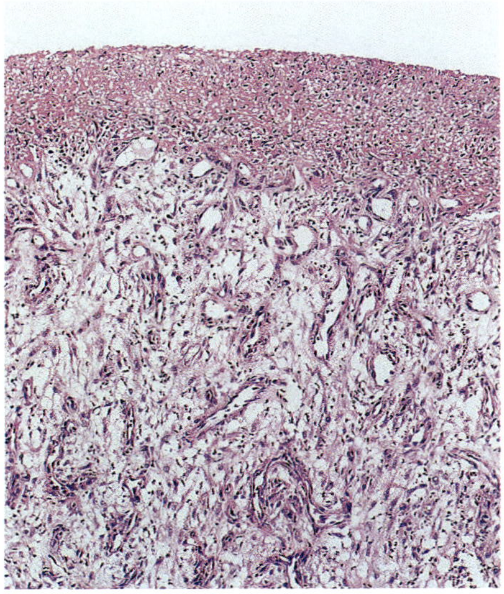

Fig. 10.2 Histological appearance of the surface layers of the excision specimen.

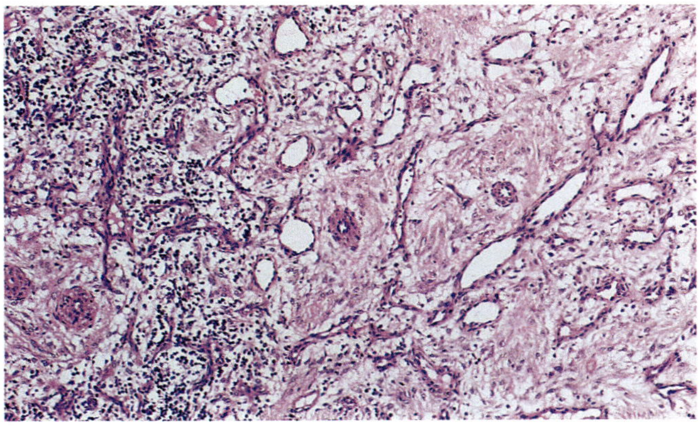

Fig. 10.3 The deeper tissue of the specimen.

Yes: elimination of the causative factors may induce considerable resolution. However, the degree of resolution varies; softer more vascular lesions shrink most and firmer more fibrous lesions hardly at all. Removal of calculus and improved oral hygiene may cause partial resolution and leave a smaller lesion which is easier to excise and bleeds much less. Such a course of action is often appropriate for treatment of pregnancy epulis, both because of the wish to avoid the procedure during pregnancy and because excision during pregnancy carries a risk of recurrence. Definitive excision may then be delayed until after parturition. Occasionally resolution is almost complete and no further treatment is required.

■ ***If, on removing the lesion, you felt bone within it, what would this signify?***

Woven and lamellar bone, sometimes quite large pieces, can lie within fibrous epulides and pyogenic granulomas. Bone may be noted on excision or on histological examination. Sometimes such lesions are referred to as mineralizing epulides (or peripheral ossifying fibroma in the US). The presence of bone seems to be of no great significance and it may indicate that such lesions arise by proliferation of the deep fibrous tissue of the periosteum. Some consider lesions containing bone more likely to recur than those without but there is no good evidence to support this belief.

Case • 11

Pain on biting

SUMMARY

A 32-year-old man presents at your general dental practice surgery with intermittent pain on biting. Identify the cause and discuss treatment options.

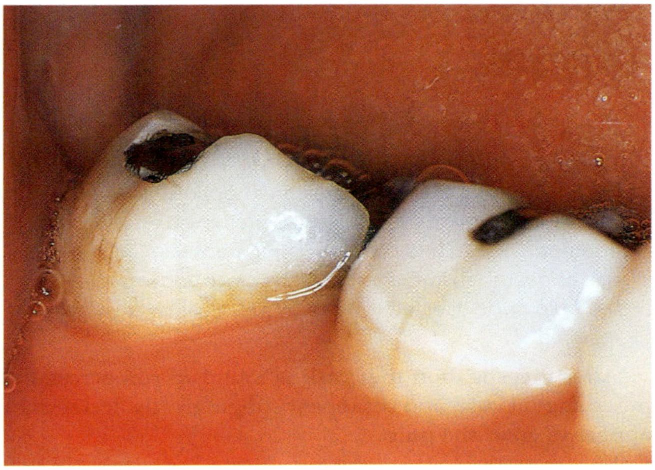

Fig. 11.1 The teeth in the lower right quadrant.

History

Complaint

He complains of pain on biting which is unpredictable, extremely painful and sharp but poorly localized. It originates in the lower right quadrant and lasts a very short time, only as long as the teeth are in contact, and is so painful that he has become accustomed to eating on the left. The pain only arises on biting hard foods or deliberately clenching his teeth. Apart from these sharp electric shock-like pains he has no other symptoms.

History of complaint

The pain is a recent phenomenon, having been first noticed a month or two ago. At first it was frequent but it has become less of a problem now that he has learnt to avoid triggering the pain. He has not noticed the pain being provoked by hot or cold.

Dental history

The patient has been a regular attender at your practice since childhood. He has a small number of relatively small restorations. At his last appointment, some 4 months ago you placed an amalgam restoration in the lower right second molar.

- ***Based on what you know already what are the likely causes? Explain why.***

A pulpal pain is the most likely cause because the pain appears to originate in a tooth and is poorly localized. Pain of periodontal ligament origin should be well localized. However, pulpitis appears not be present because there is no sensitivity to hot or cold. Pulpitis caused by placement of the recent amalgams and pain due to caries or exposed dentine can be excluded for the same reasons.

A crack in the tooth or electrogalvanic pain are possible causes suggested by pain on biting. Both are triggered by tooth–tooth contact.

Trigeminal neuralgia should be considered as an unlikely nondental cause. It causes paroxysmal stabbing or electric shock-like facial pain in distributions of the trigeminal nerve and may be initiated by touching or moving trigger zones. It usually affects the middle-aged or elderly. The history of pain on biting is almost conclusive of a dental cause but it can be difficult to exclude trigeminal neuralgia in some patients, particularly when trigger zones lie in the mouth or attacks are triggered by eating. If no dental cause is found, the possibility of trigeminal neuralgia may need further investigation.

Acute periodontitis caused by an occlusal high spot on the recently placed amalgam needs to be considered. However, although this could cause great tenderness on biting it would be expected that the pain from the bruised periodontium would be present at other times. Also, such periodontally-sensed pain would be well localized.

- ***What additional questions would you ask? Why?***

The patient should be asked about clenching or bruxing of the teeth because the additional occlusal load can cause fracture and will determine treatment options.

The patient describes a habit of nocturnal bruxism with some tenderness of masticatory muscles at times of stress.

Examination

Extraoral examination

There is a suspicion of hypertrophy of the masseter muscles on clenching.

Intraoral examination

The incisal edges of the upper and lower anterior teeth are worn and the dentine is exposed. The cusps of the posterior teeth are slightly flattened or rounded consistent with mild attrition. There is no evidence of any loss of attachment or gingival recession.

The appearance of the teeth in the lower right quadrant is shown in Figure 11.1. The lower right molars and premolars contain small- to moderate-sized MOD amalgam restorations, those in the molars having small buccal extensions. The upper molars have small separate MO and DO amalgams, the DO amalgams having buccal extensions. The upper premolars are unrestored.

■ ***What features of the restorations would you note particularly?***

The restorations should be inspected for occlusal high spots, indicated by a burnished mark on the occlusal surface. Premature occlusal contact could be confirmed with articulating paper and relieving the area might cure the pain indicating the diagnosis.

Though they are unlikely causes for this particular pain, marginal caries, poor marginal adaptation or a cracked restoration should be sought.

Differential diagnosis

■ ***What is your differential diagnosis? Why?***

The pain is almost certainly caused by a cracked cusp or crown. The presence of masseteric hypertrophy and attrition on the occlusal surfaces of the teeth would suggest a parafunctional habit that could predispose the tooth to cracking.

Galvanic pain may be excluded because there are no occluding restorations of dissimilar metals.

■ ***Which tooth would you suspect? Why?***

The lower second molar appears the most likely to be cracked. It should be investigated first because the pain seems to have started shortly after restoration. The risk of cracking depends on the size of restorations. The upper teeth have small restorations which are limited to fissures and mesial and distal surfaces. In the upper molar the ridge of enamel joining the distobuccal to mesiopalatal cusps is intact so that cusps are unlikely to be undermined.

Intact teeth can also crack, though usually only in association with increased occlusal load. The most susceptible teeth are the premolars because moderately sized amalgams undermine the lingual and palatal cusps in the small crowns. Lower first molars are also prone to crack because they tend to contain the largest restorations in the mouth.

Root-filled teeth are prone to crack but obviously could not cause a pulpal pain. Symptoms would then only be produced if the periodontal ligament were involved and the pain would be well localized.

Investigations

■ ***What tests and further examinations would you perform to identify the causative tooth? What do the results tell you?***

The investigations are described in Table 11.1.

On performing these tests you discover that all the teeth in the quadrant are vital. Biting on cotton wool on the lower second molar provokes pain that the patient identifies as the same as that on biting. No particular cusp can be identified and no crack can be found.

Treatment

■ ***What would you do next? Explain why.***

The path of the crack must be defined as far as possible because this will determine treatment options. The restoration(s) in the tooth should be removed and a further attempt made to find the crack using transillumination and dye as described in Table 11.1. If the crack appears to enter the pulp or be directed towards it, root treatment will be required.

After investigation the crack is found to run across the mesiolingual cusp and disappear subgingivally. It does not appear to enter the pulp.

Table 11.1 Identifying the causative tooth

Investigation	Significance
Tests of vitality of all teeth in the lower right quadrant should be performed, either with an electric pulp tester or a cold stimulus.	The pain must originate from a vital tooth. It is also possible that the cracked tooth might be hypersensitive. This could aid diagnosis though hypersensitivity to testing would not be expected in the absence of pain on hot and cold. Vitality might also affect the choice of treatment.
Close examination with a good light (a bright fibre optic is especially useful for transillumination). A soluble dye such as a disclosing agent may be painted onto the crown. After the excess is washed off small amounts may remain in the crack rendering it visible.	May reveal a crack.
Attempts to stimulate the pain by pressing the handle of an instrument against each cusp, preferably from more than one direction.	Pain indicates a cracked cusp and the causative cusp is identified.
Ask the patient to bite hard on a soft object such as a cotton wool roll.	This transmits pressure to the whole occlusal surface and forces the cusps slightly apart. Pain on biting suggests a cracked tooth.
Place a wooden wedge against each cusp in turn and ask the patient to bite on each.	This is a more selective test to identify the cusp or cusps which are cracked. By placing the wedge on different surfaces of the cusp it may be possible to tell in which direction the crack runs. There may be pain on biting but pain which is worse on release of pressure is said to be characteristic.
Radiograph	To exclude the possibility of caries and to assess the feasibility of root filling the tooth should it be necessary. The radiograph is unlikely to be of direct help in diagnosis and might not be necessary if other investigations successfully identify the cracked cusp.

Table 11.2 Restoration options for cracked teeth

Option	Advantages and disadvantages
No treatment	This is not an option, even if the patient is happy to put up with the pain. Cracks may propagate into the pulp, allow bacterial contamination and devitalize the tooth.
Removal of the cracked portion followed by restoration	This is unsafe. Levering of the cracked portion risks a catastrophic fracture with pulpal communication. Many cracks are incomplete and leverage may propagate them in unpredictable directions. Just occasionally the fragment will be limited to enamel and dentine of the crown, particularly where the tooth already contains a large restoration undermining the cusp, but even then a deliberate fracture is not recommended.
Full or partial coverage gold indirect restoration	This is the treatment of choice. The preparation should finish supragingivally wherever possible. Gold is malleable and allows some plastic deformation which is not possible with ceramics or composites which are more brittle. Full occlusal coverage is needed to protect the tooth from further damage and a casting can provide some splinting, reducing the potential for further cracks.
Full coverage bonded porcelain crown	Full coverage with porcelain bonded to metal has the advantage of a better appearance but the ceramic is brittle. This disadvantage may be offset by using an adhesive to lute the crown. There is then the potential for the crack to be sealed by the infiltrating cement.
Adhesive restoration	In theory an adhesive restoration would cement the crack together and prevent movement of the two fragments. However, on curing, adhesive materials undergo polymerization shrinkage which places further stress on the crack and may propagate it further.
Porcelain inlay/onlay	These suffer the same disadvantages of metal fused to porcelain crowns.

■ ***What are the treatment options for restoring cracked teeth? What are their advantages and disadvantages?***

These are listed in Table 11.2.

■ ***If the cracked portion had already been broken off at presentation and the pulp were not involved, what restoration options would have been open to you?***

Assuming no second crack were present, this would present a simple choice. One of the methods described in Table 11.2 could be used and this would have the advantage that further cracks would be prevented. In view of the history of bruxism this might be an appropriate option.

However, most cracks are single and it would also be possible to adopt a more conservative approach and restore with a composite and a dentine bonding agent or a sandwich restoration. The latter uses a glass ionomer to replace the dentine and a composite to replace the enamel. An amalgam restoration is also simple and highly effective. Both these would require the cusp to be reduced in height to reduce the occlusal load.

■ ***Suppose you had been unable to identify the causative tooth using the methods described above. What would you try next?***

Sometimes it is difficult to identify a crack. The pain is poorly localized and a first step would be to repeat the whole procedure on the upper molars and premolars in case the patient has incorrectly localized the pain.

If no crack is identified, the restorations must be removed from any further teeth that appear to be likely causes. Finally, the most suspect tooth may have a tight fitting copper band or orthodontic band cemented around it. This can be left in position for several weeks to see whether the pain is abolished, and is a particularly useful test when the pain is felt infrequently.

Case 12

A defective denture base

SUMMARY

The acrylic denture base and cobalt–chromium casting shown both have defects caused by similar mechanisms. Can you identify the problem and its causes, which are different in the two examples.

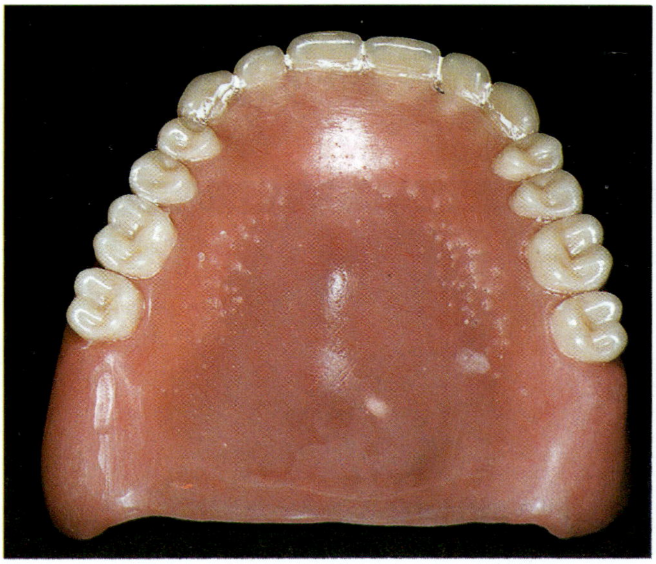

Fig. 12.1 The heat-processed 'acrylic', poly(methylmethacrylate) denture base.

Acrylic complete denture

■ ***A heat-processed 'acrylic', poly(methylmethacrylate) denture base is shown in Figure 12.1. What do you see and how do you interpret these observations?***

The denture base has a cluster of small round holes in a horseshoe-shaped distribution just inside the teeth. The defects are more frequent in areas of thicker acrylic. Each defect appears to be round, some are completely enclosed in acrylic, while others communicate with the surface via sharply defined holes.

The presence of numerous small holes or defects within the acrylic is known as porosity.

■ ***What are the types of porosity? How do they manifest and what are their causes?***

The types of porosity are presented in Table 12.1.

Table 12.1 Types of porosity

Defect	Manifestation	Cause
Contraction porosity	Porosity throughout the denture. The denture may be the incorrect shape.	Insufficient material packed into the flask, or inadequate flasking pressure. Correct use of the trial packing stage should eliminate this.
Gaseous porosity	Porosity in a localized area of the denture base, particularly in the thicker parts. Each defect is round and sharply defined.	Vaporization of monomer during processing.
Granular porosity	Porosity appears in thin sections of the denture, which often have a 'white and frosty' appearance.	Incorrect polymer: monomer ratio when producing the dough, or failing to pack the flask at the dough stage.

This denture has suffered from gaseous porosity and the appearances are typical but more extensive than usually seen.

■ ***What causes monomer to vaporize during processing?***

The boiling point of methylmethacrylate is 100.3°C at standard temperature and pressure. If the boiling point is exceeded then the methylmethacrylate vaporizes and bubbles produce porous defects. The polymerization of methylmethacrylate is exothermic and will contribute to vaporization if precautions are not taken to reduce the temperature. Because the process is heat-dependent, it is most likely to develop in thick sections of the denture and in the last portions to be polymerized.

■ ***How is gaseous porosity normally prevented?***

Methylmethacrylate should be polymerized at a low temperature and under pressure. Packing the dough under pressure raises the boiling point of the methylmethacrylate, and polymerization at 72°C for 16 hours (or 72°C for 2 hours and 100°C for a further 2 hours) followed by slow cooling gives time for the heat of the exothermic reaction to dissipate.

Cobalt–chromium casting

■ ***A cobalt–chromium denture framework is shown in Figure 12.2. What do you see and how do you interpret these changes?***

The metal has numerous small perforating holes. They are of various sizes and some have coalesced to form large defects.

■ ***What are the common defects in cobalt–chromium casting? How may they be prevented?***

See Table 12.2.

■ ***Which of these defects affects the present casting? Explain why.***

The casting defects are small and round, like those in the acrylic denture, and also appear to be caused by gas bubble formation. This is another example of porosity but it is much more extensive than is seen when the investment is too thick or gas dissolves in the alloy. In this case a more fundamental mistake must have been made and the cause is probably use of the wrong investment material.

If a framework is invested in a gypsum-bonded investment, the investment will break down at a lower temperature than the melting point of the alloy. The $CaSO_4$ binder reacts with the SiO_2 refractory to produce SO_3 gas, bubbles of which cause porosity in the casting. Gypsum-bonded investments are used for gold-based alloys and phosphate-bonded investments must be used for Co–Cr based alloys.

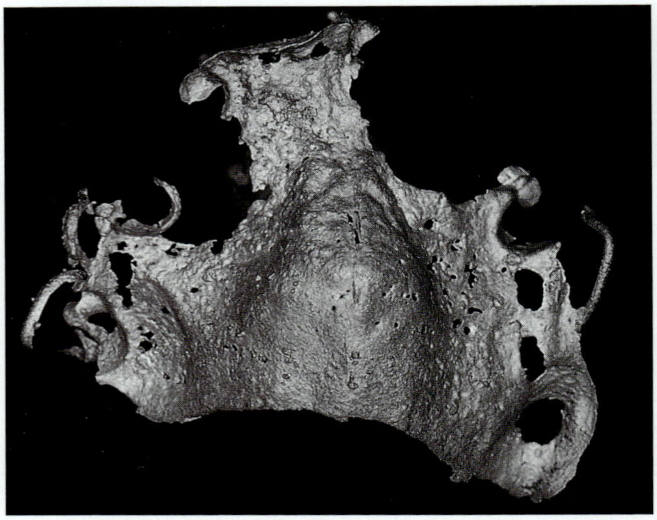

Fig. 12.2 The cobalt–chromium partial denture casting.

Table 12.2 Common defects in cobalt–chromium castings

Defect	Cause	Preventive measure
Porosity: spherical voids	Investment too thick Gases dissolve in the alloy and form bubbles on cooling	Use the correct powder: liquid ratio Do not overheat the alloy
Porosity: irregular voids	Casting shrinkage Turbulent flow of the alloy	Ensure sprues are of the correct diameter Ensure sprues are in the correct position
Incomplete cast: rounded margins	Back pressure of air in the mould	Use a porous investment or include vents
Incomplete cast: short casting	Insufficient alloy Mould too cold when cast Insufficient casting force	Use sufficient alloy Ensure the correct operating temperature Ensure the machine is correctly set up
Fins	Investment cracking	Use the correct investment and do not heat too rapidly
Rough surface	Investment breakdown Air bubbles on wax pattern	Use the correct investment and do not overheat Use a wetting agent
Distortion	Stress relief of the wax pattern	Warm the wax thoroughly before making the pattern
Cast too small	Insufficient investment expansion	Use the correct operating temperature
Cast too large	Too much investment expansion	Use the correct investment for the alloy, and the correct operating temperature

Case • 13

Sudden collapse

SUMMARY

A 55-year-old male patient suddenly collapses in your general dental practice. What is the cause and what would you do?

History

Complaint

The patient has attended for a routine dental appointment to receive some simple conservation work under local anaesthetic. He is a regular attender but dislikes injections.

Twenty minutes after injection of the local anaesthetic he suddenly becomes anxious and complains of a pain in his chest. He is breathless. When your nurse asks the patient if he is OK there is no response.

Medical history

Having checked the medical history just before starting treatment you are aware that the patient is a well-controlled insulin-dependent diabetic. He suffers hypertension and takes enalapril 20 mg daily (Innovace) and is overweight. He smokes 20 cigarettes a day and describes himself as a 'social drinker', consuming 30 units of alcohol each week.

■ ***What would you do immediately?***

Check to see whether the patient is conscious. Make a determined effort to rouse him by shaking him and asking loudly whether he can hear you.

The patient does not respond.

■ ***What causes of sudden loss of consciousness might affect a patient undergoing dental treatment?***

The important causes of unexpected loss of consciousness are:

- vasovagal attack (faint)
- hypoglycaemia
- cardiac arrest
- steroid crisis.

Loss of consciousness may also follow several other emergencies including respiratory obstruction or respiratory failure, epilepsy, stroke or anaphylactic shock, in which the cause is likely to be evident.

■ ***How may these causes of loss of consciousness be differentiated?***

Cause	Signs and symptoms
Vasovagal attack (faint)	Often associated with anxiety. Usually, though not always, some premonitory symptoms of faintness before losing consciousness. Cold clammy skin, pallor, initially bradycardia and low pulse volume followed by tachycardia and a full pulse. Rapid recovery on placing supine or slightly head down (maximum recommended inclination 10°).
Hypoglycaemia	Seen in starved patients or diabetics with relative insulin overdose caused by starvation or stress. Rapid recovery on administering oral glucose or, if unconscious, glucagon followed by oral glucose on regaining consciousness.
Steroid crisis	Seen only in those taking systemic steroids in relative insufficiency as a result of stress.
Cardiac arrest	No central pulse. Usually history of angina, coronary arterial disease, hypertension or other risk factor.

■ ***Which is the most likely cause in this case? Why?***

In this case the cause is very likely to be cardiac arrest. The symptom of pain in the chest radiating to the neck and arm is characteristic of myocardial infarction, the commonest cause of cardiac arrest, and is not seen in the other causes of collapse. Diabetes, hypertension and a high alcohol intake are all risk factors for atheromatous arterial disease and its complication of myocardial infarction.

■ ***Does cardiac arrest always follow myocardial infarction?***

No. The heart may continue to pump unless a large area of the myocardium or conducting tissue is damaged. Cardiac arrest may also follow hypoxia or respiratory obstruction.

■ ***How will you confirm your provisional diagnosis?***

For a diagnosis of cardiac arrest the patient must be:

- unconscious
- not breathing or have abnormal breathing (infrequent noisy gasps).

Examination

You place a hand on the patient's neck to feel the carotid pulse. He feels cold and clammy. Even though it is only half a minute since he lost consciousness the patient already looks grey and he is beginning to look cyanosed. He is not breathing.

■ ***What is the current protocol for assessing and managing sudden collapse?***

It is critically important to start Basic Life Support (BLS) procedures immediately without further consideration of possible causes. The current 2005 Resuscitation Council guidelines for the management of respiratory and/or cardiac arrest in an adult are:

1. Check the area for danger to yourself and victim
2. Assess responsiveness by shaking shoulders and shouting
3. Shout for help (do not call 999 yet)
4. Open the airway (tilt head and lift chin or jaw thrust)
5. Check mouth for vomit / debris and remove with finger scoops
6. Assess breathing – listen and feel for breathing while observing chest movements. Take no more than 10 seconds
7. If breathing is abnormal (infrequent noisy gasps) or absent, call emergency service on 999. You may have to leave the victim to do this
8. Perform 30 chest compressions of 4–5cm each over the centre of the sternum at 100 per minute
9. Give 2 ventilations
10. Continue compressions (30) and ventilations (2) until help arrives, the victim shows signs of life or until you are physically exhausted and unable to carry on.

■ ***What are Basic and Advanced Life Support?***

Basic Life Support (BLS) is the diagnosis and immediate management of cardiac arrest (of whatever aetiology) without the use of equipment. It represents the absolute minimum standard of resuscitation skills which all dentists, dental hygienists and dental nurses must acquire and maintain.

Advanced Life Support (ALS) is concerned with the restoration of spontaneous circulation and stabilization of the cardiovascular system. Techniques include ECG assessment, defibrillation and the administration of drugs.

■ ***What is the aim of Basic Life Support?***

To protect the brain from irreversible hypoxic damage. This develops within 3–4 minutes of cardiac arrest in a previously healthy and well-oxygenated individual. Basic Life Support delays the rate of deterioration of cerebral function and maximizes the chances of ALS being successful. Effective BLS followed by prompt ALS and hospital admission greatly increases the patient's chance of survival.

■ ***Why not dial '999' as soon as the patient loses consciousness?***

The most common cause of sudden loss of consciousness in the dental chair is a vasovagal attack (faint) which does not require attendance by the emergency services. The call for help in step 3 is intended to summon local helpers such as dental nurses or receptionist.

■ ***What is the most common cause of failure or difficulty with BLS?***

Airway obstruction in the unconscious patient is the commonest problem and is usually due to the relaxed tongue falling back to obliterate the airway in the oropharynx. This may be overcome by measures which pull the tongue forward such as head tilt (neck lift), chin lift and jaw thrust. Blood, vomit or other foreign materials (including poorly fitting or broken dentures) may also obstruct the airway.

■ ***Should dentures be removed during BLS?***

Only if they are loose or broken. Well-fitting dentures usually facilitate a good oral seal during expired air (mouth-to-mouth) ventilation.

■ ***If the patient is not breathing, can you be certain that the patient has suffered cardiac arrest?***

No. The diagnosis depends upon loss of consciousness and absence of a central pulse. However, calling 999 for professional assistance if there is respiratory arrest at this point is sensible, because cardiac arrest follows respiratory arrest very quickly.

■ ***Having dialled 999, what information should your helper give the operator?***

- your name
- address (with directions)
- your telephone number
- that a patient has collapsed with a suspected cardiac arrest.

Although this sounds simple, hurried calls may omit essential information. Response to cardiac arrest is usually provided at highest priority by a specialized team and is not a routine ambulance call. Failure to provide your telephone number leaves the emergency services unable to return your call.

Prognosis

■ ***Is it likely that your patient will recover spontaneously?***

Unfortunately not. Even with prompt ALS support from a specialist team the chances of death are greater than 50%. This may seem a poor chance of survival but if BLS and ALS are delayed, less than 2% of patients will live. In this case the patient recovered following ALS care provided by a specialist ambulance team who arrived at the practice 12 minutes after the 999 call was placed; a very rapid response.

■ ***How long would you continue to provide BLS?***

Until help arrives or you are exhausted.

■ ***How can you increase your chances of providing effective Basic Life Support?***

Only by regular practical instruction and testing the competence of yourself and your practice team. BLS cannot be learned from a book.

Case 14

A difficult child

SUMMARY

A mother brings her nervous 4-year-old daughter for treatment. How will you approach examining her and defining a treatment plan?

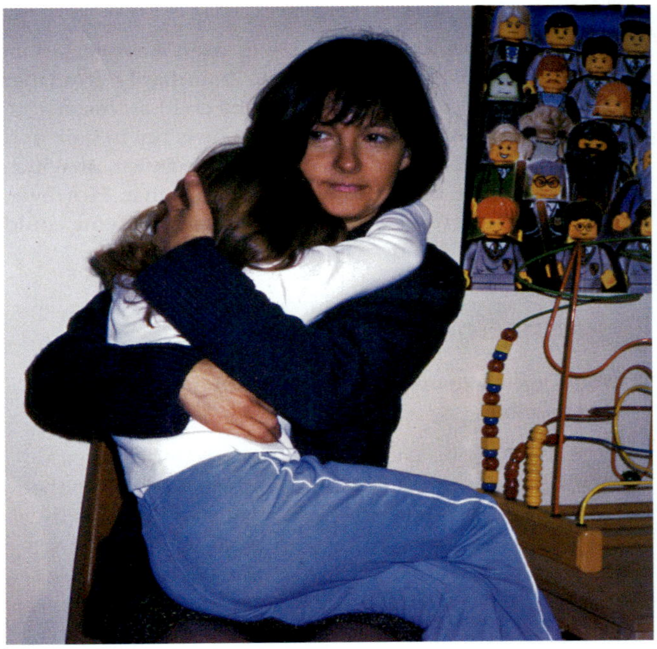

Fig. 14.1 The child and mother in your surgery.

History

Your nurse shows the child and mother into the surgery. The child is clinging tightly to her mother and will not look at you or acknowledge you.

Complaint

The child has no complaint but her mother has noticed holes in her back teeth.

History of complaint

The mother first noticed the holes 6 months ago and there has never been any toothache.

Dental history

The child has never had a dental examination or treatment before. She was taken to another dentist but became hysterical in the waiting room and refused to go in. She is only in your surgery because she has been bribed with a chocolate bar.

Medical history

The child is fit and well.

■ ***This is not looking hopeful. What must you do before you can attempt to examine the child?***

You need to encourage child to feel safe and engender feelings of trust. To do this you must establish a rapport with the child. Without some form of rapport little progress is possible.

■ ***The child appears frightened. What fears would you expect in a 4 year old in a dental setting?***

A typical 4 year old is usually scared of:

- the unknown
- pain
- new environments
- new people
- being separated from their mother.

■ ***What further questions would you ask and why?***

Does the child attend a nursery or playgroup full-time or part-time? If so for how long have they attended?
A child attending nursery will be used to dealing with people outside their home and should have greater coping skills, be more socially developed and used to being separated from the mother. They should also understand the concept of rules that have to be followed. You can be more confident of successfully managing the behaviour of such a child.

How does the mother feel about going to the dentist?
Maternal anxiety is a strong influence on the young child's reaction to dentistry. If the mother is nervous at this appointment the child will already have sensed this. Indeed if the mother is severely anxious it may be better for the father or grandparent to accompany the child. A mother who is herself very nervous may not be able to support you later on if things get difficult.

How is the child's behaviour at home? This will have to be asked very tactfully as parents usually insist that their children behave well. Try asking whether she sleeps well – perhaps the child goes to bed when she wants and also gets her own way in most other things. Find out whether the parents routinely use bribes to gain the child's cooperation. You need to find out whether the child is over indulged ('spoilt') or whether the parents are used to setting limits for their child's behaviour. Limit setting is considered good parenting practice. If the child is used to having limits set to her behaviour, she will be much easier to direct in the dental setting. If she is an only child, the parents may be inexperienced in good parenting.

Is the child genuinely nervous or just playing up? Your strategies for managing fear, shyness and naughtiness would be different. However, this is difficult to assess without observing the child's behaviour. You may not be able to make an immediate decision and, of course, it is quite possible that all factors are contributing.

You discover that the patient is an only child. She has just started part-time nursery but is having problems settling down after her mother leaves the room. The child is generally good at home and, like most children, she likes to have her own way. However, she responds well to direction and is not allowed to have her own way all the time. Her mother attends the dentist but is rather nervous of treatment. From this you can see that in addition to allaying the anxiety of both child and mother, you will also have to teach the child what behaviour is expected and appropriate at the dentist.

■ ***What can the average 4-year-old child be expected to do? How does this knowledge help?***

Some of the developmental milestones for a 4-year-old child are shown below.

Milestone
• Usually separates well from mother
• Names four primary colours
• Can state own age and address
• Listens intently to stories
• Understands turn-taking
• Starts to understand concept of obeying rules
• Washes and dries own hands
• Understands yesterday, today and tomorrow, simple past and future
• Blows nose reliably

Talking about these abilities with the mother allows you to develop a rapport with her and may alert you to any educational difficulties that the child may have. Not all parents are completely forthcoming about their child's development. If the child has learning difficulties your approach will be slower and more considered.

You discover that the child appears to have reached the normal developmental milestones for her age.

■ ***Now that you have a better appreciation of the background, how will you develop a rapport with the child?***

Make eye contact. You may catch the child's attention while talking over the previous points with the parent and already be interacting with her in some way or other. If not you must now direct all your attention to the child. Start with a compliment about the child's clothes, toys, hair or a similar topic and catch her eye. You may need to say gently 'look at me'.

Talk to the child in appropriate language. You must be able to converse at the level of a 4 year old and this takes knowledge and practice. Always use the child's first name, child friendly language and avoid potentially fear-promoting words. This is often called 'childrenese' and examples are referring to your vacuum as a hoover and the operating light as sunshine. Ask open questions that cannot be answered with a simple yes or no to promote responses. Knowledge of some current children's television characters is always useful and will provide plenty of topics of conversation.

Use nonverbal communication. Young children generally respond better to nonverbal communication, particularly touching and smiling. A pat, or stroke of the hand or hair is valued much more by a young child than a comment such as 'good girl' or 'well done'.

Be aware of body language. Children are very sensitive to nonverbal communication. Watch the child and be aware of your own body language. Are you being defensive or welcoming and friendly?

Consider engaging through play. Children learn through play so consider the use of familiar toys or puppets. Perhaps she would like to show you how she brushes her teddy bear's teeth? However, remember that toys and play alone are only a means to an end and are not a substitute for good behaviour management.

Dispel fear of the unknown. Tell the child that all you want to do today is talk to her and her mother, count her teeth and check that mummy has brushed them properly. Stress that you are going to do nothing else and continually check back with the child to involve her and ensure that she understands the limits of the planned dental experience.

Using these strategies you are able to open a conversation, though the child does not separate voluntarily from her mother. Ideally you would examine the child at this visit to assess the treatment needs. However, she is not in pain and you could delay examination until the next visit, at which time you and the surgery will be more familiar. However, the mother is worried and would prefer that you could examine the child today.

Examination

■ ***Would you try to use the dental chair for this first examination?***

Not necessarily. The child may be examined initially on the mother's lap, on an ordinary chair, or standing between the mother's knees, all of which are more familiar than the dental chair. Place the mother where your dental light can be used if the child will tolerate it. If the child does not allow her teeth to be examined in these positions then you must consider an examination under more controlled conditions.

■ ***How could you safely examine the child without frightening her further?***

If you decide to perform a full examination on a reluctant child it must be done in a controlled, caring and confident manner with experienced nursing support and with the consent and cooperation of the mother. You must explain to the mother exactly what you are going to do, seek verbal consent and repeat to the child that you are just going to count teeth. Then:

- Align the chair in a fairly upright position.
- Ask the mother to sit in the chair as if she is being examined – the child will probably come with her.

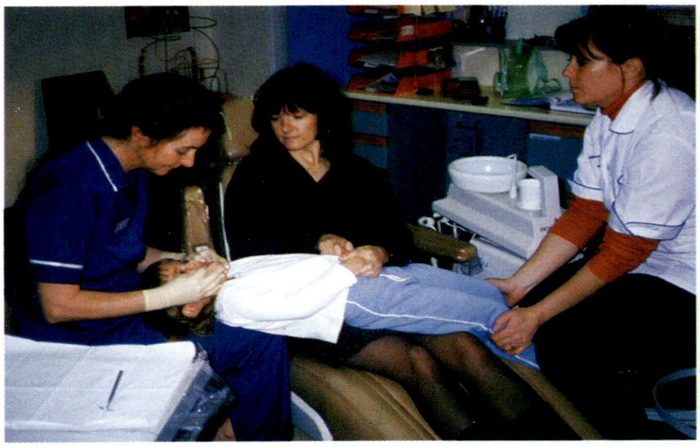

Fig. 14.2 Controlled examination technique.

- Ask the child to sit on the mother's lap.
- Explain to the child what you are going to do.
- Ask the mother to turn the child so that she is sitting across the mother with her head at the 10 o'clock position.
- Ask the mother to control the arms and hands.
- Your nurse will gently control the feet.
- Slowly and calmly lower the child's shoulders and head onto your lap, explaining what you are doing.

The technique is shown in Figure 14.2. Note how hands and legs are gently held and the child remains in close contact and able to see her mother. This position is useful not only for mild degrees of anxiety but also to examine severely frightened children in pain who are determined to resist. Understandably the child sometimes cries, but not always. Although not ideal, crying often allows good access to the mouth. If the child will not open their mouth, your nurse tickling their stomach will usually have the required effect. Your nurse will need to position the operating light carefully as light in the child's eyes is often upsetting.

Keep the examination short and immediately afterwards, whether the child is upset or not, reward her with words, (a 'soft' reward) and a sticker or balloon, (a 'hard' reward). This will encourage the child to allow examination at the next visit. However, be careful not to give inappropriate praise for poor behaviour and inadvertently give the impression that bad behaviour is acceptable.

In your brief examination you see the appearances shown in Figure 14.3.

■ *The appearances on examination are shown in Figure 14.3. What do you see and what do the appearances indicate?*

- Caries in the occlusal pits and fissures of the second primary molar
- Caries in the distal of the first primary molar, the marginal ridge has collapsed
- Reasonable gingival condition with some interdental marginal inflammation.

The key feature is the collapse of the marginal ridge of the first primary molar. The pulp is either directly involved by caries or compromised in the great majority of primary molars once the ridge collapses. This tooth will require a

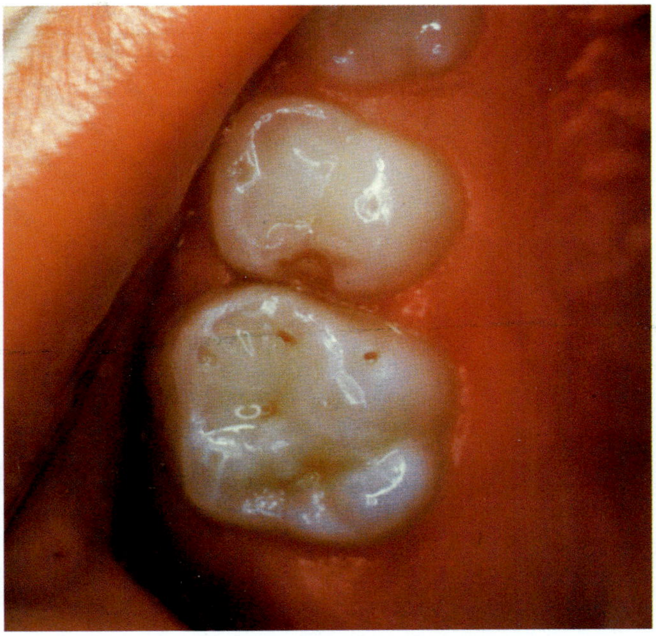

Fig. 14.3 Appearances on examination.

pulpotomy or extraction. Following pulpotomy, a preformed metal crown will be the restoration of choice because they have been shown to be more durable than an intracoronal restoration. However, in an anxious child with limited cooperation it might be appropriate to stabilize the lesion with a temporary intracoronal restoration and delay the definitive restoration for a few months.

■ *What would you do next at this appointment?*

Nothing further is to be gained from this first visit. However, it is essential that you prepare the child for the next visit. Ask her to bring her toothbrush next time and introduce the concept of future visits and a radiograph ('photograph').

Discuss your findings and proposed approach, possible treatment needs and preventive advice with the mother including a 3-day diet diary.

During this period your nurse should take the initiative to talk informally with the child, introduce the dental chair and equipment in a play-like manner and allow the child to take the lead in exploring the surgery. Some children respond very well to this indirect approach by a second person.

■ *How will you plan treatment taking the child's nervousness into account?*

The child requires a range of treatment ranging from oral hygiene instruction to a pulpotomy and a preformed metal crown. You must teach the child to accept the more complex treatment by leading her along a graded pathway of increasing challenge.

If treatments are listed in order of increasing difficulty for any child, the challenge scale would look something like Figure 14.4.

The speed at which you progress along the scale will depend on the individual child's ability to cope with each procedure.

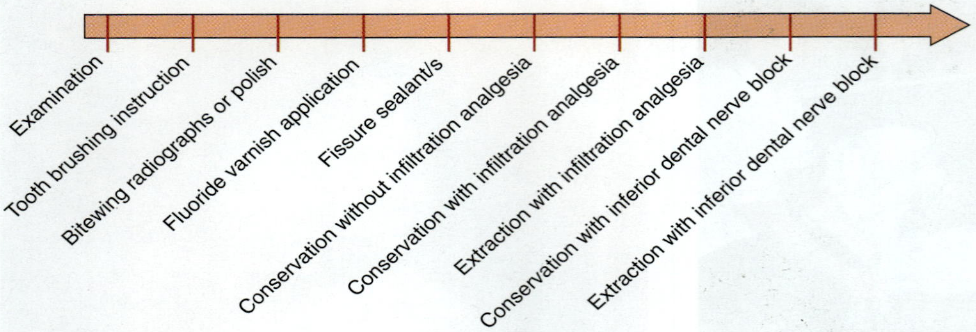

Fig. 14.4 Treatments in order of increasing difficulty.

Table 14.1 Behaviour management strategies

Technique	Comments
Tell–show–do	An important part of shaping the child's behaviour, effective for many children and widely taught. Explain what you are going to do, show the patient how you will do it and only then do it.
Behaviour shaping	Introducing the child to new experiences in a number of small stages or approximations. This involves using tell–show–do. Backtrack if the desired behaviour is not forthcoming and only progress to next behavioural challenge after the child has accepted each stage in the build up. Use prevention to get you started and work along the scale of challenge above.
Voice control	Consider repeating an instruction in a slightly different way if you sense that the child is not responding, perhaps with a different tone of voice, eye contact, facial expression or touch.
Use of empathy	Question to elicit the patient's feelings, for instance: 'Is that OK?', 'How is that feeling?','Is that better now?'. One of the most useful tools in child management; empathic statements have been shown to reliably lessen anxiety in children. They make the child feel that you are genuinely concerned about them. On the contrary **reassurance** is much less effective. Comments such as 'It will be all right', 'That's fine', 'You are doing well' are frequently used but it would be much better to make an empathic statement.
Provide sense of control	A child who feels helpless will feel anxious. Minimize this by establishing a sense of control for the child. Arrange stop signals and give the child choices. Stop signals are particularly effective. Tell the child to raise their hand if they want to tell you something or if something is worrying them. Watch out for children who abuse this power. Limit unpleasant treatment, such as use of the air rotor, to short bursts of defined length and count out loud as you use up the time. Agree the number of seconds that is acceptable with the child and gradually extend the time period.
Specific reinforcement	Use specific reinforcement for any behaviour; tell the child what they are doing well and also what you find to be unhelpful behaviour.
Soft rewards	Keep rewarding the child verbally throughout; most children like to be told how clever they are. Say how well the child is trying and reward them for doing their best.
Hard rewards	These are items such as stickers or balloons. Rewards work best when they are consistent, immediate and relevant to the child. They need to be matched to the child's age and gender.
Modelling	Using another child of similar age, perhaps an older sibling or a video, to demonstrate good behaviour can sometimes be helpful, but it is of limited use in young anxious children.

You need to monitor the child's reactions continually to check that you are not progressing too fast.

Items in the treatment plan should be arranged as far as possible in order of increasing challenge. A child may accept a challenging treatment when in pain but subsequently might only accept a lower rated treatment.

What behaviour management strategies, tips and tricks might you use during examination and treatment of nervous children?

A range of methods are given in Table 14.1. All may be appropriate at various times.

Are there strategies you should avoid?

Yes, the following will almost certainly make the situation worse. Try not to:

- use bribes or coercion – these only work in the very short term and reinforce bad rather than good behaviour.
- use bland reassurance such as 'Well done', 'That's fine'. Be more specific, tell the child what was helpful and they will usually try to help again in most instances.
- belittle the child or tell them they are behaving like a baby. This lowers their self-esteem and poor self-esteem is often linked to anxiety in children.
- send the parent of a child this age outside. Removing the main source of security for a young child is counterproductive.
- fall back on the skills that you may use to control your own children or young relatives in a social setting. It is important to maintain a professional distance and follow behaviour management strategies that are based on sound principles.
- lose your cool or raise your voice. It can be stressful treating anxious children and you need to recognize this.

If these strategies fail, what other options might be open to you?

With skilled behaviour management many normal but anxious children can accept the more challenging treatments listed below. However, sometimes a child will be too anxious and alternatives may need to be considered. If a child is not showing the desired behaviour by the second or third visit you should consider referral to a specialist paediatric dentist or use of nitrous oxide-inhalation sedation. Inhalation sedation usually works best in children aged 5 and above though occasionally younger children are receptive, depending on their emotional maturity and ability to cooperate. Intravenous sedation is unpredictable in children and not recommended. If all else fails treatment under general anaesthetic is a last resort but this must be carefully planned, definitive and completed in one visit to avoid the need for further episodes of general anesthesia.

How could you have made the first appointment easier?

If you had known that a new nervous child patient was booked, a pre-appointment questionnaire could have provided much useful information, such as likes and fears, personality, previous experiences, nicknames, preventive habits and the names of favourite toys or pets. The form could also give information to the parent on your approach to children's dental care and the concept of introducing the child to dentistry in a measured way through prevention. This allays maternal anxiety. At the opposite end of the spectrum, it helps to avoid the situation where the mother asks why you are not going to do a filling at the first visit.

You would also have greeted the child and parent in the waiting room, reception area or office as this reduces anxiety in children. You also need a child-friendly environment with comics, computer games, toys or music and videos. These confirm to both the parent and the child that they are in a caring and understanding practice.

The use of modelling, whereby a cooperative child is used or shown in a video can sometimes be helpful in allaying moderate anxiety in some children.

Are you at a disadvantage dealing with nervous children if you are male?

There is no good evidence that children prefer female dentists. However, most preschool or nursery children will be much more familiar with female carers and may take more time to settle with a male dentist. There is no need to refer small children specifically to female dentists.

Some male dentists feel uncomfortable about the use of touch as part of their nonverbal communication approach; indeed for some it is culturally unacceptable. This could be a handicap for treating very young children. If you are male and are worried that touching children may be misconstrued by the parent, it is important to touch only head and hands and always in the presence of a chaperone.

Case 16

A numb lip

SUMMARY

A 68-year-old man presents to you in general dental practice complaining that his lower lip has become numb. How would you investigate and manage this symptom?

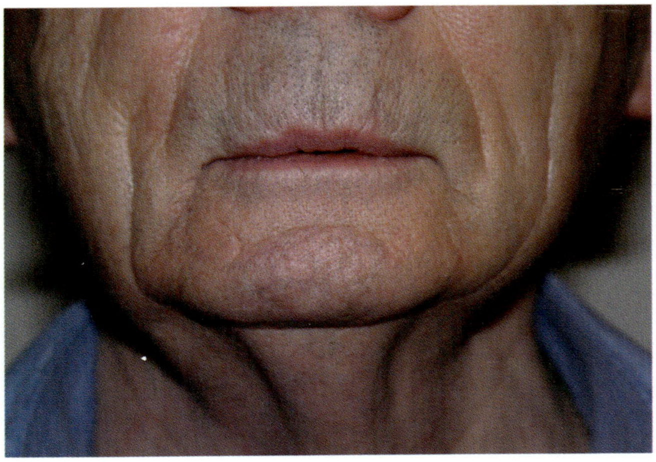

Fig. 16.1 The patient on presentation.

History

Complaint

He complains of sudden onset of numbness of the lower right lip. It feels cold, as if he had had an injection for dental treatment (Figure 16.1).

History of complaint

The patient noticed the numbness immediately he woke up the previous morning. His jaw has been aching for some months and he has noticed some tingling in the lip, which he ascribes to recent dental treatment.

Dental history

You are seeing the patient for an emergency appointment. He is normally under the care of one of your colleagues and his records and radiographs are available.

A series of appointments over the last few months have addressed pain from the lower right quadrant. The tingling in the lip was noted 3 months ago. The lower right first molar had been considered to be the cause. Your colleague placed a root filling 4 months ago but the pain did not resolve completely. Three weeks ago the lower right second premolar was extracted as a likely cause of the pain. However, discomfort continued.

Medical history

The patient reports that he is fit and well. He takes 50 mg atenolol daily for mild hypertension. In the past he has suffered depression and was treated with antidepressants in the past.

■ ***What is the sensory nerve supply to the lip?***

The sensory nerve supply to the face is shown in Figure 16.2. The three divisions of the trigeminal nerve supply most of the face. The greater auricular nerve is formed by the ventral rami of the cervical nerves C2 and C3.

The lower lip is supplied by the mental nerve.

■ ***What is the course of the nerve supply?***

The trigeminal nerve starts in the pons where its sensory and motor roots arise. The ophthalmic and maxillary branches leave the skull via the superior orbital fissure and the foramen rotundum respectively. The mandibular branch leaves the skull at the foramen ovale to enter the infratemporal fossa, where it divides into an anterior group of mostly motor branches and a posterior group of sensory branches.

The anterior group of branches includes the nerves to lateral pterygoid, deep temporal nerves to masseter and the sensory long buccal nerve. There are three posterior branches, including the auriculotemporal nerve, which is given off almost immediately. This passes backwards to innervate the side of the scalp and part of the ear. The main nerve then divides into the lingual nerve, which passes to the tongue

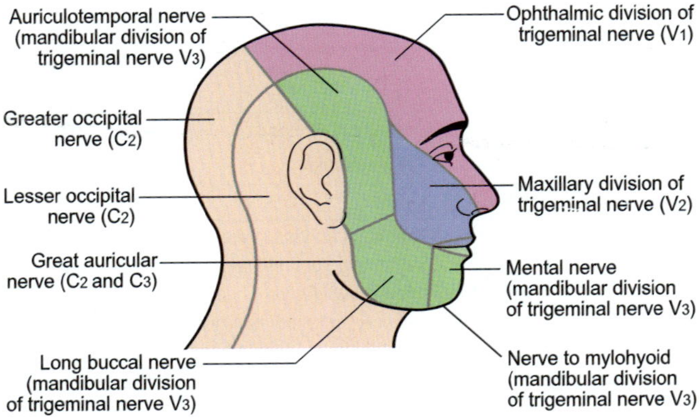

Fig. 16.2 Sensory nerve supply to the face.

along the lateral pterygoid, and the inferior alveolar nerve, which gives off the small motor branch to mylohyoid and then enters the mandibular foramen in the mandibular ramus. It emerges from the mental foramen to provide sensation to the lip.

Unlike many other areas of sensory innervation, those on the face are well defined and sharply delineated. Though there is some slight variation between individuals, there is little overlap of the areas supplied by different nerves.

What are the causes of numbness of the lip?

Numbness may be constant or temporary/intermittent, depending on the cause. The main causes are shown in Table 16.1, and each may affect the nerve at different parts along its course.

Examination

Extraoral examination

The appearance of the patient is shown in Figure 16.1. He appears normal; the lip is of normal colour and shows no distortion or drooping to suggest a motor nerve lesion.

When you examine him you find that there is only a very mild swelling of the posterior right lower jaw. There is no detectable mass, but the patient is tender in the right submandibular area. There is normal movement of the lip.

How will you test for sensation? Why is this necessary?

A sensation of numbness may be central in origin, denote damage to the peripheral nerve or be psychosomatic. Only by testing sensation can the exact area affected be defined and this will help define the cause.

Table 16.1 Major and more frequent causes of a numb lip

Infection	Osteomyelitis Apical infection causing pressure on nerve in mandibular canal
Tumour	Primary malignant neoplasm of bone such as osteosarcoma, chondrosarcoma Primary malignant neoplasm of mucosa invading bone such as oral squamous cell carcinoma Primary malignant neoplasm of brain or tissues along path of nerve Metastatic malignant neoplasm to brain or tissues along path of nerve Benign tumour of brain such as meningioma or nerve schwannoma
Trauma	Mandibular fracture Direct trauma to nerve at mental foramen
Autoimmune	Peripheral neuropathy Multiple sclerosis
Vascular	Vascular compression of nerve root
Psychological	Tetany from hyperventilation
Metabolic	Tetany from alkalosis
Iatrogenic causes	Intraneural injection of local anaesthetic Direct trauma to the inferior dental nerve at the lingula or mental foramen from dental injection Trauma to the inferior dental bundle from dental extraction (particularly third molars), apicectomy or implant placement Injury to the mental nerve during surgical extractions/apicectomy Injury to the inferior alveolar nerve by extruded root filling material or caustic endodontic agents

Tests of sensation may include light touch (with a wisp of cotton wool or a Von Frey hair – fine filaments of calibrated rigidity for testing touch), pain (with a sharp and blunt point), vibration, temperature and two-point discrimination. A cotton wool fibre and a sharp point such as a hypodermic needle are usually sufficient for a dental setting. Outline the area affected, making sure that hand movements cannot be seen by the patient so that the results are objective. Test and retest if the results are unclear.

If the results are abnormal, it will be necessary to test the other cranial nerves, because these may be affected if a lesion is present in the brain or along the common paths of the cranial nerves.

How will you test cranial nerve function?

The cranial nerves' main head and neck functions may be tested as described in Table 16.2.

When you do this, the skin of the patient's lip is found to be almost completely without light touch and pain sensation in the area below the vermilion border and on its mucosal surface. There is a sharp cut-off in the midline and the skin below the chin has normal sensation.

How do you interpret the findings so far?

The extraoral findings are relatively subtle. There is mild swelling of the mandible that suggests a local mandibular cause. The tenderness in the right submandibular area might represent infection or reactive lymphadenopathy.

The fact that the area of anaesthesia is sharply delineated suggests a peripheral nerve cause. It also almost excludes a psychosomatic origin, as psychosomatic sensations do not tend to follow neurological or vascular distributions. The fact that lip movement is normal indicates normal facial nerve function. As the roots and paths through the base of skull of the trigeminal and facial nerves are close, this would suggest that a central or base-of-skull lesion is not the cause.

The distribution on the lower-lip skin suggests injury or compression of the inferior alveolar nerve. The normal sensation under the chin is significant. This area is supplied by the nerve to mylohyoid, given off the inferior alveolar nerve just above the lingula, to supply a thumbprint-sized patch of skin under the chin. Therefore, the cause must lie between the start of the inferior dental canal and the lip.

Intraoral examination

The oral mucosa is healthy apart from the lower right second premolar extraction site. The socket opening is swollen and filled with granulation tissue that is growing out slightly above the alveolus. There are no sequestra and no sinus or pus at the socket mouth.

The remaining teeth appear healthy and none is tender to percussion.

How should a healing socket appear 3 weeks after extraction? Is this socket normal?

The initial clot starts to be replaced by granulation tissue growing in from the periphery a few days after extraction. By

Table 16.2 Methods to test the functions of cranial nerves in the head and neck

Cranial Nerve	Test	Comment
I Olfactory	Check each nostril individually with easily recognized non-pungent smells	If the smell is pungent or irritant it will trigger a pain response via the trigeminal nerve as well
II Optic	Pupil reactivity to light and visual acuity	Test each eye separately
III Oculomotor IV Trochlear VI Abducens	Check eye movement in each gaze (up/down/lateral/medial and each oblique gaze), asking the patient to follow a finger with the eyes – the finger should be 25 cm from the patient's eyes	Check both eyes together and individually
V Trigeminal	Check sensation in each division by touch, comparing each side. Ophthalmic division can also be tested with corneal reflex. Check motor component of mandibular division by asking patient to clench teeth	
VII Facial	Ask the patient to raise the eyebrows, tightly shut the eyes, smile and purse the lips	Compare left and right sides for asymmetry
VIII Auditory	Check to see if the patient can hear fingers being rubbed together close to the ear, a ticking watch or whispering	Distance from the ear is important
IX Glossopharyngeal X Vagus	Ask the patient to say 'aaah' and look for symmetrical movement of the soft palate	Functions of IXth and Xth nerve in the head and neck are intermingled so these nerves are effectively tested together
X Vagus	Vocal cord movement/hoarseness	
XI Accessory	Ask the patient to press the chin downwards on to your hand and the bulk/power of the sternomastoid and trapezius muscles can be compared. Then ask the patient to turn the head against your hand. Finally ask the patient to shrug the shoulders	Weakness is demonstrated in the muscle *opposite* to the direction of head turning
XII Hypoglossal	Ask the patient to stick out the tongue	The tongue deviates to the affected side

8–10 days, even a large molar socket should be filled with granulation tissue. At 3 weeks there should be an intact layer of epithelium over the granulation tissue. This socket is not epithelialized. The granulation tissue growing out from the socket indicates a process of frustrated healing that could have many causes. This socket has failed to heal.

■ *What are the causes of failed or delayed socket healing?*

General causes

- Age
- Diabetes
- Steroids and other immunosuppressants
- Bisphosphonate therapy
- Malnutrition
- Cancer chemotherapy

Local causes

- Impacted food debris
- Foreign bodies – bony sequestra, root fragments
- Dry socket
- Infection, including tuberculosis
- Oroantral fistula formation
- Previous radiotherapy to the site
- Sarcoidosis
- Local malignancy.

■ *How do you interpret the findings now?*

There would appear to be a local cause in the body of the mandible causing compression or injury to the inferior alveolar nerve. Inflammation or infection from nonvital teeth or the nonhealing socket could involve the nerve. Alternatively another process may cause both nerve injury and have prevented socket healing.

Investigations

■ *What investigations should you perform?*

The remaining teeth in the affected quadrant should be tested for vitality.

A radiograph is required to assess the extraction socket, the adjacent teeth, the whole height of the slightly expanded mandible and the full length of the inferior dental canal. Either a dental panoramic or an oblique lateral radiograph would be an appropriate view.

The lower first molar is root-filled. The second molar is vital, but the lower right incisors, canine and first premolar appear nonvital.

■ *The panoramic tomograph is shown in Figure 16.3. What does it show?*

Several teeth are heavily restored. The lower first molar is root-filled and there is a poorly defined radiolucency about 2 cm in length extending from the distal root of the second molar to the premolar socket. The cortical bone outline of the inferior dental canal cannot be seen in this region. The recent extraction socket still has the lamina dura present, though it appears slightly more indistinct than normal, consistent with infection or another process causing resorption. No sequestra or root fragments are present in the socket, though a plain periapical view would have been

Case 17

A loose tooth

SUMMARY

A 25-year-old man presents in your general dental practice with a loose tooth. Identify the cause and summarize the treatment options.

Complaint

The patient complains of a loose tooth and points to his upper left lateral incisor which is crowned. He says it is uncomfortable when it moves and has become so mobile that he thinks it may fall out.

History of complaint

He has noticed that the tooth has become progressively looser over the last few months and would like a replacement. There has been no pain associated with the tooth but he is aware of an unpleasant taste which appears to emanate intermittently from his upper front teeth.

Dental history

The patient had been a regular attender at another dental practice for many years until he moved to your area. He is motivated and does not wish to lose any teeth.

Four years previously, the lateral and central incisors had been fractured in an accident at work. Both teeth sustained class II coronal fractures but were initially left untreated. Several months later another dental practitioner provided some restorations on both teeth and shortly afterwards the patient asked for the lateral incisor to be crowned because he was unhappy with the appearance.

Medical history

The patient has insulin-controlled diabetes. Otherwise he is fit and well and is taking no medication.

Examination

Extraoral examination

No submandibular or cervical lymph nodes are palpable.

Intraoral examination

The patient has an extensively restored dentition with a crowned upper left lateral incisor that is grade II mobile buccolingually but not vertically. There is generalized but mild redness and delayed bleeding on probing around the gingival margin associated with a small amount of plaque at the crown margin. However, there is no increase in probing depth around this tooth. There is no evidence of caries on any teeth and generally the periodontal condition is good. The adjacent teeth are firm. No sinuses are present to explain the bad taste and no pus is detected on periodontal probing.

■ ***What additional questions might you ask?***

Did you notice the mobility suddenly increase or hear a crack from the tooth? The marked mobility without evidence of periodontitis suggests a root fracture.

The patient has noticed no sudden increase in mobility.

■ ***How would you clinically assess the possibility of root fracture?***

By determining the axis of rotation of the mobile crown. Apply pressure forwards and backwards to identify how far down the root the axis of rotation appears to be.

When you do this you find that the crown appears to rotate about a point 2–3 mm below the gingival margin. If rocking the crown produces bubbles of saliva at the gingival margin this would be an indicator of a root fracture communicating with a periodontal pocket or the gingival crevice. No such bubbles are seen.

■ ***Based on what you know so far, what are the likely causes?***

Having excluded mobility caused by periodontitis and coronal bone loss, the two possibilities which remain the most likely are resorption or root fracture. The mobile tooth is rotating about a point just below the gingival margin so either process must affect the coronal part of the root.

Resorption of the apical half of the root would move the axis of rotation of the remaining tooth coronally. There would have to be extensive resorption to cause this degree of mobility and raise the axis of rotation so far. Resorption is a recognized complication of trauma to teeth and so this would be the most likely cause.

Root fracture is possible. No fracture was noted but the marked mobility would be consistent with the root fracture of the coronal part of the root. If there is a root fracture it would appear to be independent of the original trauma. Teeth which suffer coronal fractures do not usually suffer root fractures as well because most of the energy is absorbed by fracturing the crown. However, if a root fracture had been present for the last 4 years it might have triggered slow resorption, combining both possible causative factors.

An unsuspected lesion has destroyed the bone and/or the tooth root apically, leaving support only coronally; this is a remote possibility. The tooth would then be mobile about the remaining intact periodontal ligament. The commonest

Table 17.1 Investigations to be carried out

Test	Reason	Problems
Vitality test	To check the vitality of all four upper and lower incisors and canines (excluding any known root-filled teeth). Late loss of vitality is a complication of trauma and any one of these teeth could have periapical infection and be the cause of the bad taste. The vitality of the lateral incisor needs to be known, to plan treatment once the diagnosis is established.	Electric pulp tests are notoriously difficult to perform on crowned teeth and the results must be interpreted with caution. The lateral incisor has a metal ceramic bonded crown and the ceramic will insulate the tooth while the metal layer will diffuse the applied voltage and conduct the stimulus to the gingiva. The patient may mistake a gingival sensation for a vitality response.
Periapical radiograph	To detect the possible causes and assess bone levels around the teeth. To determine the pulp canal morphology in case root canal treatment is required, and the root morphology in case extraction is necessary.	Root fractures may be difficult to identify if the fragments are not separated. A second view at a slightly different angle may allow detection of a root fracture invisible in the first. However, this tooth is so mobile that any root fracture should be readily identified.

lesion to do this would be a radicular cyst arising on a nonvital tooth.

However this seems most unlikely as there is no expansion and the adjacent teeth are not displaced or mobile. A different lesion remains a remote possibility.

Investigations

■ ***What investigations would you carry out? Why? What are the potential problems?***

See Table 17.1.

On performing the tests of tooth vitality you find that it is impossible to obtain a response from the upper left central and lateral incisors. All other anterior teeth appear vital.

■ ***The periapical radiograph is shown in Figure 17.1 What do you see?***

The left lateral incisor is crowned but not root filled. A large oval radiolucency fills the middle third of the root and extends laterally to replace the full width of the root and communicate with the periodontal ligament. The margins of the defect are smooth and sharply defined. The lamina dura around the apex appears intact. The bone level mesially and distally is coronal to the defect and there is no evidence of either horizontal or vertical bone loss. Very little root dentine remains below the crown and gingival margin.

The upper left central incisor is root filled. The filling appears well condensed and extends very close to the ideal level. The root appears to have a curve at the apex. There is a poorly defined radiolucency around the apex mostly on its mesial side, where the lamina dura is missing.

The canine has mesial caries and its apical lamina dura is indistinct. However no obvious apical radiolucency is present.

■ ***What is wrong with the radiograph in Figure 17.1?***

A regular pattern is superimposed over the whole film. This is a developing artefact caused by some film processors (e.g. Velopex) which use woven nylon bands to transport the film between solutions. If these bands are dirty or worn their surface texture transfers an imprint onto the film. A less marked example of the same artefact is shown in Figure 35.3.

Another uniform artefactual pattern results from exposing the wrong side of an intraoral film packet to the beam. The embossed metal backing foil casts a patterned shadow onto the film and the shielding causes an additional underexposure, differentiating this artefact from the one illustrated.

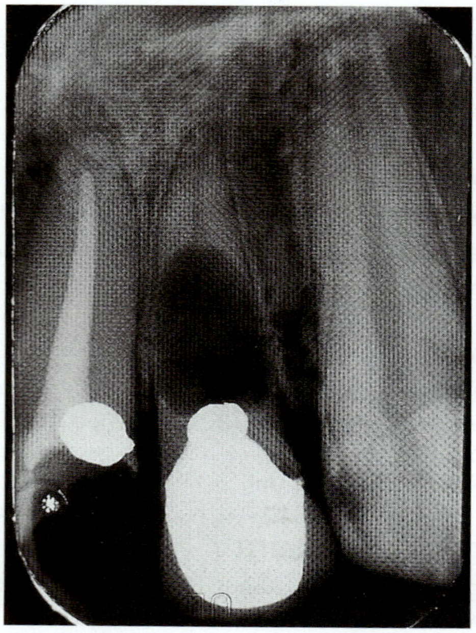

Fig. 17.1 Periapical radiograph of the mobile lateral incisor.

Diagnosis

■ ***What is your diagnosis?***

There is extensive internal resorption of the lateral incisor. The central incisor has a failed root filling with a periapical granuloma or abscess. The cause of the taste could be intermittent drainage of pus from this periapical lesion, plaque trapped in the resorption defect or caries on the mesial surface of the upper left canine.

■ ***What types of resorption are there? What are their characteristic features?***

Resorption is the process of removal of dental hard tissues by osteoclasts. There is usually some form of repair, either by reactionary dentine or bone, and repair may lead to ankylosis. All resorption is identical in its basic process, but it is convenient to subdivide resorption into clinically relevant types. Resorption may be classified as inflammatory or replacement types, or alternatively as internal or external types. All types may be transient or progressive.

Inflammatory resorption is associated with detectable inflammation and may be internal or external (apical or cervical). Inflammation may be evident radiographically, as radiolucency in the adjacent bone, or clinically as redness. The inflammatory type of resorption has the positive aspect that treatment of the cause of the inflammation may halt the resorption.

Unfortunately this is not entirely predictable. Many cases of so-called inflammatory resorption, both internal and external, are not associated with significant inflammation clinically or histologically and are perhaps better regarded as idiopathic.

Replacement resorption is resorption accompanied by progressive replacement of the tooth by bone. It is often associated with ankylosis and is a complication of luxation injuries, particularly intrusion and avulsion. Inflammation is absent, so that treatment, which is difficult, must be directed at the resorption itself.

Internal resorption starts on the pulpal aspect of the dentine. It typically affects the middle third of the root and forms a well-demarcated defect with a smooth symmetrical shape. Internal resorption indicates that the pulp is vital and that, provided the lesion has not perforated the root, the process will be halted by root canal treatment.

External resorption starts on the surface of the tooth, usually on the root but occasionally on the crown in unerupted teeth. A microscopic degree of superficial external root resorption is normal and is usually repaired by cementum. Greater apical resorption may be seen radiographically on teeth that have been moved orthodontically. Extensive apical resorption may accompany periapical inflammation or infection on nonvital teeth. A nonvital pulp may also trigger external resorption of the root coronally by producing noxious products which diffuse outwards to the periodontal ligament along the dentinal tubules. Cervical resorption usually starts just below the gingival margin and may affect one or many teeth. Radiographically, the early stages may mimic the appearance of an infra bony periodontal pocket. All types of external resorption are irregular in outline and extensive lesions often spare a thin layer of dentine around the pulp so that the pulp can remain vital until a late stage, even if the defect communicates with a pocket.

What causes resorption?

Resorption and repair are physiological processes on the external surface of the root. On the pulpal surface resorption is pathological but repair is one of the pulp's responses to injury. External resorption is known to follow damage to the cementum layer or loss of vitality of cementum and this is thought to be why avulsion injury is so commonly followed by resorption. Cervical resorption is assumed to be primarily inflammatory in aetiology, caused by the periodontal flora, though this does not explain cases where multiple lesions affect several teeth.

Internal resorption must follow loss of the pre-dentine layer separating pulp from dentine, but the causes of this loss are unknown. A degree of inflammation or increased pulpal pressure are probably factors.

What are the features of resorption?

- Asymptomatic (unless an inflammatory cause is symptomatic)
- Internal resorption is only active in vital or partially vital teeth
- External resorption may develop on vital or nonvital teeth
- Resorption itself does not compromise vitality until the pulp communicates with the mouth
- Usually slow and intermittent, occasionally very rapid
- Mobility or pathological fracture
- 'Pink spot': pulp visible through the crown
- Ankylosis (continuity of tooth and bone)
- Radiolucency and loss of tooth substance.

What are the signs of ankylosis?

- Lack of normal mobility
- High pitched metallic percussive sound
- Infra occlusion (in the growing jaw)
- Sometimes identifiable radiographically as a bridged periodontal ligament
- Patchy 'moth-eaten' root surface/lamina dura.

What is your diagnosis?

Internal resorption, probably as a late sequela of the previous trauma or restoration of the teeth. Resorption is advanced and the root has suffered a pathological fracture making the coronal fragment very mobile.

The upper central incisor has a persistent periapical periodontitis despite root canal treatment.

Treatment

How would you manage this problem in the short and long term?

The prognosis for the lateral incisor is poor and it requires extraction. It cannot be restored because the resorption has involved the periodontal ligament around much of the tooth circumference. A tooth with a more localized perforation might be repaired surgically. However, in combination with the necessary root canal treatment, this would be heroic treatment with an unpredictable chance of success. Repair is more likely to be practical for external cervical resorption.

Time must given for alveolar remodelling before the definitive restoration is made and a temporary replacement will be required.

What are your options for a short-term replacement?

- Every-type or spoon acrylic denture
- Immediate insertion of an adhesive/minimal preparation bridge
- In the very short term, the existing crown might be splinted to the adjacent teeth pending extraction.

What are your options for the long-term replacement?

Minimal preparation simple cantilever bridge replacing the lateral incisor with a retainer on the canine. This would require the carious lesion in the canine to be small and sufficient occlusal clearance for the retainer.

A conventional simple cantilever bridge using the canine as the abutment.

A conventional simple cantilever bridge using the upper left central incisor as the abutment. This would require a parallel-sided, cast or preformed post and core to support a single cantilever replacing the lateral incisor. Such a retainer is not ideal because using a post crowned tooth as a single abutment has a relatively high failure rate; indeed post retention is best avoided in all bridge designs. The failed root filling in the central incisor is also a problem. Retreatment would not produce a better root filling than the existing one which appears well condensed and as close to the apex as possible. Apicectomy will have to be considered for this tooth and if it is performed the root length available for a post will be reduced. Taken together with the time necessary to ensure apical healing, these factors exclude a replacement retained by the central incisor in the short term.

In the longer term this incisor might be usable as an abutment and if it were, the design could be further strengthened against rotation by using the mesial cavity in the canine for an inlay to act as a minor retainer for a fixed movable bridge.

A single tooth implant would be possible but a cautious approach is prudent in diabetes. This is not a complete contraindication to implants, but the possibility of delayed healing in diabetes, and the maxillary site (where implants have a reduced survival rate), mean that an implant might not be recommended. Further discussion of anterior single tooth implants will be found in case 35.

Case • 18

Oroantral fistula

SUMMARY

A 42-year-old man presents with pain following extraction of an upper first molar. What is the cause and how will you treat him?

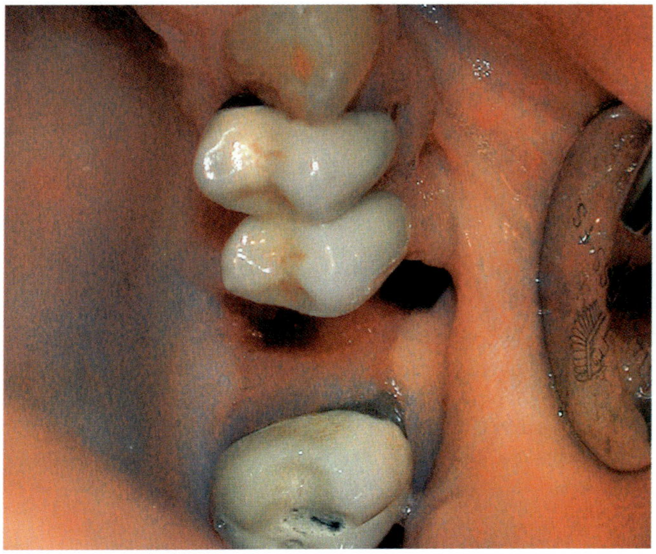

Fig. 18.1 The extraction socket on presentation.

History

Complaint

The patient is suffering dull throbbing pain in his upper jaw and face on the left side only. Pressure below his eye is painful and all his upper teeth on the left are tender on biting. He has a nasal discharge and blocked nose on the left.

History of complaint

He has had the pain for 2 weeks following extraction of the upper left first molar by his dentist. The extraction was difficult and the roots required surgical removal. There was little pain immediately afterwards but pain has slowly developed so that it is now preventing him from sleeping. The pain is constant.

Medical history

He gives a history of smoking 20 cigarettes a day for 24 years but considers himself fit and healthy.

Examination

Extraoral examination

He is a healthy looking man with no facial swelling or lymphadenopathy. There is a lightly blood-stained discharge from the left nares and halitosis.

Intraoral examination

■ ***The appearances on presentation are shown in Figure 18.1. What do you see and how do you interpret the features?***

There is a large defect in the alveolus at the site of the first molar socket, the socket appears empty and the oral mucosa has grown to line the visible sides of the socket. After 2 weeks the oral epithelium should have proliferated to cover the socket mouth but there must have been a failure of clot formation and/or organization. One possibility is that the patient has a dry socket (see Case 15). No bone is visible in the socket but it could be exposed apically. However, dry socket is rare in the maxilla and it is more likely that the socket is communicating with the maxillary antrum.

Differential diagnosis

■ ***What causes for this pain are possible and why?***

Sinusitis secondary to oroantral fistula. An oroantral communication itself causes little or no discomfort but usually induces a degree of sinusitis. The nature and distribution of pain and presence of nasal discharge are typical of sinusitis. This seems the most likely diagnosis. Fistula formation is most commonly associated with extraction of maxillary first and second molars.

Dental pain. Before jumping to conclusions, it is worth considering whether the wrong tooth may have been removed. If the extraction was performed for pulpitis (which is often poorly localized), it is possible that at least some of the symptoms may arise from the adjacent teeth. You will need to check whether additional symptoms suggest pain of dental origin.

■ ***What is an oroantral fistula?***

An oroantral fistula (OAF) is a persistent epithelialized communication between the maxillary antrum and the mouth, present for more than 48 hours. The epithelial lining of the fistula grows from the gingival epithelium, periodontal pocket lining or the antral lining and it may take up to 7 days for the epithelium to completely line the walls of the communication. If the tract is not lined by epithelium it is known as an oroantral communication or perforation.

Oroantral communications either close spontaneously or become epithelialized and persist as fistulae.

What is the aetiology of oroantral fistula?

The vast majority of oroantral fistulae result from dental extraction. Up to 10% of upper molar extractions may create oroantral communications but very few, only 0.5%, persist to become fistulae. Other causes include malignant neoplasms arising in the oral cavity or antrum.

What factors predispose to formation of oroantral fistulae following extraction of teeth?

- Proximity of roots to maxillary antrum, large sinus
- Difficult extraction, unfavourable root morphology
- Periapical lesions such as apical granulomas or cysts
- Bone loss due to periodontitis or periapical–endodontic lesion
- Hypercementosis
- Local infection or sequestrum
- Predisposition to infection (e.g. diabetes)
- Dry socket or other poor healing
- Advanced age
- Pre-existing diseases in the sinus, though this is probably not a very significant factor.

What are the signs and symptoms of OAF?

The symptoms depend on the size of the fistula. Initially there may be persistent pain localized to the tooth socket but later, when inflammation has subsided, the fistula will be painless. If pain is a prominent symptom, some additional element such as infection must be suspected. The socket may present as an empty cavity or as a prolapse of antral lining through the socket into the mouth.

The most characteristic symptoms are the escape of fluids from the mouth into the nose on eating, or air or fluid into the mouth on blowing the nose. Passage of saliva, food and bacteria into the antrum causes sinusitis and the symptoms experienced will depend on its severity. Unilateral nasal obstruction, a feeling of fullness, pain over the maxilla and tenderness on pressure are typical.

Investigations

What investigations would you carry out, how and why?

Investigations need to be performed to confirm the communication with the antrum, to check for associated complications and to exclude the possibility that a malignant neoplasm is the cause of either the antral communication itself or the failure of the socket to heal. Investigations are summarized in the Table 18.1.

The periapical radiograph of the socket is shown in Figure 18.2. What do you see?

The first molar socket is indistinct. The lamina dura has been resorbed, probably as a result of inflammation or infection. The tract of a fistula is not visible. This is usually the case because the cortex is intact buccally and palatally, providing most of the radiodensity of the socket. The floor of the antrum is just visible and a root fragment approximately 3 mm long lies on the sinus floor (outlined in Fig. 18.7). The second molar has an inadequate root canal treatment, probably associated with loss of apical lamina dura and a small periapical radiolucency. A pin has perforated the distal root.

What else do you need to know about the root fragment?

Whether it is loose in the antrum or trapped under the sinus lining or in granulation tissue. The root will have to be removed and if it is under the lining or trapped, it should be possible to remove it through the socket. If it is loose in the antrum, removal in this way may prove impossible, necessitating a later elective surgical procedure such as a Caldwell–Luc approach.

How will you decide where the root is and whether it is mobile?

If the fistula opening is large you might try to visualize the fragment directly. If not, a second radiograph at right angles to the periapical, such as an occipitomental view, would help to localize it. A further view with the patient's head tilted would reveal whether or not the root moves.

Table 18.1 Summary of investigations

Aim of investigation	Methods
To demonstrate communication between antrum and mouth, the definitive test for oroantral fistula if there is no history of fluid or air passing between sinus and mouth.	If the fistula is large it may be possible to see into the antrum or pass a probe or large gutta percha point through into the antrum. If not, the patient can be asked to blow air into their nose while pinching the anterior nares closed and keeping their mouth open. You may see air bubbles, hear a hissing noise or detect air movement with a wisp of cotton wool at the socket opening.
To detect retained root fragments or sequestra in the socket. To exclude the possibility of other lesions such as malignant neoplasms.	Radiographs of the socket, ideally a periapical view, possibly also a panoramic tomograph.
To detect root fragments displaced into the antrum and exclude other antral disease.	Radiographs of antrum, usually a panoramic tomograph or standard occipitomental view is sufficient. However, it is difficult to visualize the whole antrum in any one view without superimposition of other structures. Cone beam computerised tomographic imaging is the best way to examine the sinus if a root fragment is suspected but cannot be detected on other views. However, it requires a higher X-ray dose, is expensive and only available in some centres.
To eliminate dental causes for any pain.	Vitality tests (thermal and/or electric) and examination for mobility of adjacent teeth.
To exclude malignancy or identify other causes for impaired socket healing.	Biopsy. Not usually required but if there is a worrying radiographic appearance or solid tissue in the socket, biopsy is indicated.

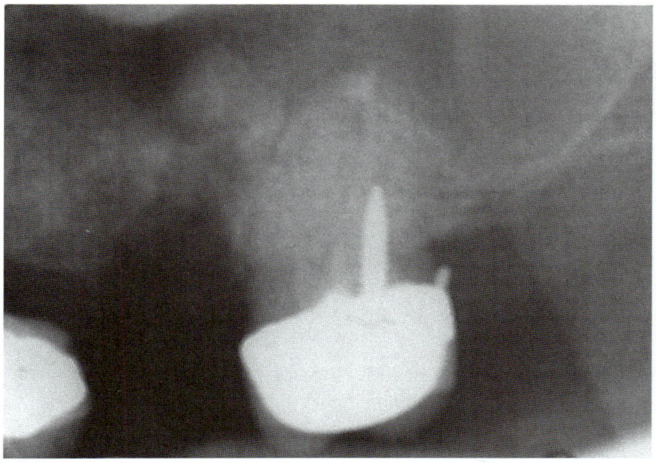

Fig. 18.2 Periapical view of the socket on presentation.

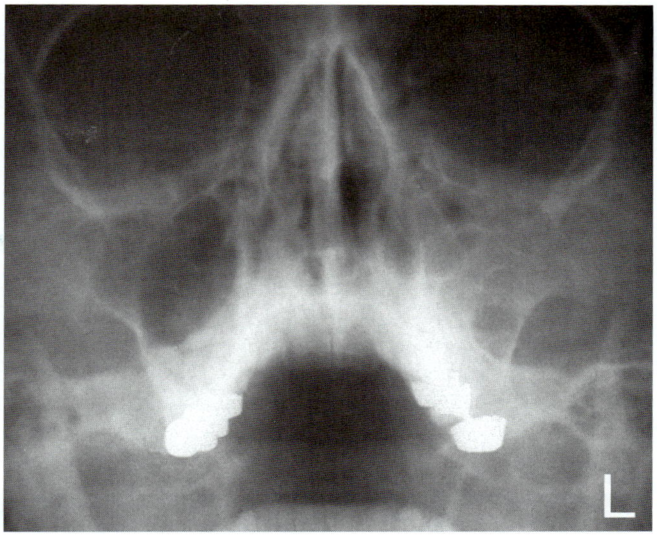

Fig. 18.3 Part of the occipitomental view.

■ ***A section of the occipitomental view is shown in Figure 18.3. What do you see and how do you interpret the appearances?***

The sinuses and facial bones are symmetrical and there is no expansion of the maxillary antrum. However, the sinus on the left is much more radiopaque than that on the right indicating oedema and thickening of the sinus lining or exudates within it. There is no fluid level visible. The root fragment is not visible because it lies on the sinus floor and is obscured by the superimposed alveolus.

Diagnosis

■ ***What is your final diagnosis?***

Sinusitis secondary to oroantral fistula caused by extraction of the upper first molar. A root fragment has been displaced into the sinus. Apical periodontitis of the second molar may also contribute to the sinusitis but this is a chronic problem and a lower priority for treatment.

Treatment

■ ***How would you treat this patient?***

- If pus is present in the fistula or if symptoms are severe, consider treating the sinusitis first and closing the fistula later after the sinusitis has partially resolved (it will not resolve completely until the fistula is closed). If there is long-standing infective sinusitis, this must be treated prior to surgical closure otherwise healing will be compromised
- Excise the fistula, otherwise remnants of the epithelial lining may proliferate to reform the tract
- Remove the root fragment from the sinus
- Close the oroantral communication surgically.

■ ***Would you treat this patient in general practice?***

Provided you are confident of your ability to remove the root fragment, there is no reason why this cannot be dealt with in a general practice situation. However, if the root is mobile in the antrum, the patient should be referred to hospital.

■ ***How would you excise the fistula and remove the root?***

Under local anaesthesia, incise around the edge of the socket from gingiva right down into the antrum, removing all the soft tissue in the socket as a cylinder or cone-shaped piece and draw it into the mouth. Depending on the size of the bony defect and the amount of bone resorption (usually greater in long-standing fistulae) this opens up a large hole into the sinus. With suction, good light and direct vision try to identify the root fragment and remove it with fine forceps, sucker tip or other instrument. Take care not to displace it into the sinus. If it becomes displaced it may be possible to wash it out by flushing saline into the sinus. Alternatively, better surgical access to the sinus may be achieved using a Caldwell–Luc approach under general anaesthesia. This is the main reason for referring patients with mobile fragments to hospital.

Send the excised tract for histopathological examination in case of unexpected underlying lesions.

■ ***How will you close the defect?***

The buccal mucoperiosteal flap with advancement (buccal advancement flap) is the most commonly used technique and it has more than a 90% success rate. The technique is shown in Figure 18.4. After excising the fistula, as above, proceed as follows:

Make two incisions buccally, anterior and posterior to the socket, passing parallel up the attached gingiva and then splaying to provide a wider base to ensure a good blood supply for the flap. The line of the incisions must be compatible with the flap sliding palatally to cover the defect in the alveolus.

Elevate the mucoperiosteal flap you have outlined by lifting the soft tissues in the plane beneath the periosteum.

Advance the flap. The flap cannot yet be pulled across the defect because the periosteum cannot be stretched. Fold the

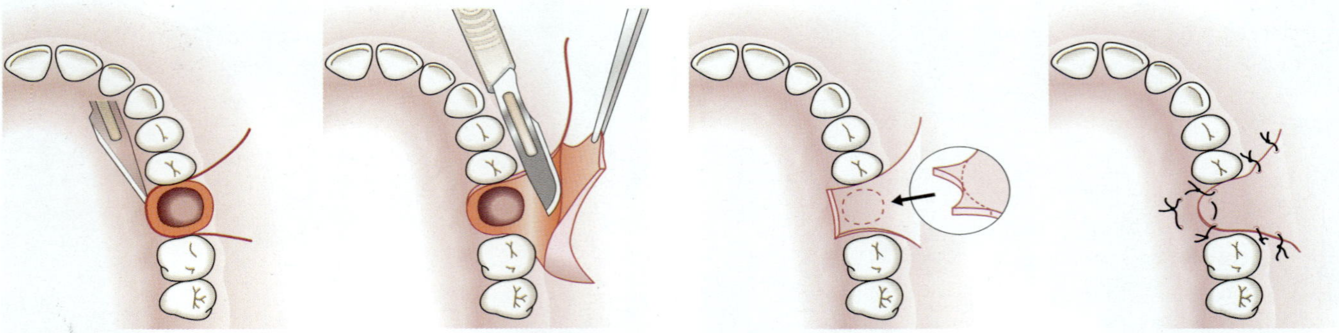

Fig. 18.4 The buccal advancement flap. Note how the relieving incisions buccally flare widely, shallow incision of the periosteum, trimming of the flap apex to ensure a good fit palatally and the rim of palatal bone on which it lies.

Table 18.2 Local flap design

Local flap design	Indications/advantages	Contraindications/disadvantages
Buccal advancement flap (see Figure 18.4).	Relatively simple, no flap donor site to heal, suitable for local analgesia.	Not ideal for large defect, advancing the flap reduces the depth of the residual buccal sulcus. Alveolar rather than masticatory mucosa advanced onto the ridge. Flap may break down if under tension.
Buccal fat pad transfer. As above and the buccal fat pad is dissected from under the buccal flap on a pedicle and secure in the socket.	As above, able to fill a larger defect.	General anaesthesia required for fat pad dissection, sulcus loss.
Palatal flap.	Possible when buccal flap has failed or would have insufficient length to cover a palatally placed bone defect. Covers the defect with masticatory mucosa.	The flap is of thick tissue and is difficult to mobilize. The donor site is left to granulate and this is painful until healed.

flap back to expose its periosteal surface and make several shallow parallel incisions across the flap that penetrate only the periosteum (about 0.25–0.5 mm in depth). This must be done very carefully with the flap under slight tension. As the periosteum is incised the flap will be felt to stretch. Do not perforate the flap or it will either be cut off or have a compromised blood supply. Make sufficient incisions to lengthen the flap so that it can reach across to the palatal side of the defect with minimal tension.

Prepare the palatal aspect of the alveolar defect. Refresh the margin of the palatal side to expose a narrow bony rim at least 1 mm wide, preferably 2 mm. The flap must be sutured into place at a site that has bony support.

Suture the flap in place using slowly resorbable sutures (for instance 3/0 vicryl) or nonresorbable sutures. Place several sutures around the apex of the flap (mesial, distal and central) and buccally. The flap must not be under tension and sufficient sutures must be placed to ensure an airtight and watertight seal supported by underlying bone. Ensure haemostasis. The sutures must remain in place for 10–14 days.

■ *What alternative flap designs are possible?*

The buccal advancement flap may not be possible when the bony defect is very large or when a previous attempt at repair has failed.

A number of other flaps are possible including the palatal island flap, submucosal palatal island flap, combined buccal and palatal flaps and even pedicled grafts from the tongue. However, most of these techniques are complex and have been superseded by the buccal fat pad technique. Diagrams of the rotated palatal flap technique, the second most commonly used method, are shown in Figure 18.5. Alternative methods to close oroantral fistulae are noted in Table 18.2.

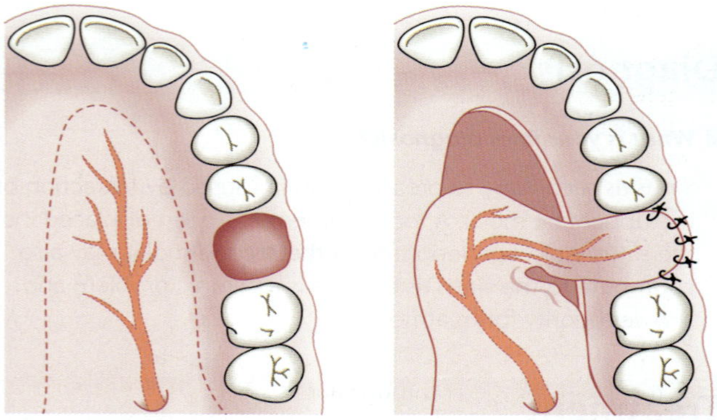

Fig. 18.5 The palatal rotation flap. Note how the flap derives its blood supply from the palatal artery within It. The difficulty of folding the thick flap is clear. The exposed bone will granulate and should be covered with a pack during healing.

■ *What postoperative instructions are required?*

In addition to the routine instructions given after extraction, the patient must be placed on an *antral regime* to reduce inflammation and prevent a rise in air pressure in the antrum. The upper first molar is situated in the lowest point of the maxillary sinus. Persistent infection or inflammation will induce exudates that will drain to this point and cause breakdown of the clot. Increased air pressure in the sinus, for instance from sneezing or blowing the nose, will force air or exudate through the alveolar defect as well as physically disrupting the clot and flap. Decongestants maintain the patency of the opening of the sinus to favour drainage to the nose.

A suitable antral regime would be:

- an absolute ban on blowing the nose for 48 hours
- sneeze allowing pressure to escape through the mouth
- nasal decongestant (such as ephedrine nasal spray 0.5%)
- decongestant inhalant (e.g. Karvol).

In addition, chlorhexidine mouthwash should be given. The repair will fail if there is leakage of saliva and bacteria past the flap from the oral aspect. No rinsing should be performed for 24 hours.

Other possibilities

How might formation of oroantral communication be prevented?

The risk of oroantral communication should be assessed routinely on a radiograph before extraction of upper molars. If the risk is high, an experienced surgeon should remove the tooth. Surgical extraction, possibly with elective sectioning of the tooth, reduces the chances of disrupting the maxillary floor.

The preoperative radiograph is shown in Figure 18.6. What do you see?

Several features in the list of risk factors above are evident. There is a low antral floor in contact with the roots, there is little alveolar bone height and there is loss of lamina dura around the tooth root apices.

How could an oroantral communication be confirmed at the time of extraction? How might this help?

If an antral communication is present, an echoing 'wind tunnel sound' will be heard if a small suction tip is held in the socket, the result of air being sucked from the antrum as well as the mouth. If the communication is large you may be able to see into the antrum or identify nasal regurgitation of your irrigation fluids or blood from the extraction site. Do not ask patient to blow through their nose while holding it. The sinus lining may still be intact but would be burst by the pressure and a small communication might be enlarged.

If a communication is suspected, stabilization of the clot, closure of the socket with resorbable sutures and appropriate warnings to the patient about blowing the nose should prevent a fistula developing. This is likely to be effective if the diameter of the communication is 4 mm or less. If it is larger, it should be repaired immediately using a suitable flap technique to avoid sinusitis and infection developing.

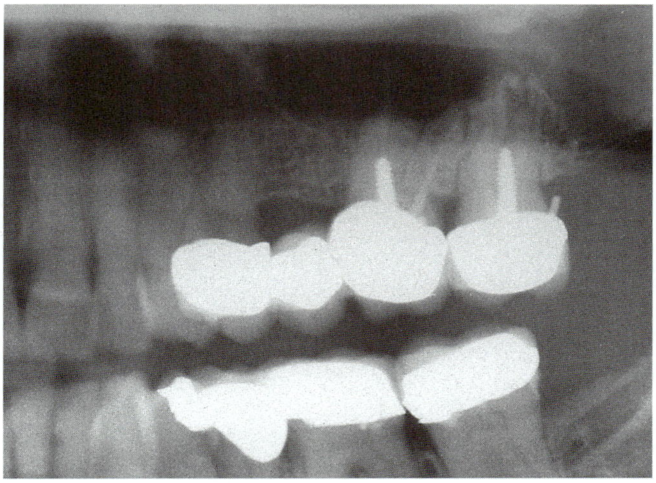

Fig. 18.6 Preoperative radiograph.

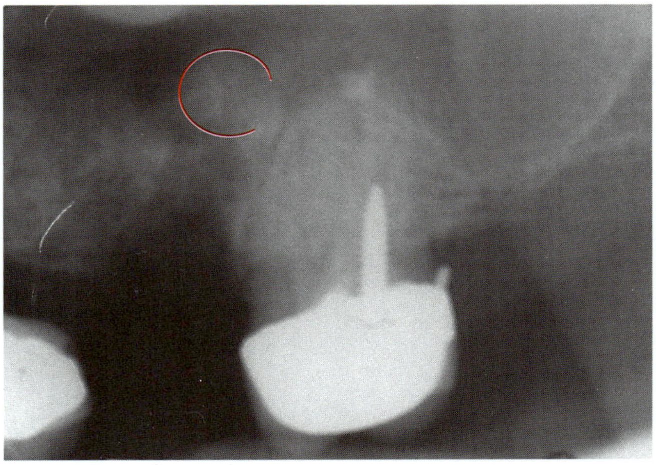

Fig. 18.7 The root fragment outlined on Figure 18.2.

Other possibilities

Case • 19

Troublesome mouth ulcers

SUMMARY

A 38-year-old woman with mouth ulcers has noticed a recent exacerbation in their severity. You need to make a diagnosis and decide on suitable investigations and treatment.

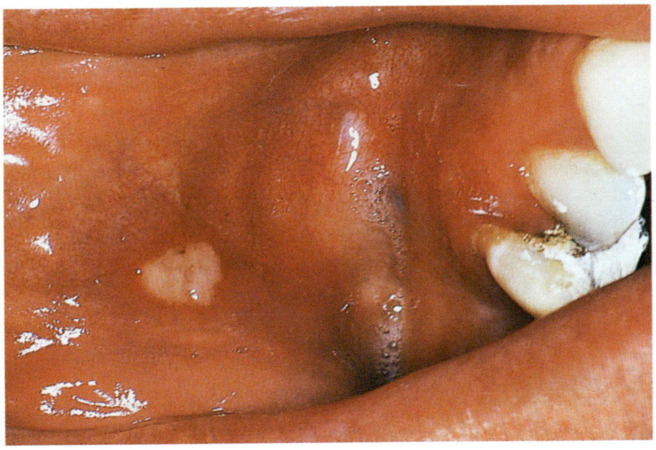

Fig. 19.1 The appearance of one ulcer.

History

Complaint

The patient complains of mouth ulcers which have been troubling her recently.

History of complaint

She has suffered from occasional mouth ulcers, usually small, one at a time, over a period of more than 20 years. However, recently they seem to have become worse and she now has several. Normally she ignores them but, because she was attending your surgery for a filling, she thought she would ask whether anything could be done.

Medical history

The patient is otherwise fit and well.

■ ***The patient has already provided several pieces of information of value for differential diagnosis. How do you assess her ulcers on the basis of the information available?***

The patient has noted an outset of ulceration early in life with recurrent attacks of single ulcers or small crops of ulcers. There are very many causes of oral ulceration but these ulcers appear to be **recurrent**, that is they appear periodically and heal completely between attacks. Recurrent ulceration has relatively few common causes.

■ ***What are the common causes of recurrent oral ulceration?***

- Recurrent aphthous stomatitis (RAS)
  - Minor type
  - Herpetiform type
  - Major type
- Erythema multiforme
- Occasional cases of traumatic ulceration
- Ulcers associated with gastrointestinal disease.

■ ***How will you differentiate between these conditions?***

Almost entirely on the basis of the findings in the history. Some features of the examination, blood tests or a biopsy may be helpful in certain cases, but the history is most important.

■ ***What features of the ulceration would you ask about to determine the diagnosis? Explain why for each.***

See Table 19.1 This patient's answers are shown in the right-hand column.

■ ***How are major and minor RAS differentiated?***

By severity rather than by any one feature alone. RAS may be labelled as major because of the size of the ulcers, their long duration or because they develop scarring on healing.

■ ***From which type of ulcers does the patient appear to be suffering?***

She would appear to have typical minor RAS which has increased in severity recently.

Examination

Intraoral examination

■ ***The appearance of one ulcer is shown in Figure 19.1. What do you see?***

There is an obvious ulcer on the anterior buccal mucosa. It is shallow, a few millimetres in diameter and has a slightly irregular but well-defined margin. The surrounding mucosa appears normal with only a narrow rim of erythema around the ulcer. There is a temporary restoration in the upper right first premolar and the ulcer would lie in approximately this region at rest.

Table 19.1 Features of ulcers

Feature	Reason	This patient's ulcers ...
Site	Recurrent aphthous stomatitis (RAS) almost exclusively affects nonkeratinized mucosa. Erythema multiforme affects predominantly the vermilion border of lip, buccal mucosa and anterior mouth. Recurrent traumatic ulceration usually recurs at the same site, often close to a sharp tooth.	... affect the labial mucosa and anterior buccal mucosa, especially in the sulci behind the lips. They never occur on the dorsal tongue or palate.
Size	Recurrent aphthous ulcer size depends on type. Minor ulcers are usually up to 8 mm in diameter, herpetiform 0.2–3 mm, and major ulcers are larger than 1 cm, sometimes up to 3 or 4 cm in diameter.	... are usually 3–5 mm in diameter.
Duration of each ulcer	Minor RAS ulcers heal in approximately 10 days. Herpetiform ulcers may heal in about the same time or sometimes a shorter period (they are often smaller). Major RAS lesions may fail to heal for weeks or even months. Erythema multiforme is variable depending on severity and heals in 10–21 days.	... last a week or so before each ulcer heals.
Number of ulcers	Minor RAS lesions usually appear singly or in crops of 4–5 ulcers; major RAS lesions are fewer in number, often only one or two; herpetiform ulcers are numerous, from 30 to 100 at a time.	... are normally single, occasionally 2–3 develop at once. Recently there have been up to 5 at once.
Frequency of attacks	Frequency of attacks of RAS varies with severity. Ulcers may appear almost continuously or just once a year. Sometimes they coincide with menstruation. Erythema multiforme classically recurs at 6–8 week intervals in severe cases but the frequency may be only one or two attacks in a year.	... are usually confined to one or two attacks a year but she has had three crops in the last 4 months.
Shape	RAS ulcers are usually round or oval and sharply defined, especially in the early stages. They may become more irregular as healing takes place. Herpetiform ulcers coalesce to form irregular shapes. Ulcers in erythema multiforme are irregular and ragged and often poorly defined, merging with inflamed surrounding mucosa. Those on the lips are often covered by bloody fibrin sloughs.	... are round or oval.
Whether multiple ulcers develop synchronously or asynchronously	In RAS, ulcers may develop in crops within a few days of one another, or asynchronously. One crop may appear before another has healed. Herpetiform RAS lesions usually appear in crops together. In erythema multiforme all the ulcers develop synchronously.	... usually appear within a few days of one another.
Are ulcers preceded by vesicles?	The presence of vesicles indicates possible viral infection or vesiculobullous disease. This fact may be helpful in the differential diagnosis of herpetiform ulcers, which resemble viral ulcers but are not preceded by vesicles.	... have not been preceded by any vesicles, at least as far as the patient has been aware.
Age of onset	RAS usually has onset before or around adolescence. Erythema multiforme typically develops in the second or third decade.	... started with occasional ulcers in childhood and she has had occasional ulcers throughout her life.
Family history	Often present in RAS; not found in erythema multiforme.	... or ulcers like them do not appear to affect her parents. The patient's 7-year-old son occasionally has ulcers.
Exacerbating or relieving factors	None is usually detected for RAS, though an ulcer may develop at a site of minor trauma, complicating the differential diagnosis if the ulcers are very infrequent. Stress often appears to precipitate attacks of RAS. Erythema multiforme may be triggered by a drug, viral or other infection, classically 10 days before the ulcers appear. Often no trigger is identified.	... occasionally develop where she bites herself or knocks her mucosa with a toothbrush.

When you examine the patient you find two more ulcers. One is 2 mm in diameter and lies in the lower labial sulcus on the alveolar mucosa adjacent to the lower right canine. A third ulcer, also 3 mm in diameter, lies on the upper left buccal mucosa anterior to the parotid papilla. They appear to be identical to the ulcer shown.

■ *What can you deduce from these appearances?*

The appearances are not particularly helpful in differential diagnosis but are typical of those seen in minor recurrent aphthous stomatitis. The slightly irregular outline of the largest ulcer indicates early healing. The ulcers are not at all suggestive of erythema multiforme.

If you were able to examine the mouth you would find that there is no evidence of scarring in the common ulcer sites, which would have suggested the major form of RAS. The mucosa is otherwise healthy excluding the possibility of chronic ulceration in a mucosal disease, such as lichen planus or a vesiculobullous disease. The normal mucosa at sites of previous ulcers confirms that the ulceration is indeed recurrent.

Diagnosis

■ *What is your diagnosis and what would you do next?*

The diagnosis is recurrent aphthous stomatitis of the minor form. The next step is to exclude the possibility that the ulcers are associated with an underlying condition.

■ *With what underlying conditions/causes may RAS be associated?*

- Iron deficiency
- Vitamin deficiency, particularly B_{12} and folate
- Gastrointestinal disease
- Behçet's disease
- Smoking cessation.

■ *What features of the ulcers themselves might indicate the presence of an underlying predisposing condition?*

Any feature in the history or examination which is atypical for the type of RAS should raise suspicion of an underlying condition. In particular, the following should trigger a search for underlying predisposing causes:

- Onset after the second decade
- Increase in ulcer size, duration, symptoms or severity
- Marked periulcer erythema.

How would you investigate the possibility of an underlying condition?

Iron deficiency is relatively common. Check for known history of anaemia. Question the patient about common causes of iron-deficiency anaemia, including menorrhagia and gastrointestinal bleeding (peptic ulcer, hiatus hernia, inflammatory bowel disease and haemorrhoids). Check that a balanced and varied diet is consumed, even though dietary deficiency is rare. Perform blood tests or refer the patient to her medical practitioner to check for microcytosis and to determine haemoglobin and red cell/haemoglobin indices. Ulcers may be associated with minor degrees of iron deficiency that are insufficient to cause anaemia and sensitive tests for iron depletion are required. Serum ferritin, which reflects body iron stores, is the ideal test.

Vitamin deficiencies associated with aphthous stomatitis are usually of folate or B_{12}. Check that a balanced and varied diet is consumed and that there is no gastrointestinal disease to reduce absorption of folate. Exclude dietary deficiency of B_{12} by asking about pernicious anaemia and gastrointestinal disease and confirming that the diet is adequate, particularly if a strict vegetarian diet is consumed. Perform blood tests for mean cell volume (increased in vitamin deficiency) and assay serum or erythrocyte folate level and serum B_{12}.

Gastrointestinal disease exacerbates RAS because of reduced absorption of iron, folate and B_{12}. Ask about both diarrhoea and constipation, abdominal cramps, weight loss and blood in stools and check the medical history.

Gastrointestinal diseases are also associated with other types of oral ulceration. Sometimes these ulcers are recurrent but their appearances are usually characteristic and they are most unlikely to be mistaken for ulcers of RAS. Large leathery ulcers, multiple pustules and irregular haemorrhagic ulcers are very occasionally seen in ulcerative colitis, linear ulcers with hyperplastic margins in Crohn's disease and herpetiform-type ulcers in coeliac disease.

Behçet's disease is rare but can present with oral ulcers as the most significant problem. Patients may suffer from a broad spectrum of signs and symptoms and should be questioned about genital ulcers on mucosa or skin, rashes including erythema nodosum or pustules, arthritis of large and small joints, venous thrombosis and bowel symptoms. Ocular signs including uveitis and conjunctivitis are found in a minority of patients and these, and central nervous system symptoms, are serious. There are no specific tests for Behçet's disease (though HLA typing may help identify those at risk from ocular disease). A biopsy of an oral ulcer may be helpful because it can demonstrate the underlying vasculitis that accounts for many of the manifestations.

Smoking cessation is excluded by questioning. It sometimes exacerbates ulceration but starting smoking again does not usually induce remission.

Treatment

What treatments are available and which would you suggest?

Many treatments are available. Unfortunately none is highly effective in all patients and treatment must be selected to suit individual cases. Reassurance is an important part of treatment in minor RAS. Tell the patient that RAS is very common, but is a 'nuisance' condition rather than serious or infectious and warn her that:

- no one treatment is consistently effective;
- she may need to try several treatments before she finds one which works well for her;
- treatments are not completely effective, and they should only be expected to moderate the symptoms and sometimes the frequency of ulcers;

Table 19.2 Treatments for minor RAS

Treatment	Indications
No treatment	Probably the best option for occasional ulcers.
Covering agents, e.g. Orabase	Good for infrequent ulcers anteriorly in the buccal and labial mucosa, ideally single ulcers. Use is difficult and the patient must be capable of some dexterity.
Anti-inflammatory/analgesic mouthwash, e.g. benzydamine Antiseptic mouthwash, e.g. chlorhexidine	Both types of mouthwash are useful when ulcers affect a range of oral sites not accessible to covering pastes. In general not highly effective but may reduce pain directly or by reducing infection of the ulcer surface. Popular with most patients.
Low potency topical steroid pellets such as hydrocortisone (Corlan) and steroid in Orabase such as triamcinolone (Adcortyl in Orabase)	Ulcers must be at sites where the pellet can be left to dissolve or Orabase applied, usually in the sulci. Useful first-line treatments if the ulcer-free period is longer than 1 month and may reduce frequency in some patients.
Steroid mouthwashes, e.g. betamethasone	Used when ulcers affect a range of sites and are of sufficient severity to merit a therapeutic treatment. Potent, not available to general dental practitioners in the UK. Patients must dissolve tablets to make fresh mouthwash.
Steroid aerosols, e.g. budesonide	Useful when a more potent steroid must be delivered to a single site. Potent, not available to general dental practitioners in the UK.
Systemic drugs, steroids, colchicine, azathiaprine, thalidomide	For severe cases and Behçet's disease refractory to other treatments. Potent, not available to general dental practitioners in the UK.
In addition, simple advice may help to make ulcers bearable: avoid spicy foods, acidic fruit juices and carbonated drinks; consider drinking with a straw when ulcers are present; avoid sharp foods such as crisps, and astringent toothpastes or those with irritant flavourings or detergents.	

- the aim of treatment should be to make the ulcers bearable.

If an underlying condition such as iron deficiency is detected, its correction will probably reduce their severity but will not cure the ulcers completely.

Treatments available are shown in Table 19.2.

For this patient, the most important factor is to exclude underlying causes and iron deficiency is the most likely. Treatment of underlying deficiency may reduce the ulcer severity so that the patient can again ignore her ulcers. In the meantime a mouthwash or hydrocortisone pellets would appear to be suitable as a first-line treatment though the patient might also be encouraged to try some of the many nonprescription preparations available.

■ ***The patient asks whether the buccal ulcer could be caused by the temporary restoration in the adjacent tooth. What is your opinion?***

No. This is most unlikely. The history of RAS is so typical that the diagnosis is not in doubt. Reactions to dental materials are not associated with ulcers of this type. However, recurrent aphthous ulcers often develop at the sites of minor trauma. Trauma either during restoration, from a sharp edge or from biting while the mucosa was anaesthetized might well explain the location of this particular ulcer.

Case 20

A lump in the neck

SUMMARY

A 55-year-old man presents to your oral and maxillofacial surgery department clinic with a lump on the left side of the neck. You must make a diagnosis.

History

Complaint

The patient complains of the lump and notices some discomfort on swallowing, as if something is stuck in his throat. He assumes the lump is the cause.

History of present complaint

He thinks he first noticed the lump about 3 months ago. It has always been painless and is slowly enlarging. The discomfort on swallowing is of recent onset.

Medical history

The patient is otherwise fit and well. He smokes 20 cigarettes per day and drinks 10 units of alcohol each week as beer.

Examination

Extraoral examination

The appearance of the swelling is shown in Figure 20.1.

■ ***What do you see? What is the likely origin of the mass?***

There is a swelling just anterior to the anterior border of the sternomastoid muscle and below and behind the angle of the mandible. It is several centimetres in diameter and extends forwards below the angle of the mandible towards the submandibular region. The overlying skin does not appear to be inflamed.

The lesion lies over the deep cervical lymph node chain and could well arise from a cervical lymph node. It is too low and too far posterior to be arising from the submandibular gland and too low to have arisen in the lower pole of the parotid gland. Other soft tissues of the neck could be the origin, but a lymph node is the most likely cause.

If you could palpate the lesion you would find that it is approximately 8 cm by 6 cm in size and feels firm on palpation, possibly slightly fluctuant. It is mobile, not fixed to the overlying skin or deep structures. The patient does not notice any tenderness on palpation. There are no other swellings or enlarged lymph nodes palpable on either side of the neck.

Intraoral examination

The submandibular glands are palpable bimanually and appear symmetrical. Both are mobile and clearly separate from the swelling, which lies posterior to the gland.

The patient's mouth has been well restored in the past but suffers from recent neglect and several carious cavities are visible. There is no significant periodontal disease

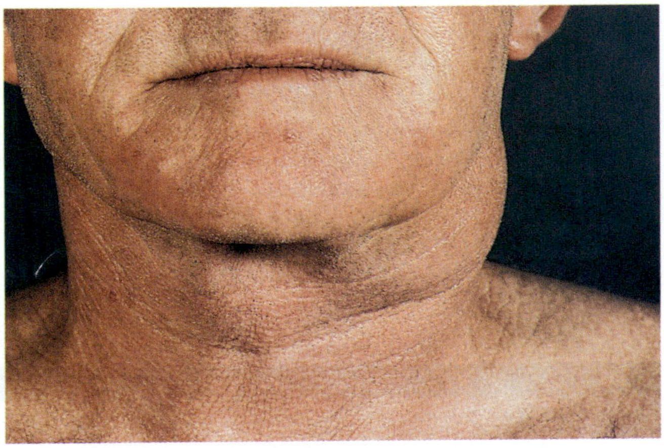

a

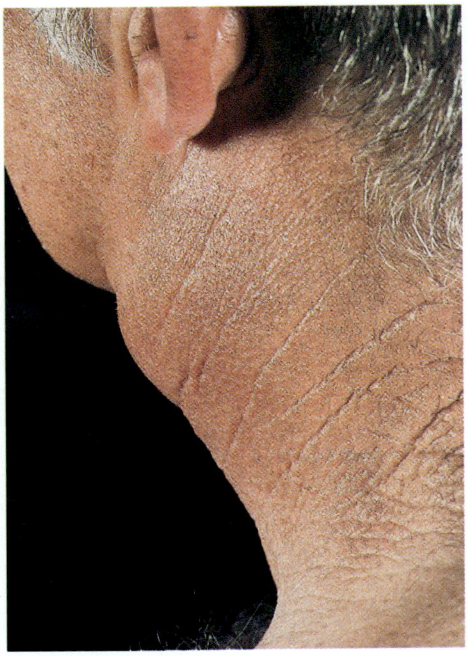

b

Fig. 20.1 **a** and **b** The appearance of the swelling.

with most probing depths less than 5 mm and no mobile teeth. The lower left first permanent molar has lost a large restoration and has extensive caries. There is no soft tissue swelling, sinus or tenderness in the sulcus adjacent to the apices of the roots. The tooth is not tender to percussion. The oral mucosa appears normal, and the tonsils appear to be symmetrical.

Differential diagnosis

■ ***What are the most likely causes of the lump and why?***

Metastatic malignancy appears likely and this lesion is so typical of a cervical lymph node metastasis that it must be considered to be malignant until proved otherwise. The combination of features suggestive of metastasis is the patient's age (should be considered a possible cause in any patient aged over 45), the site (consistent with a cervical lymph node), the firm consistency and lack of tenderness. Fixation to the skin or other structures would be almost conclusive of malignancy but is a late sign. The patient is a smoker and drinker and so has an increased risk of malignancy. Either a squamous carcinoma or adenocarcinoma is likely. Melanoma and other malignancies are further possible causes.

Lymphadenitis secondary to a local cause is common and so must be considered. However there is no tenderness on palpation to suggest an inflammatory cause. If this were a reactive inflammatory enlargement, the most likely source of infection would be a dental, pharyngeal or skin infection. The patient has a potential source of dental infection in the lower left first permanent molar but the tooth is not tender to percussion nor associated with overt infection, making it an unlikely cause.

Tuberculosis needs to be considered both as a possible diagnosis and as a factor affecting management. Most patients with cervical lymph node enlargement caused by tuberculosis have reactivation ('secondary' or post-primary) tuberculosis in which a previous quiescent infection becomes reactivated. This localized infection may or may not be accompanied by pulmonary disease though there may be radiologial evidence of past tuberculosis on chest radiograph. Cervical tuberculous lymphadenitis is common in those from the Indian subcontinent. Atypical mycobacterial infection is a disease which often affects the cervical lymph nodes but is almost always seen in children or the immunosuppressed.

■ ***Which additional but less likely causes need to be considered whenever a patient complains of an enlargement at this site? Why are they unlikely causes in this case?***

Numerous lesions could arise at this site and it is not useful to list them all. A number of possible causes (Table 20.1) merit consideration, because they are common, easily excluded or cause significant morbidity.

Table 20.1 Further possible causes of the enlargement

Cause		Reasons
Developmental causes	Branchial cyst	Branchial cysts develop at this site. They usually present in childhood or early adulthood but can on occasion be asymptomatic for many years and present late with infection. However, 55 years of age would be extremely late and a metastatic malignancy is a much more likely cause. Cystic change in metastatic carcinoma in lymph nodes is a well-recognized finding and fluctuation can be misinterpreted as indicating a benign cyst such as a branchial cyst. Branchial cysts are *rare*.
Infectious causes	Cat scratch disease, toxoplasmosis, brucellosis, glandular fever	These are less common causes of cervical lymphadenopathy in this age group. All usually cause enlargement of several nodes, often bilaterally. Toxoplasmosis and glandular fever usually affect young adults. Cat scratch disease may present with a single markedly enlarged node. Exposure to cats or other pets or history of a primary skin infection at the site of a scratch aids diagnosis. Serological tests allow the diagnosis of cat scratch disease, toxoplasmosis and brucellosis. Of these conditions, only cat scratch disease is a conceivable cause for this swelling and the likelihood is low.
	HIV infection	Should always be considered in chronic lymph node enlargement but causes generalized lymphadenopathy. May be accompanied by signs of immunosuppression. A most unlikely diagnosis for this presentation.
Inflammatory causes	Sarcoidosis	Another cause of generalized lymphadenopathy or enlargement of a group of nodes. More common in the 20–40 age group. African-Americans, West Indian and Irish immigrants to the UK are at particular risk. Usually accompanied by other signs which aid diagnosis. An unlikely cause for this patient's swelling.
Benign neoplasms	Salivary gland neoplasm	The tail of the parotid gland extends low into the neck, to just below and behind the angle of the mandible. This lesion does not appear to be in the correct site for a parotid gland origin but the possibility of a benign salivary neoplasm might be considered. A Warthin's tumour or pleomorphic adenoma would be the most likely possibillities because they are commonest.
	Carotid body tumour (paraganglioma)	These arise from the carotid body at the carotid bifurcation and cause a swelling just in front of the sternomastoid muscle but slightly higher than the present swelling. They are rare, affect the 30–60-year-old age group and are sometimes bilateral. Though an unusual cervical swelling, the accompanying pulsation, thrill or bruit from the carotid blood supply aids diagnosis. The lesion is mobile horizontally but not vertically because it is attached to the carotid artery. An unlikely cause for this patient's swelling.
	Other benign soft tissue neoplasms	Many are possible, arising from muscle, nerve, fat or fibrous tissue. None merits singling out as a possible cause in this case.
Other primary malignant neoplasms	Lymphoma	An enlarged lymph node in the deep cervical lymph chain could be the first presentation of lymphoma. Non-Hodgkin's lymphoma would be the most likely type in a patient of this age. However, enlarged lymph nodes in lymphoma are almost always multiple and feel rubbery. The presence of such a large discrete lesion without other enlarged lymph nodes almost completely excludes lymphoma.

Table 20.2 Techniques for obtaining tissue

Investigation	Advantages	Disadvantages
Fine needle aspiration biopsy/ cytology (FNA or FNAC)	The least invasive procedure which can provide a sample of the lesional tissue. FNA does not risk seeding tumour or tuberculosis into the tissues of the neck. Rapid. Readily repeated if fails. Leaves no scar.	It is possible to miss the lesion when inserting the needle. If this is likely to be a problem, the procedure can be performed under ultrasound or radiological guidance. Provides only a small sample and definitive diagnosis on cytology may not be possible (though a sufficiently accurate diagnosis to plan treatment may be provided).
Incisional biopsy	Readily performed and provides a large tissue sample which will almost certainly be sufficient for diagnosis. In lymphoma, a lymph node is usually required for classification of disease. (However, the neck is not the favoured site for the resulting scar and another node would probably be sampled).	If the lesion were malignant it would probably be spread into the tissues of the neck, making subsequent surgical treatment very difficult, if not impossible. This complication can be minimized by taking the biopsy from an area which would later be excised. However, spread into the tissue planes of the neck cannot be reliably prevented. Risk to adjacent structures in the neck.

Table 20.3 Other investigations

Investigation	Reason
Vitality tests	To search for dental causes of infection.
Radiographs of teeth on left side	To search for a dental infectious cause and provide information to plan necessary dental treatment.
Sialogram	To determine whether the mass is within the submandibular or parotid glands, unlikely in this case.
Chest radiograph	To search for metastasis in lungs, or for evidence of tuberculosis.
Serology	Viral titres and specific tests to determine potential infectious causes such as cat scratch fever.
Ultrasound scan	To determine the lesion's relationship to the salivary glands; determine its extent, and whether it is cystic; to find out whether other masses or enlarged lymph nodes are present.
CT/MRI scan/PET scan	To localize the lesion and its relationships to normal tissues. Unnecessary at this stage. May be required later to plan treatment when diagnosis is established.

Investigations

■ ***What is the most important investigation? Which methods might be used and what are their advantages and disadvantages?***

The critical requirement when malignancy is suspected is to obtain tissue speedily for microscopic diagnosis. All other investigations are less important at this stage. Two techniques are in common use; the fine needle aspiration biopsy and the surgical incisional biopsy (Table 20.2).

■ ***What other investigations might be performed, either now or at a later date? Why?***

See Table 20.3.

In this case a suitable combination of investigations would be fine needle aspiration, dental radiographs, vitality tests and possibly ultrasound scan. The sialogram would have been performed if a salivary origin had been thought possible after clinical examination.

The lower first molar was nonvital and a periapical radiograph revealed apical radiolucency. The smear from a fine needle aspirate is shown in Figure 20.2.

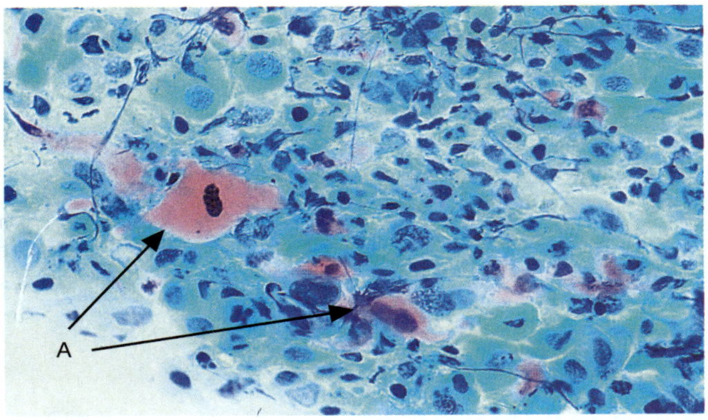

Fig. 20.2 Fine needle aspirate from the lesion.

■ ***What does the fine needle aspirate show and how do you interpret the appearances?***

The aspirate shows cells from the lesion spread as a single layer and stained with the Papanicolaou stain. This stains nuclei dark blue, keratin orange and the cytoplasm of nonkeratinized epithelial cells turquoise. The cells are almost all epithelial as shown by their prominent cytoplasm and by the presence of keratinization (arrowed A) in some of them. The larger cells have angulate polygonal cytoplasm typical of squamous epithelial cells. The nuclei of the cells range markedly in size from small hyperchromatic nuclei to very large irregular nuclei. At higher power the chromatin pattern is coarse. These features indicate malignancy and the keratinized cells indicate that this is a squamous carcinoma. Many normal lymphocytes were found elsewhere on the slide. This indicates that the carcinoma is in a lymph node and is therefore a metastasis.

Diagnosis

The patient has metastatic squamous carcinoma, almost certainly in a cervical lymph node.

■ *What are the possible sites for the primary malignant neoplasm?*

Any site in the drainage area of the lymph node in which squamous carcinoma may develop:

Oral mucosa, particularly ventrolateral tongue, floor of mouth, soft palate, fauces or retromolar mucosa
Pharynx, nasopharynx or oropharynx
Tonsil
Maxillary sinus
Facial skin and scalp
Salivary glands

■ *What would you do to localize the primary carcinoma?*

- Check history for previous known malignant disease
- Re-examine for symptoms or signs of possible primary carcinomas at all these sites
- Upper aerodigestive tract endoscopy under general anaesthesia
- Computerised tomography, magnetic resonance imaging or positron emission imaging

In this case, endoscopy revealed an ulcerated mass in the pharynx near the base of the tongue, and biopsy revealed squamous cell carcinoma.

■ *What would you do if a primary carcinoma is not identified?*

During endoscopy, blind biopsy of the nasopharynx and ipsilateral tonsillectomy may reveal an unsuspected small carcinoma. If this fails to identify the primary then the search will have to be widened, initially to other common sites for squamous carcinoma, such as lung, and then to the whole body. Very occasionally no primary lesion is found and the patient is said to have an occult primary.

Treatment

■ *What are the treatment options assuming a primary is identified in the head and neck?*

The treatment of choice for most primary head and neck squamous carcinoma with lymph node involvement is surgical resection, with subsequent radiotherapy in selected cases to eradicate any possible residual disease. Radiotherapy is always given if the carcinoma is found to have spread outside the capsule of lymph nodes in which metastases have seeded (extracapsular spread). Radiotherapy alone would be used in selected cases such as small tongue, tonsil or laryngeal carcinomas, for palliation in advanced carcinoma or when patients refuse surgery. Surgery would usually involve the en bloc removal of the primary site and lymph nodes from the deep cervical chain in continuity (block dissection of neck). Reconstruction using local, distant or free flaps may be required.

Chemotherapy and immunotherapy are of little benefit in squamous carcinoma of the head and neck. Further information is included in Case 57.

Another possibility

■ *If the fine needle aspirate had shown adenocarcinoma or poorly differentiated carcinoma, which possible primary sites would have required investigation?*

Adenocarcinoma (carcinoma showing glandular differentiation) might well have arisen in the breast, lung or prostate. The thyroid, salivary glands and minor mucous glands in the upper aerodigestive tract would also be possible primary sites. A poorly differentiated carcinoma could have metastasized from any of the squamous carcinoma or adenocarcinoma primary sites.

The stomach is a further possible source and a low cervical metastasis on the left side is a recognized presentation. However, in this case the swelling is too high in the neck to have arisen from the stomach.

■ *Why does a gastrointestinal carcinoma sometimes metastasize to the left side of the neck?*

Lymph from the oesophagus and the upper part of the stomach drains upwards in the thoracic duct which enters the lower end of the internal jugular vein. There is a rather variable anatomy at the site and often the subclavian and internal jugular lymph trunks join the thoracic duct rather than the internal jugular vein. In this situation, malignant cells draining up the thoracic duct can be carried a short distance into the lymphatics of the neck by retrograde flow (because the lymphatics are at a low and fluctuating pressure). Such cells can seed metastases in the lymph nodes just above the clavicle (Virchow's node).

Case 21

Trauma to an immature incisor

SUMMARY

An 8-year-old girl has fractured her upper right permanent central incisor tooth.

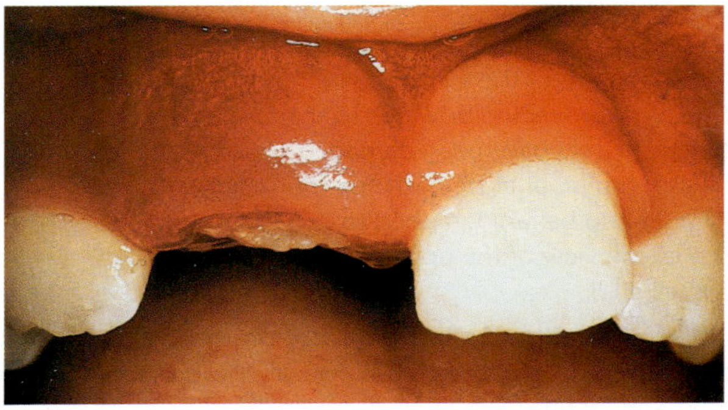

Fig. 21.1 The patient's anterior dentition on presentation.

History

Complaint

The child is brought in as an emergency by her mother, complaining of a broken front tooth.

History of complaint

Two hours prior to presentation the child had slipped at school, hitting her mouth. One front tooth appears to be broken.

Medical history

The child has mild asthma, but is otherwise healthy.

Dental history

The child has attended the dentist irregularly, has no caries and no experience of operative dentistry. Her mother states that the broken tooth had not appeared normal and may have been decayed.

■ ***What additional questions would you ask and why?***

Did the patient lose consciousness? This would indicate a relatively severe blow to the head and might indicate significant intracranial trauma. If the patient lost consciousness, even for a short period, they should be referred to hospital where they would almost certainly be admitted for 24 hours of observation. In this case the patient did not lose consciousness.

Was a piece of the tooth broken off and was it found? Missing fragments of teeth may have been inhaled, swallowed, embedded in the lip or lost. If a fragment has been found it must be matched to the fracture to determine whether other pieces remain missing and the patient investigated to locate and remove the pieces. In this case no fragment was found.

Has the patient suffered trauma previously? Previous trauma to this tooth could have resulted in arrested root development, disturbed crown formation or pathological mobility prior to this incident, depending on the age and stage of dental development at the time. Such changes could affect treatment and might explain the parent's observation that the tooth was not normal. In this case no previous trauma could be recalled by the parent.

Was the damaged tooth fully erupted before the accident? In early mixed dentition, incisors on opposite sides of the mouth may be at different stages of eruption. At this age it would be expected that eruption would be complete but there is wide variation in eruption date and rate. It would be possible to misinterpret incomplete eruption as an intrusion injury if the original degree of eruption were not known. In this case, the child's mother reported that both front teeth were fully erupted.

What object or surface did the child hit with her mouth? Injury on surfaces such as playgrounds, roads and pavements carries the risk of contaminating the wound with dirty particulate material. Sometimes such foreign material even enters intraoral wounds. Thorough debridement would then be required. It would also be necessary to check the child's immunization status for tetanus prophylaxis and arrange a booster dose if required. In this case, the child hit the edge of a table.

Examination

Extraoral examination

The child is distressed but is readily examined. There is some slight swelling of the upper lip but no external abrasions or lacerations.

Intraoral examination

■ ***The appearances of the teeth are shown in Figure 21.1. What do you see?***

The gingival tissues labial to the upper right permanent central incisor are erythematous and swollen. The crown of the tooth appears to be missing and less than 1 mm of the tooth is visible above the level of the gingiva. The visible fragment appears to be an intact incisal edge rather than a fractured enamel or root surface. The lateral incisors show mild hypomineralization of the labial enamel in the incisal third of the crown.

If you were able to examine the patient you would find that the palatal gingiva of the upper right central incisor is also red and swollen. The remainder of the dentition is caries-free. There are no lacerations in the mucosa of the inner aspect of the lip.

■ ***What additional examination(s) would you perform?***

Injury to the adjacent incisors and teeth in the lower labial segment should be investigated. Vitality, mobility, tenderness to percussion and fractures should be noted. A periodontal probe should be gently inserted into the labial gingival sulcus to confirm or exclude the presence of a deep pseudo-pocket which would indicate traumatic displacement.

■ ***Having completed the examination, what question should the examining dentist keep in the back of their mind? Explain why.***

Are the injuries seen consistent with the history given? If not, inconsistencies in the history should be probed by further gentle questioning. While children are often reluctant to offer an accurate account of minor accidents, significant inconsistencies or evasive responses by the parent or child should raise suspicion of nonaccidental injury. Further details are given in problem 36.

■ ***What features in the history and examination would lead to suspicion of nonaccidental injury?***

History of repeated trauma (dental and facial injury, but also limb fractures)
Presenting injury not consistent with history given
Child's account varies significantly from parental account
History changed over course of initial consultation or review visits, evasive answers to questions
Delayed presentation
Bruises, abrasions or other soft tissue lesions apparently sustained over a period of time (for instance at different stages of healing) which are not accounted for by the presenting injury

Differential diagnosis

■ ***What is your initial differential diagnosis?***

There are two main possibilities, either the central incisor has been almost completely intruded (intrusive luxation) or its crown has been fractured horizontally at gingival level. The appearance in the figure indicates that this is an intrusion luxation because the visible tooth is an intact incisal edge rather than a fractured root.

Investigations

■ ***What investigations would you perform? Explain why for each.***

Radiographs are required to visualize the intruded/fractured tooth and to assess damage to it and the adjacent teeth. Periapical views should be taken of all upper incisors to detect possible root fracture and to assess the stage of root development of the incisors. In intrusion injuries the force of the blow is directed upwards so that it is unlikely that the lower incisors have been damaged. However, if the upper incisor turns out to be fractured then the lower incisors should also be radiographed to exclude root fracture. The periapical view of the upper right central incisor is shown in Figure 21.2.

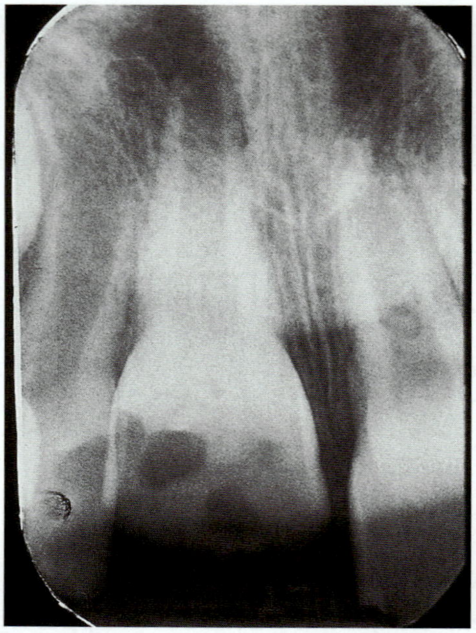

Fig. 21.2 Periapical radiograph.

Tests of vitality of all incisors are required. If the patient is sufficiently composed to allow it, all the incisors should be checked for vitality, preferably by electric pulp testing. Teeth recently subjected to trauma may not respond to testing ('concussion') and testing teeth with open apices may give an artificially low reading. However, it is important to take a baseline reading soon after the injury so that if vitality does not recover, treatment may be instituted without delay.

■ ***The periapical radiograph is shown in Figure 21.2. What does the radiograph show?***

The radiograph shows a severe intrusive luxation of the maxillary right permanent incisor. The periodontal ligament space is indistinct or obliterated in part. There is no crown or root fracture visible, and the root is immature with a wide open apex. A peculiar feature on the film is the small circular radiolucent areas on the crown of the intruded tooth. These are well demarcated and smooth in outline.

■ ***What could these radiolucent areas be?***

The lesions are relatively radiolucent and lie towards the incisal edge where enamel rather than dentine is responsible for the radiopacity of the tooth. This suggests that missing enamel is likely to be the cause. The patient's mother mentioned that the tooth had always appeared decayed and causes predating the current injury are the most likely. A number might be considered:

Cause	Merits as a diagnosis
Loss of enamel/dentine as a direct result of the trauma	Such an injury would be unusual and the circular pattern is difficult to explain.
Dental caries	Caries in this distribution also seems unlikely. Labial surface caries is usually found following the gingival margin in individuals with poor oral hygiene. This child is caries free and has good oral hygiene.
Enamel hypoplasia or hypomineralization	Could affect single or multiple teeth. Hypomineralization was noted in the incisal third of the enamel of the adjacent teeth. Hypomineralization could not result from the present injury because the teeth were erupted.
Resorption defects	These are a possibility but the distribution would be unusual and some cause, such as previous injury, might be expected. Resorption could not occur so rapidly after the current intrusion but may be seen on the root surface some months following an intrusive luxation.

Enamel hypoplasia or hypomineralization would appear to be the most likely cause.

■ *Why is there a horizontal dark line on the radiograph across the crown of the upper left central and upper right lateral incisor?*

It is the edge of the soft tissue shadow of the upper lip.

Diagnosis

■ *What is your final diagnosis?*

The patient has an intrusive luxation to the permanent central incisor. This tooth also has several discrete hypoplastic enamel defects that were present before the accident.

Treatment

■ *What types of tissue injury result from intrusion and what are their complications?*

Injury	Complication
Crushing and rupture of the periodontal fibres	Bacterial infection or inflammation tracking along the periodontal ligament. Increased risk of root resorption. Weakened periodontal attachment.
Crushing, devitalization and scraping off of cementum	Transient surface root resorption with the possibility of more extensive external resorption and ankylosis in the longer term.
Crushing of the apical neurovascular bundle (and the pulp itself in immature teeth)	Loss of pulp vitality.

■ *Will the tooth re-erupt or should it be surgically repositioned?*

All mature teeth (closed apex) and over 60% of immature teeth become nonvital as a result of intrusive luxation. Therefore, it is advisable to reposition the tooth as rapidly as possible so that access to the pulp chamber can be facilitated before pulp necrosis occurs. Intruded teeth with open apices do have the potential for re-eruption, but if this has not commenced within 1 week, intervention is required. There is at present no evidence to indicate the optimal treatment for the intrusive luxation of permanent teeth. Given sufficient cooperation, immediate surgical repositioning of the tooth will immediately restore the appearance. This should be followed by a short period of splinting of 7–10 days. This option may, however, increase the likelihood of external root resorption and loss of marginal bone support. Relatively rapid orthodontic extrusion over a period of 3–4 weeks is considered less traumatic and less likely to induce resorption.

■ *What immediate treatment is indicated?*

Immediate treatment aims to prevent subsequent external root resorption, preserve marginal bone support and prevent sepsis. Teeth with a closed apex should be treated by immediate pulp extirpation and placement of a non-setting calcium hydroxide root canal dressing. Immature teeth should be monitored for spontaneous re-eruption and loss of vitality. A 5-day course of systemic antibiotics should be prescribed, and the false gingival pocket surrounding the intruded crown gently irrigated with chlorhexidine.

■ *What follow up should you arrange?*

Follow-up period	Reason
1 week	To monitor spontaneous eruption and vitality of immature teeth, or to remove the splint and change the calcium hydroxide paste in a tooth treated by immediate repositioning.
3 weeks and 6 months	To continue monitoring spontaneous re-eruption of an immature tooth. Replace calcium hydroxide dressing. Radiograph.
6-monthly and then annually for several years	To observe for delayed onset of external root resorption.

In this case, spontaneous eruption was awaited, but was very slow. Electric pulp testing indicated early pulp necrosis. The tooth was then extruded rapidly with a simple orthodontic appliance engaged on to a bracket attached to the labial surface of the intruded tooth. As soon as there was adequate access to the pulp chamber, the necrotic pulp was extirpated, the canal cleaned and obturated with non-setting calcium hydroxide paste. The appearance of the extruded tooth is shown in Figure 21.3 and it confirms the diagnosis of enamel hypoplasia made radiographically.

■ *How would your management have differed if the patient had been a 3-year-old child with an intruded primary incisor?*

Mild intrusive luxation injuries in the primary dentition may be treated with reassurance and observation though parents should always be warned that damage to the permanent successor is common. Partial or sometimes total re-eruption over the following months is usual.

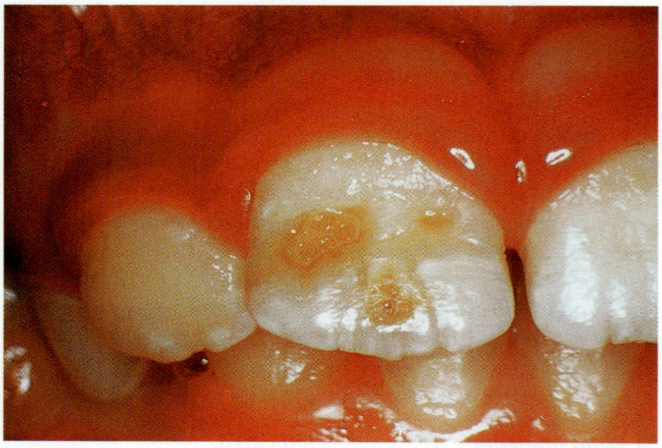

Fig. 21.3 Appearance of the extruded upper right central incisor.

However, extraction should be performed without delay if a combination of periapical and lateral radiographs demonstrate that the deciduous tooth has impinged on the follicle of the underlying tooth or if there is subsequent loss of vitality. As in the permanent dentition, vitality must be monitored carefully if the apex is closed at the time of injury. Pulp tests in young children are often unreliable because of lack of understanding, and a close watch must be kept for colour change.

Case 22

Hypoglycaemia

SUMMARY

A 55-year-old man collapses in your general dental surgery. What is the cause and what would you do?

History

Problem

The patient appears to become distant and incoherent towards the end of a treatment session.

Medical history

Having re-checked the medical history before commencing the treatment, you are aware that he is an insulin-dependent diabetic. He has had diabetes mellitus for 40 years and is currently taking insulin 20 IU in the morning and 15 IU at night. In addition he has peripheral vascular disease resulting in intermittent claudication and angina, for which he takes glyceryl trinitrate (GTN) spray when necessary.

Dental history

This gentleman has been a regular patient at the dentist for a number of years. On this occasion he has attended during his lunch hour for routine dental treatment involving simple periodontal treatment and the preparation of a six-unit bridge under local anaesthesia.

■ ***What is the likely diagnosis?***

Hypoglycaemia.

■ ***Why was this particular diabetic at risk of hypoglycaemia?***

The patient is an insulin-dependent diabetic. He has an absolute deficiency of insulin and requires insulin to control his blood glucose. Hypoglycaemia is an effect of the insulin rather than the diabetes itself.

■ ***What are the underlying events leading to the clinical presentation?***

The patient said he had taken his insulin as normal. This has mobilized glucose from the blood into the tissues, reducing the blood glucose level. The patient must eat to replenish his blood glucose otherwise the level will continue to fall. Glucose is almost the only energy source for the brain but it stores little and requires a constant supply in the blood. Reduction in blood glucose starves the brain and results in abnormal brain activity. This may present as altered behaviour, including aggression and confusion.

■ ***What would you do immediately?***

- Reassure the patient
- Assess vital signs, blood pressure, pulse and respiratory rate.

Examination

The patient is conscious. However, he is becoming increasingly confused and is sweaty and has tachycardia.

■ ***What other signs would you look for?***

Signs of sympathetic nervous system activity may accompany hypoglycaemia as the body tries to mobilize glucose. This could lead to the patient being sweaty and tachycardic. However, neuropathy and vascular disease are common complications of diabetes and may prevent signs of sympathetic activation being apparent until a late stage. It is important not to waste time looking for other signs to confirm your diagnosis for the following reasons:

- the condition can worsen quickly;
- the history of diabetes and presentation are diagnostic;
- treatment cannot cause any significant adverse effects – raising blood glucose in the short term is safe.

Treatment

■ ***What treatment would you provide?***

Give a glucose drink (20 grams of glucose) quickly as the patient may otherwise become unconscious in minutes. Alternatively, the equivalent amount of glucose gel, sugar lumps or a proprietary glucose drink may be used.

Unfortunately there is a delay finding and dissolving the glucose and the patient lapses into unconsciousness before he is able to drink it.

■ ***How may this cause of loss of consciousness be distinguished from other similar causes?***

Cause	Symptoms and signs
Vasovagal attack (faint)	The commonest cause of collapse and often associated with stress. There are usually premonitory symptoms before loss of consciousness. Cold, clammy skin, pallor, initial bradycardia and low volume pulse followed by tachycardia and a full pulse. Rapid recovery on placing supine or slightly head down (tilt not greater than 10°).
Steroid crisis	Usually only seen in patients taking, or who have recently taken, systemic steroids. Arises as a result of relative insufficiency during periods of stress.
Cardiac arrest	Usually a history of cardiovasular disease in the form of angina, hypertension or previous myocardial infarction. No central pulse.

What treatment would you now commence?

In this situation there are three options:

Give 1 mg of glucagon intramuscularly. This will cause mobilization of glucose from the last stores of glycogen in the patient's liver, sufficient for him to regain consciousness. It is not a definitive treatment, but a way of producing a conscious patient who can swallow oral glucose. Glucagon works for about 15 minutes and is easy and safe to administer. As soon as the patient is alert and able to swallow, oral glucose should be given. Without this further treatment the patient will lapse back into a hypoglycaemic coma and a second dose of glucagon will be ineffective because all the liver glycogen will have been metabolized.

***OR* give 50 ml of 50% glucose intravenously.** This is a difficult treatment to use and impossible if you cannot cannulate a large vein with a large intravenous cannula. 50% glucose is like thick syrup and very difficult to inject. It is also very irritant and will irreversibly damage the vein into which it is injected.

***OR* give 100 ml of 20% glucose intravenously.** This still requires venous access, but is easier to inject and less likely to cause vein damage.

Only the first option is usually feasible in a general dental practice setting. The presentations of drugs useful in the treatment of hypoglycaemia are shown in Figure 22.1.

How would you proceed once the patient has recovered?

- Abandon dental treatment
- Continue to monitor the vital signs
- Arrange transfer of the patient to an appropriate secondary care facility
- Advise the patient of the need for formal review of their diabetic control.

Other possibilities

Can this happen to a patient with noninsulin-dependent diabetes mellitus (NIDDM)?

Yes. NIDDM is managed by diet control, oral hypoglycaemic drugs, insulin or a combination of these. Both oral hypoglycaemic drugs and insulin could potentiate hypoglycaemia if there is a relative deficiency of glucose, for instance if the patient does not eat despite having taken their normal dose of medication.

What could have been done to minimize the risk of such an event?

The timing of the appointment should have taken account of the need for the patient to avoid disturbances in their normal daily routine. Routine treatment under local anaesthetic should be undertaken at a time that allows for completion of

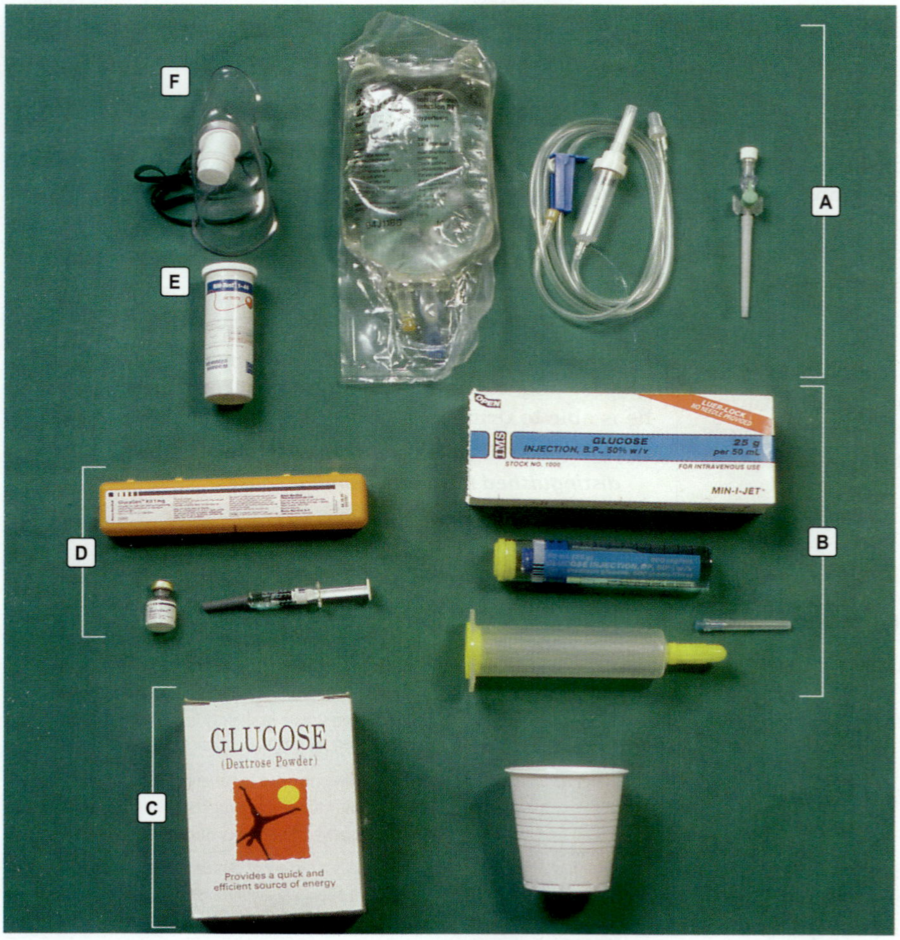

Fig. 22.1 Typical presentations of drugs used to treat hypoglycaemia.
A. Infusion set with 20% glucose.
B. Glucose 50% in Min-I-Jet format. The yellow plastic cover is removed from the back (left hand end) of the syringe barrel and front of the glass cartridge and the cartridge is screwed into the syringe barrel. Available in two types, with needle fitted and with luer lock fitting for a conventional needle (shown). After removing front cover and fitting needle, if required, use as a conventional syringe.
C. Glucose powder, dissolve 20 grams in up to one cup of water.
D. Glucagon emergency set with vial of lyophilised powder. Dissolve by injecting water for injection already in the syringe, and draw up for injection.
E. Blood glucose dipstick test strips.
F. Oxygen mask, give 5 litres/minute.

the procedure and recovery before the next food intake is due. In this way the possibility of a hypoglycaemic episode can be minimized. It is also advisable to avoid appointment times at the end of the day when medical assistance may be less readily available in the event of a complication. In this instance the patient had delayed his lunch to undertake a long appointment.

A more rapidly accessible glucose formulation might have helped. Glucose powder is useful for nonurgent uses but a ready-to-use solution is best for emergency use.

Further points

■ ***What are the oral complications of diabetes?***

Oral complications of diabetes include:

- Reduced resistance to infection. Infection requires effective treatment early
- Increased severity of periodontal disease and susceptibility to periodontal abscess
- Xerostomia, as a result of dehydration, may also be a problem and may further predispose the patient to oral candidosis
- Sialadenosis (salivary gland swelling for hormonal, metabolic or nutritional reasons) may also be seen
- Oral hypoglycaemics may be associated with the development of lichenoid reactions
- Peripheral mononeuropathy in the oropharyngeal area is a very rare effect.

Case 23

A tooth lost at teatime

SUMMARY

A 78-year-old female patient has lost a tooth while eating. What is the cause and what will you do?

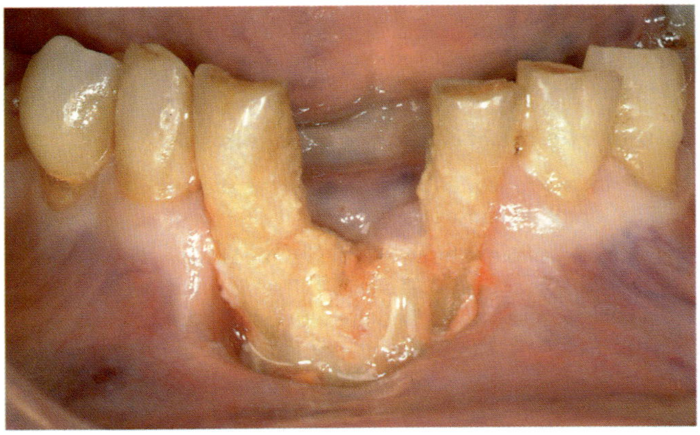

Fig. 23.1 The patient on presentation.

History

Complaint

The patient reports that one of her front lower teeth has been loose recently. The tooth simply fell out yesterday when she bit a biscuit. There was no pain before, during or after losing the tooth.

History of complaint

This woman has attended your practice for many years and has a well-cared-for mouth, a low caries rate and minimal periodontal disease. She is concerned that a healthy tooth has come out so easily and also that she has had no pain or bleeding from the area since.

Medical history

Five years ago she fractured her arm in a fall and a diagnosis of osteoporosis was made. She takes calcium supplements daily and alendronate (Fosamax) weekly.

Examination

Extraoral examination

Oddly, there is no lymphadenopathy, no tenderness to palpation over any of the facial skeleton and no obvious halitosis.

Intraoral examination

The patient is partially dentate and wears dentures. Her mucosa is normal, the mouth is not dry, there is no active caries and no pocket depths exceed 3 mm.

There is an area of exposed bone in the anterior mandibular alveolus and a socket from which a lower incisor has been lost, as shown in Figure 23.1. The adjacent teeth in the exposed bone are mobile in their sockets and are also in danger of spontaneous exfoliation.

The attached gingiva in the region is missing and the buccal soft-tissue margin of the lesion is lax and can be lifted to allow a dental probe to be inserted down almost to the patient's chin. No pus is present.

■ ***How do you interpret the findings so far?***

The lack of bleeding and sensitivity suggest that the bone is necrotic and the teeth non-vital. Despite bacterial plaque and debris accumulating on the exposed bone there seems to be no infection, even though there is a deep soft-tissue pocket extending to the chin. The surrounding mucosa is hardly inflamed, suggesting that local trauma and infection are not responsible.

The appearances are very characteristic and it is possible to make a fairly confident diagnosis without any further investigations.

Diagnosis

■ ***What is your diagnosis?***

Bisphosphonate-related osteonecrosis is almost certainly the diagnosis on the basis of asymptomatic necrosis of bone without pain. The patient has taken alendronate, a bisphosphonate drug, for several years and this is a recognized complication.

■ ***What alternative diagnoses have you excluded and why?***

Chronic osteomyelitis would seem a possibility but the presentation is not correct for this diagnosis. Relatively mild pain or discomfort would probably be present, as would bad taste, discharge of pus indicating infection and possibly sequestration of the nonvital bone. There would also normally be both a cause and a predisposing factor. If dental infection were the cause, it would be evident clinically or radiographically, or there might be a history of trauma such as a fracture or dental extraction. Patients who develop osteomyelitis usually have some systemic predisposing condition such as diabetes mellitus or immunosuppression. It seems that this option is most unlikely, though a radiograph would help exclude or confirm it.

Acute osteomyelitis is even less likely. Acute infection would be accompanied by the cardinal signs of inflammation

– pain, erythema and swelling. There is a severe, deep boring pain in acute osteomyelitis with systemic signs of infection.

Necrotizing periodontitis could cause necrosis of soft tissue with exposed bone but would be associated with other signs and symptoms. It is almost exclusively found in severe immunosuppression, usually late or untreated human immunodeficiency virus (HIV) infection. Necrotizing periodontitis is usually painful and limited to the gingiva and alveolar margin. It would not cause extensive soft-tissue separation from bone as here.

Cancrum oris (noma) is a necrotizing mixed bacterial infection sometimes developing from acute ulcerative gingivitis. It causes tissue necrosis of large parts of the face or other tissues, including bone. The disease is almost confined to malnourished and debilitated children below the age of 8 years in developing countries.

What is the difference between osteomyelitis, osteitis and osteonecrosis?

Osteomyelitis is an *infection in the medullary cavity* of the bone. It is usually bacterial. The resulting increased pressure in the medullary space and the inflammatory reaction devitalize the marrow by compressing its blood supply and parts of the bone undergo necrosis. After an acute and intensely painful phase, pus drains and osteoclasts separate the necrotic bone to form sequestra. If the sequestra can be shed, the bone may heal. If not, infection persists in the sequestrum and is difficult to treat, the disease becomes chronic and the surrounding bone becomes sclerotic.

Osteitis is a superficial inflammation of bone, such as is seen in the exposed bone of dry socket (see problem 15). Small sequestra may form but infection does not penetrate into or spread within the medullary cavity.

Osteonecrosis is death of bone. The causes are usually loss of blood supply, vascular or bisphosphonate drugs. The dead bone is sterile, at least initially, and only becomes colonized by bacteria once exposed to the exterior. Osteonecrosis can follow irradiation of bone because this induces endarteritis, narrowing of the blood vessels with eventual necrosis. Osteonecrosis is increasingly recognized in patients taking bisphosphonate drugs for prevention or treatment of osteoporosis, management of bone metastasis in cancer or for metabolic bone diseases.

What are bisphosphonate drugs and why are they used?

Bisphosphonate drugs reduce bone turnover. The drugs are adsorbed on to bone surfaces where they remain bound for a prolonged period. They are taken up by osteoclasts at sites of bone resorption, and interfere with adenosine triphosphate (ATP) metabolism or membrane function. Osteoclasts either die or become unable to resorb bone. Bone formation then exceeds bone resorption, remodelling is slowed and bone density increases or stabilizes.

The drugs have a variety of uses:

- To prevent further bone loss in osteoporosis
- To prevent malignant tumours in bone releasing excess calcium into the blood stream
- To prevent bony metastases from enlarging by inhibiting bone resorption around them
- To reduce bone turnover in Paget's disease of bone
- To increase bone mass in osteogenesis imperfecta.

Are all bones affected equally?

No, the effects are systemic but the effects are much more pronounced in the mandible and the maxilla. Why this should be is not clear, but they may be subjected to higher drug levels because of their good blood supply. They are also close to the surface so that the bone is readily exposed. Bisphosphonate-induced osteonecrosis affects the mandible twice as often as the maxilla, but is almost never seen in other bones.

Why does the tissue die?

It is not completely clear. The drugs interfere with inter- and intracellular signalling and inhibit growth of new blood vessels. The tissue of the marrow becomes avascular and dies. The bone also becomes depleted of both osteoclasts and osteoblasts because the two cell populations are interdependent. Osteocytes are not replaced by maturing osteoblasts and eventually die. Both bone and soft tissue undergo slow necrosis without symptoms.

As the overlying mucosa relies on blood partly from the bone and periosteum and partly from mucosa, it may also die. This is most commonly seen to happen in areas where the mucosa is very thin, typically over mandibular tori and on the posterior lingual aspect of the mandible, where there are few muscle attachments.

What is the risk of developing osteonecrosis?

The risk is very low and depends on the drug, the dose and duration of administration.

The many different bisphosphonate drugs have different potencies, as shown in Table 23.1. The non-nitrogenous drugs cause osteoclast death and the nitrogenous drugs inhibit osteoclast function. The more potent drugs are much more likely to cause osteonecrosis of the jaws. This is especially so when given in high doses intravenously, as for metastatic malignancy.

The proportion of patients taking bisphosphonates affected by osteonecrosis is estimated to be only 0.05%. However,

Table 23.1 Bisphosphonate drugs and their relative potency

Drug	Relative potency
Non-nitrogenous	
Etidronate	1
Clodronate	10
Tildronate	10
Nitrogenous	
Pamidronate	100
Neridronate	100
Olpadronate	500
Alendronate	500
Ibandronate	1000
Risedronate	2000
Zoledronate	10 000

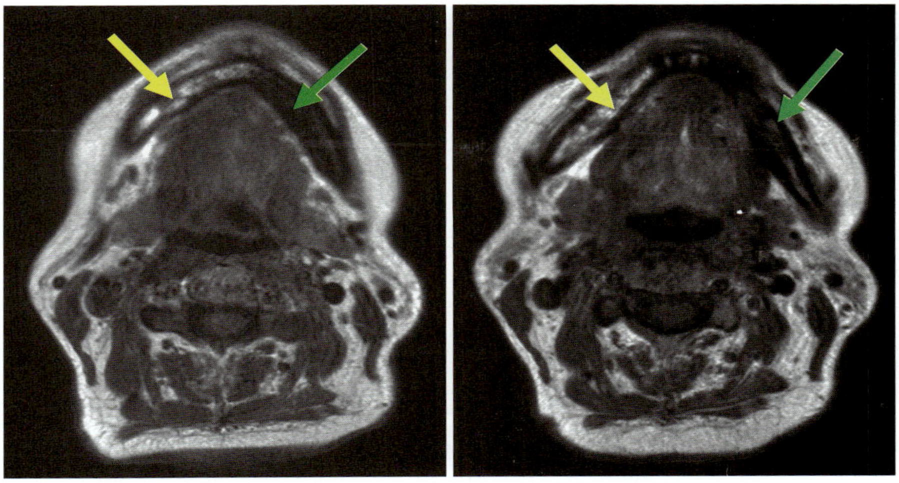

Fig. 23.2 Two adjacent axial magnetic resonance imaging scans through the body of the mandible. The normal bright marrow signal is indicated by the yellow arrow, the abnormal avascular marrow in the osteonecrotic bone by the green arrow.

these are commonly prescribed drugs. It is estimated that 3 years of oral administration is required before there is a significant risk of osteonecrosis: the risk becomes significant after 6 months of intravenous administration.

Investigations

What investigations would you perform?

Investigations are not helpful in diagnosis but may provide useful information for treatment. The vitality of the teeth in and around the exposed area of bone must be determined.

Radiographs of the area might seem a logical next step. However, if you take radiographs you will find that the mandibular bone appears completely normal. This is because the osteonecrosis is caused by loss of soft tissue in the marrow spaces. The disease does not alter the mineralized component that is responsible for the radiographic image. This is very different from chronic osteomyelitis, in which there is patchy radiolucency and sclerosis with separation of sequestra.

There is no completely satisfactory method for showing which areas of bone are dead in a patient with osteonecrosis. This is unfortunate because it would be useful to know the extent of necrosis in case extractions or surgery are required in other parts of the jaw.

Can more specialized investigations help?

Radioisotope scans are a measure of bone turnover and should show lack of uptake in osteonecrotic bone, but the resolution of the imaging is too poor to be useful.

Magnetic resonance imaging (MRI) is probably the most useful investigation, but it is expensive and only available in hospitals. Different types of MRI scan define vascularity and fat content. MRI shows clearly the loss of the marrow in affected areas, as shown in Figure 23.2 where the normal marrow has a high signal (bright) and the affected marrow appears dark. This is currently the best method to identify the extent of osteonecrosis but it is only useful in the mandible, because the maxilla has little medullary space.

Table 23.2

Serum CTX value	Osteonecrosis risk
>150 pg/ml	Minimal
150–100 pg/ml	Moderate
<100 pg/ml	High

CTX, C-terminal telopeptide of type 1 collagen.

It has been suggested that serum levels of the bone turnover marker C-terminal telopeptide of type 1 collagen (CTX-1) reflect the bone suppression by bisphosphonates. This small peptide is released into serum when collagen in bone is resorbed. It provides an indication of bone turnover in the body as a whole, but whether this is a useful reflection of the risk of osteonecrosis in the jaws remains unclear. The currently proposed risk values are shown in Table 23.2, but even a high value cannot guarantee that an extraction is completely without risk.

You decide that no investigations are likely to be useful at this stage. You find that the teeth in the exposed bone do not respond to any tests of vitality. The adjacent teeth give an equivocal result.

Treatment

What will you do for the teeth in the exposed bone?

The teeth each side of the socket are painfree but mobile. They are best extracted before problems develop and to allow proper cleaning of the area. If the teeth were firm, they might be left in situ but would probably cause problems in the future. It is not clear whether teeth in osteonecrotic bone retain their own independent blood supply. If they do not respond to any tests of vitality, the prognosis is likely to be poor.

What should be done for the exposed bone?

Once the teeth are removed the patient should be instructed to keep the mucosa and exposed bone as clean as possible using simple oral hygiene measures and topical chlorhexidine

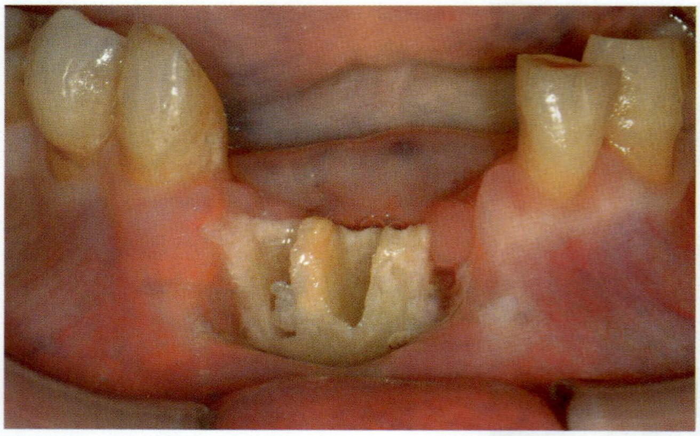

Fig. 23.3 The patient after extractions and debridement.

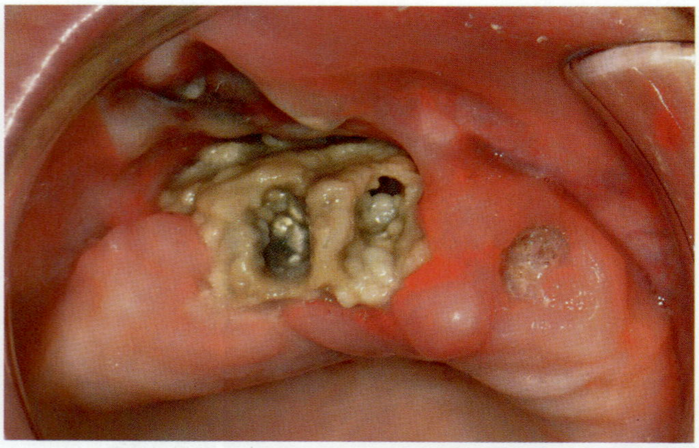

Fig. 23.4 A different patient who has developed extensive infection in the soft tissues surrounding a zone of maxillary osteonecrosis.

as needed. Any prominent bone or sharp edges can be trimmed and removed without local anaesthesia. This should prevent trauma to the oral soft tissues and make the area easier to clean (Figure 23.3).

The treatment aim in bisphosphonate osteonecrosis is very different from that in osteomyelitis or osteoradionecrosis. In these latter conditions necrotic bone is limited in extent and its removal exposes healthy, vital bone that can heal. In bisphosphonate osteonecrosis the area of bone involved is very extensive, cannot be removed and is not surrounded by healthy bone. The MRI scan of this patient (Figure 23.2) suggests that the entire anterior and one body of mandible is involved. Trimming back the bone and attempting soft-tissue closure surgically usually results in wound breakdown.

Will the exposed bone get infected?

Infection can develop but is surprisingly infrequent. The bone will have been colonized by the oral flora as soon as it was exposed but this is a contamination rather than an infection. The bone is not invaded by the bacteria and there is no host response in the avascular tissue, no inflammation and no immune response.

Simple cleaning and topical antiseptics are the most effective methods of keeping the flora at bay. Antibiotics are ineffective. Drugs cannot enter the bone because it lacks a blood supply.

Sometimes a more aggressive infection will develop in the soft tissues at the margins of the wound and this must be treated according to conventional principles. A microbiological sample should be taken for culture and sensitivity before commencing empirical antibiotic therapy. In most cases metronidazole is an appropriate choice, but this can be supplemented by amoxicillin if needed.

Very rarely there is extensive sequestration of bone and an aggressive perilesional infection, such as that shown in Figure 23.4. Open surgical debridement is then required and the antibiotics may need to be given intravenously.

What would you do if the site became painful?

To feel pain requires an intact nerve and blood supply. The bone is insensitive and any pain must arise from the mucosa. Significant infection must be suspected and excluded, but the cause is usually a local problem with tissue hygiene and it can be managed with simple cleaning and topical antiseptics.

Will the bone ever heal? Should the bisphosphonate be stopped?

The continuation of the bisphosphonate drug must be reviewed with the patient's medical practitioner or specialist clinician. When the drug is given for malignant disease it may not be possible to stop it without risking major adverse effects.

If the bisphosphonate can be withdrawn, the bone will gradually recover with no intervention other than cleaning. This recovery is very slow and it may take many months to see an improvement. However in 1–2 years most lesions will show significant improvement. Detached periosteum will reattach and the mucosa will grow to cover the revascularizing bone. Figure 23.5 shows regrowth of mucosa to cover exposed bone around a defect in the maxilla. An oroantral fistula remains but the bone is now protected from infection.

Those patients who continue to need medication may be switched to an alternative drug such as strontium ranalate or teraparatide, which do not seem to cause osteonecrosis.

Is dental treatment safe in a patient on a bisphosphonate drug?

The risk is best avoided by an effective preventive regime for caries and periodontitis. An enhanced programme of oral hygiene improvement, dietary instruction and topical fluoride preparations would be appropriate for all patients on bisphosphonates.

The safe period of 3 years after starting oral bisphosphonates and 6 months after starting an intravenous regimen gives a window of opportunity to deal with any sepsis or teeth of dubious prognosis and initiate prevention.

Routine restorative dentistry can be performed without problems. It may be a sensible precaution to use a local anaesthetic without a vasoconstrictor for infiltration anaesthesia, but this is not based on any sound evidence.

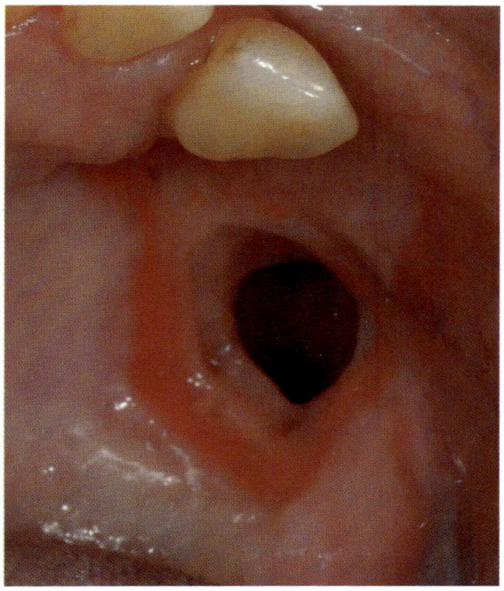

Fig. 23.5 A different patient with resolving osteonecrosis.

Oral surgery and dental implants are best avoided if the patient has taken bisphosphonates for a prolonged period of time.

What do you do if a tooth needs extraction from a patient at risk?

Most patients will have no problems following an uncomplicated extraction. Just under 1% of patients are reported to develop complications. Extractions should be performed as atraumatically as possible and flap surgery avoided.

Emergency extractions can proceed after having informed the patient of the small complication risk. Where the extraction can be postponed for a period the risk can be assessed by the use of a CTX-1 assay if it is available.

Temporarily withdrawing the bisphosphonate for a period of 3 months before and 3 months after the extraction is thought to improve the bone's healing potential and reduce the risk of bone necrosis developing. This short 'drug holiday' does not seem to put the patient at increased risk of complications of osteoporosis.

When the risk is considered high, every effort should be made to avoid extraction by root-filling teeth and retaining decoronated roots in a similar fashion to overdenture abutments. Temporary solutions such as this may allow time for a drug holiday before extraction.

All patients taking bisphosphonates should be expected to have slowly healing extraction sockets, even when no osteonecrosis develops.

Could I be considered negligent if osteonecrosis develops?

No, provided the risk has been identified and managed appropriately and the patient has been informed of the risks and has given consent for the extraction. Good record keeping will provide evidence of this.

Dental extractions or surgery appear to be a precipitating factor in one-third to one-half of cases. However, this is a complication of drug treatment, not of dental surgery. The bone may well have been necrotic without symptoms for some time; dental extraction simply unmasks the process by exposing the bone.

Should antibiotic prophylaxis be given for extractions in patients taking bisphosphonates?

No. The disease is not caused by bacteria and drugs do not penetrate the bone because it has no blood supply. Using antibiotics risks adverse effects and microbial resistance for no benefit. Similarly, chlorhexidine mouth rinse will not prevent problems with the bone, though it may help keep the soft tissues disease-free during the – sometimes slow – healing process.

Case • 24

A problem overdenture

SUMMARY

A 67-year-old lady is referred to your general dental practice complaining that her denture has never 'seemed right' from the day it was fitted.

History

Complaint

The patient complains that a small filling has recently been lost from one of the upper canine roots below her overdenture. However, it quickly becomes clear that this has caused no symptoms (the tooth is root-treated) and that she is dissatisfied primarily with her upper complete overdenture. She can wear the denture in the morning, but by about three o'clock in the afternoon it becomes too uncomfortable and if she is at home she likes to take it out.

History of complaint

The patient successfully wore an acrylic upper partial denture until 6 months ago, but failure of restorations and root treatments led to loss of several upper teeth. She was provided with an upper overdenture on the two retained upper canine roots. The denture was fitted 3 months ago, reviewed on four occasions and minor adjustments were made to the base extension. The patient is happy with the retention and fit of the denture. It does not move during eating. She reports no problem with her lower teeth.

Medical history

The patient is taking low dose aspirin (75 mg/day) following a myocardial infarction and a statin for raised serum cholesterol.

Examination

Extraoral examination

There is no lymphadenopathy. The temporomandibular joint is free of crepitus and clicks, and no muscle tenderness can be elicited in the muscles of mastication. With the denture in place, there is no facial asymmetry. The patient has a slightly open lip posture at rest.

Intraoral examination

The patient has a well-developed upper alveolar ridge with limited resorption consistent with the relatively recent loss of several upper teeth. There is slight redness of the palate under the denture-bearing area, but the ridge is not tender on palpation at any site and there is no bleeding on probing around the canine roots and no detectable sinus. One of the root-treated canine teeth has lost a small restoration from the access cavity. The remainder of the oral mucosa is normal.

There is an almost complete lower arch of natural teeth. These are adequately restored, many with large amalgam restorations, and there is no caries. The occlusal plane is relatively even. There has been slight mesial tipping of the lower second molars as a result of loss of both first molars.

The denture appears clean and without obvious defects and there is a definite post dam along its posterior margin.

■ ***On the basis of what you know so far, what are the likely diagnoses and why?***

The patient has successfully worn a denture and the transition to an overdenture from an upper acrylic partial denture should have been relatively straightforward. It might have been more difficult if the previous denture had been metal based. If the patient has persevered for 3 months without success she almost certainly has a valid complaint.

There appears to be no problem of displacement of the denture during eating, speaking or other facial movements. This makes it unlikely that the overdenture is poorly adapted, overextended or that the teeth lie outside the neutral zone. Occlusal discrepancies of some kind would appear to be the most likely cause and the vagueness of the complaint, predominantly inability to tolerate the denture, is consistent with an occlusal problem. A further reason to suspect an occlusal problem is the difficulty arising from a complete upper denture occluding against a lower natural arch.

It must also be borne in mind that some denture patients are particularly conscious of appearance and the construction of dentures that satisfy the expectations of such patients can be very demanding. Sometimes a mismatch between the denture appearance and desired facial self-image may manifest as dislike of the denture or complaints about relatively minor features. There is always a potential cosmetic problem of an overcontoured labial flange when canine roots support an upper overdenture because the roots preserve the labial aspect of the alveolar bone.

■ ***What specific features of the dentures would you examine and how?***

All features of the denture should be reviewed (Table 24.1). Denture complaints may be multifactorial and only by examining all features can an accurate diagnosis be made.

Having examined the patient you find that the denture is correctly extended, stable and retentive. The denture was not displaced on lateral excursion. This leaves the vertical dimension as the most likely cause of an occlusal problem.

Table 24.1 Examination of the denture

Feature	Method
Check base extension. Is the denture correctly extended into the sulcus?	This is done visually where possible, checking the relationship between the denture border, sulcus depth and soft tissue mobility at rest and under tension. In less visible areas, such as lateral to the tuberosity, palpation may be required.
Does the posterior border extend back to the vibrating area?	Identify the vibrating area by observing the soft tissue moving when the patient says 'Ahhh' and/or apply pressure with a blunt instrument such as a ball-ended burnisher to define the extent of displaceable tissue.
Is the denture retentive?	Check by pulling down on the upper denture in the premolar region. Check retention of the post dam by trying to displace the denture with forward pressure behind the anterior teeth.
Is there close adaptation of the denture base to the mucosa?	Look at the fit surface and check for voids between tissue and denture with a disclosing material such as a low viscosity silicone.
Make an assessment of the occlusal vertical dimension and patient's rest vertical dimension	Measure the facial height at rest and with the denture in occlusion. Subtract to identify the freeway space. (See below.)
Is the occlusion correct in retruded position?	Check whether the denture meets the natural teeth correctly in retruded position. Are there any premature contacts?
Are the natural teeth affecting the occlusal plane significantly?	Check the occlusal plane to ensure that the natural standing teeth do not place excessive destabilizing forces on the prosthesis. Assess in particular whether the denture is stable on lateral excursive movements.
Appearance	Check tooth shade, shape and set up. Carefully question the patient as to whether they are satisfied with the appearance. Check the soft tissue support provided by the denture, particularly over the canine roots.
*If there were a **lower** complete denture, you should check to ensure that the teeth lie in the neutral zone, and for denture stability. (Not directly relevant in this case.)*	*Look at the denture when the patient's mouth is half open. Is the lower denture displaced by the tongue or lips?*

What methods can be used to assess vertical dimension? What are their problems?

Initially it is most straightforward to simply observe the vertical dimension with the denture removed (Fig. 24.1) and in place (Fig. 24.2).

Note the open lip posture (Fig. 24.2) when the denture is inserted. This is an important indicator that there may be an error in vertical height and a more accurate assessment must be made.

There are three common methods which might be used, the first two of which are essentially similar and suffer some of the same problems. These both measure the lower facial height at rest and with the dentures in occlusion. The difference between these measurements is the freeway space. The head must be in a natural vertical position supported by the neck muscles. A fixed support can alter the freeway space. In most instances these methods are satisfactory and readily applied, but sometimes it may be appropriate to use all three methods to establish the correct vertical dimension.

Dividers/calipers method. Marks or adhesive markers are placed on the chin and nose and their distance apart is measured with calipers or dividers. One problem is that the markers are fixed to the skin and may move through muscle activity, particularly pursing of the lips. All suitable sites on the skin may move to some degree so that it is necessary to check that the patient remains relaxed during the procedure.

This method is shown in Figures 24.1 and 24.2. The calipers are set to the resting face height (Fig. 24.1). When the denture is inserted (Fig. 24.2) the increase in vertical dimension is clearly seen and is about 3–4 mm.

Willis bite gauge. This measures lower face height from the lower border of the nose to the lower border of the mandible. It is important to use the same pressure when recording rest and occlusal height, otherwise compression of the tissues will affect the reading. More importantly, the instrument has to be used at a consistent angle at the base of the nose. This is particularly difficult when making complete dentures against lower standing teeth, because removing the upper denture to record rest height removes the denture support of the upper lip which is used as a landmark.

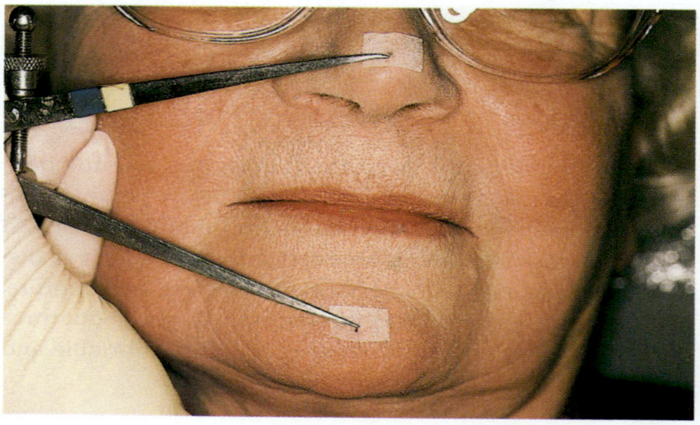

Fig. 24.1 Rest vertical dimension with the upper prosthesis removed.

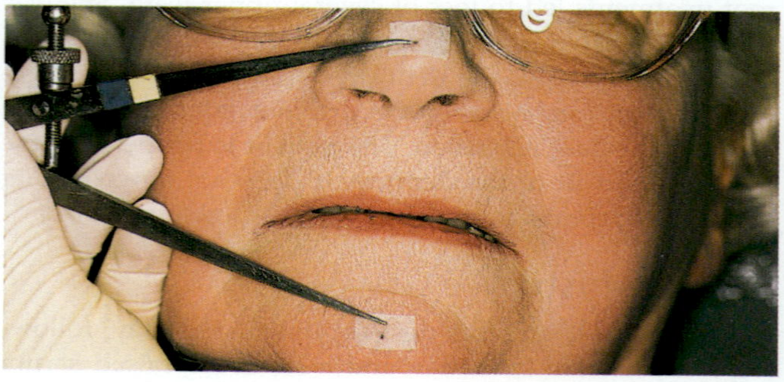

Fig. 24.2 Vertical dimension with the upper overdenture in place.

Closed speaking space method. This method provides a rough estimate of the presence of a freeway space but does not involve direct measurement. The patient is asked to say words that include prominent 'ss' sounds, such as 'Mississippi' and 'Tuesday'. These sounds are more difficult to make in the absence of freeway space. Unfortunately patients adapt their speech to both an increased or decreased occlusal height and this method can only be considered an adjunct to the more accurate methods above.

■ ***How large should the freeway space be?***

This depends on the patient. The average freeway space is 2–4 mm measured in the premolar region, and dentures may be constructed to this dimension for most patients. However, there are some circumstances in which this clearance needs to be increased. Some patients become habituated to an increased freeway space, either because of worn artificial teeth or because of faulty denture construction. In some cases the freeway space may exceed a centimetre and it would be unreasonable to expect such patients to accommodate rapidly to the normal freeway space. Provided the increased freeway space is not associated with any problems a compromise increased freeway space is appropriate.

Diagnosis

■ ***What is your diagnosis and why is this the most likely possibility?***

Error in occlusal vertical dimension. There is clearly an increased occlusal vertical dimension, based on the measurements described above, and this is beyond the tolerance level of most patients. This fault is frequently associated with a history of being able to cope with the denture for a few hours and then having to remove the prosthesis. The open lip posture is also often associated with an increased occlusal vertical dimension. Some patients naturally have an open lip posture, so this sign is only an indication of potential problems. Until the fault is corrected, it is not really possible to consider any alternative explanation.

■ ***What possible diagnoses have you excluded? Explain why for each possibility.***

Error in retruded position. Dentures with this fault produce pain on the ridge and pain on eating. If this were suspected it would be necessary to take a precontact occlusal check record and to remount the dentures on an articulator to make a definitive diagnosis. Adjustment of the occlusion to the correct record should cure the symptoms and this will confirm the cause. This possible error needs to be kept in mind in all such cases. If the occlusion is ignored and the denture base adjusted, the area of soreness will move to another area with each adjustment, progressively destroying the fit surface of the denture.

Difficulty in becoming accustomed to acrylic palatal coverage. Three months is normally a sufficient time for a patient to become accustomed to a new denture design, even when there is a change to acrylic palatal coverage. In the very elderly, or those who have worn a denture for many years, this period may need to be extended, and a minority of patients need training bases or simple acrylic partial dentures before definitive complete dentures or overdentures. However, no patient should be expected to become accustomed to a denture with an increased vertical dimension.

Denture-related stomatitis. There was redness of the denture-bearing area and this almost certainly indicates denture stomatitis (chronic atrophic candidosis). However, this condition is asymptomatic and not normally noticed by patients.

Patient's expectation of appearance has not been met. Both men and women may be embarrassed to admit that their dentures do not fulfil their cosmetic expectations. This may not just be the fault of the denture but also result from a patient's seeking to recapture their youthful appearance. While this may not be unreasonable, it may be physically impossible. Sometimes hurtful comments from relatives, friends or acquaintances may change the patient's opinion about an otherwise satisfactory denture. This problem may be manifest by repeated minor complaints that do not make sense clinically, or, as in this case, a dislike or complete rejection of the denture. This problem can only be diagnosed by careful and considerate questioning.

In the present case this possible diagnosis is unlikely given that there is a fault in the vertical dimension and the patient appears happy with the appearance of the denture.

Miscellaneous and other unusual complaints. These include complaints of irritation from a high residual monomer content in an incorrectly processed denture base, or the very rare hypersensitivity to acrylic. In both cases the denture-bearing area, and sometimes the whole mouth, would be sore. This patient has inflammation of the denture-bearing area but this is much more likely to be related to denture plaque or perhaps candidal infection and these should be excluded before considering the alternative causes. Another complaint sometimes unfairly ascribed to dentures is the symptom of mucosal burning in an otherwise healthy mouth. This is usually psychogenic and associated with depression. Nothing in the history suggests this diagnosis.

■ ***How would you manage the case?***

Replace the missing restoration in the canine root to prevent caries.

To solve the denture problem, the denture must be remade with an appropriate freeway space, but first the denture stomatitis must be treated to improve support for the new prosthesis. A smear from the palate or fitting surface of the denture should be performed to detect candidal infection, unless the appearances are typical in which case treatment may be instituted immediately. Treatment will involve improving denture hygiene, ceasing night wear, if appropriate, and provision of a short course of antifungal treatment such as amphotericin lozenges (which must be sucked with the dentures removed from the mouth). The possibility of an underlying condition predisposing to candidosis should be considered, especially if the infection involves other parts of the mouth or lips or if treatment fails despite good denture hygiene.

Case • 25

Impacted lower third molars

SUMMARY

A 24-year-old gentleman is referred to you in your oral surgery-orientated practice for a second opinion on the need to remove his lower third molar teeth. Is this the correct decision, and if it is, how should it be achieved?

History

Complaint

The patient has no complaint at present but has been advised by his general dental practitioner to have his lower third molars extracted. He is very nervous about the extractions and requests a second opinion before deciding on treatment.

History of complaint

The patient has had two episodes of pericoronitis around the lower left third molar. The first was relatively mild but the second, about 3 months ago, was associated with inability to open the mouth and slight facial swelling and required a course of oral antibiotics.

Medical history

The patient is fit and well. He has had a general anaesthetic previously to reduce and fix a compound fracture of his arm which has been permanently plated. He has had no problems with bleeding following trauma.

Examination

Extraoral examination

The left submandibular lymph nodes are palpable but not tender. There is no facial asymmetry.

Intraoral examination

■ ***What particular features of the intraoral examination are important and why?***

See Table 25.1.

In this case the patient has normal mouth opening, a full unrestored dentition without evidence of caries, periodontal disease or poor oral hygiene. The lower third molars are partially erupted and appear vertically orientated and there is mild inflammation of the attached gingivae surrounding both crowns. The upper third molars are overerupted and nonfunctional. The patient has a pronounced gag reflex when the teeth are examined.

Investigations

■ ***Would you take radiographs? If so, which views would you take and why?***

Yes, radiographs are required to assess root morphology, degree of bone impaction, proximity to inferior dental nerve and the possibility of associated disease (e.g. cysts, hypercementosis and periodontal bone loss).

Table 25.1 Important features of the intraoral examination

Feature	Reason
Interincisal opening	One feature determining access for surgical removal and affecting the difficulty of extraction. Trismus may also reflect infection or inflammation in the muscles of mastication.
Condition of rest of dentition	If the first or second molars have a poor prognosis through caries or are extensively restored, transplanting the third molars in their place might be considered.
Oral hygiene	Poor oral hygiene increases the risk of dry socket, soft tissue infection and delayed healing.
Position of lower third molars	The degree of eruption, angulation and proximity to the second molars are important. Partially erupted vertical or distoangular lower third molars are more at risk of pericoronitis than mesioangularly impacted ones.
Position of upper third molars	Nonfunctional upper third molars may overerupt and traumatize the operculum over the lower third molar or erupt buccally and traumatize the cheek. Both situations might contribute to symptoms.
Position of external oblique ridge	If this lies close behind or over the impacted tooth, access is poor and considerable bone removal may be required if the tooth is large or impacted.
Condition of lower second molars	The lower second molar is at risk of iatrogenic damage during surgical removal of the third molar. Crowns or large restorations, especially those involving the distal surface, will be at risk and may increase the difficulty of the extraction.
Presence of pericoronitis	Has the same effect as generalized poor oral hygiene except that the risk of adverse effects is higher. Surgery should not be performed in an infected field.
Miscellaneous features	Factors such as a pronounced gag reflex, poor patient compliance and anxiety may all affect treatment.

The views to be possibly taken are listed, with their advantages and disadvantages, in Table 25.2.

There is little to choose between these radiographic views in terms of radiation dose, provided fast films and appropriate intensifying screens are used.

In this case the patient's gag reflex prevented the taking of paralleling technique periapicals and so a panoramic radiograph was taken. It is shown in Figure 25.1.

What does the radiograph show?

The patient is fully dentate with no restoration or caries visible on the film. The lower third molars are vertically orientated and impacted against soft tissue rather than the second molars. The impacted teeth are of normal size and the surrounding bone appears to be of normal density. The roots of both teeth appear to be closely related to the inferior dental nerve canal, there is darkening but no narrowing or deflection of the bony wall of the canal, suggesting that it does not contact or pass through the tooth root.

You now have sufficient information to decide whether the third molars should be removed or not. What are the indications for removal?

There has been much debate about indications for removal of third molars, and those for removal of asymptomatic third molars are particularly contentious. Mandibular impacted third molars (MITMs) are very common, affecting approximately 75% of 20–30-year-old patients. Surgery is unpleasant, carries risks and is expensive to state or patient; thus, following accepted guidelines is essential.

The suggested indications for removal are:

- Recurrent pericoronitis and pericoronitis with acute spreading infection
- Unrestorable caries of MITM or adjacent teeth

Table 25.2 The radiographic views

View	Advantages	Disadvantages
Periapicals of upper and lower third molars	Provided the periapicals can be taken with a paralleling technique these are the ideal views. They provide a geometrically accurate projection with true relationships to the adjacent structures. They are also convenient for single extractions. These views are the first choice.	Unfortunately it may not be possible to obtain films using the paralleling technique because of patient tolerance. Placement of the film in the ideal position, showing the teeth and inferior dental nerve canal, is uncomfortable. If films are angled then a degree of distortion is inevitable.
Oblique laterals	Readily taken without specialized equipment. Show both upper and lower third molars without superimposition. Give a good view of the surrounding bone when adjacent lesions (e.g. cysts) are present. It is the second-best option.	Suffer a degree of distortion as the beam is angled upwards, so that the relationship to adjacent structures is not accurate.
Panoramic radiograph	Convenient survey film if equipment available. Gives a good view of the surrounding bone when adjacent lesions (e.g. cysts) are present. Though only third choice on technical merit, panoramic films are often used and in practice usually provide sufficient information to assess extractions.	Poor image quality because the view is a tomograph. In addition there is superimposition of the opposite angle of mandible over upper and lower third molars. The upward beam angle distorts the relationship between teeth and adjacent structures and the image is magnified. Root morphology often cannot be assessed on panoramic films.
Lower oblique occlusal	Useful when the lower third molar lies horizontally and is seen end-on in a periapical view. Provides information on buccolingual orientation. Useful if tooth lies out of the line of arch. Used only rarely.	
Cone beam computerised tomography	Low dose computerised tomography available in a dental setting, high definition 3D imaging showing accurate relationships between tooth and ID canal and other structures. For example, see the final image in this problem.	Not yet widely available.

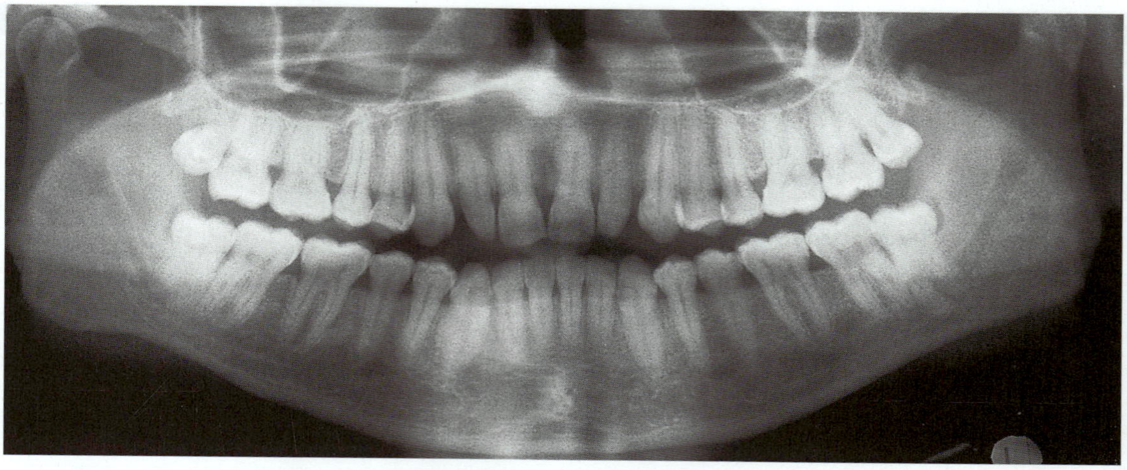

Fig. 25.1 Panoramic radiograph.

- Untreatable periapical inflammation
- Periodontal disease associated with the MITM or adjacent teeth
- Internal or external resorption of MITM or adjacent teeth
- MITM in fracture line
- Associated cysts or neoplasm
- For tooth reimplantation.
- For orthognathic surgery or restorative treatment
- Prophylactic removal may be advised in specific medical conditions

Should this patient's teeth be removed and why?

Yes, he has suffered two episodes of pericoronitis. There is increasing risk of future episodes as the number of attacks rises, and they are likely to become more frequent and more severe.

How will you decide whether extraction of this patient's third molars is within your ability?

Easier extraction	More difficult extraction
Young patient	Patient aged over 30
Female patient	Male patient
European/Asian racial group	African racial group
Superficial impaction	Deeply buried
Mesioangular or vertical impaction	Distoangular or horizontal impaction
Small crown	Wide crown
Conical root	Multirooted, divergent roots
Lying buccally in relation to line of arch	Lying lingually in relation to line of arch
Clear path of delivery, usually forward and upward	Vertical or distal path of removal required, possibly requiring tooth section
External oblique ridge well posterior to tooth	External oblique ridge overlies tooth
Sound second molar	Crowned, root-treated or heavily restored adjacent molar
Normal second molar root morphology	Conical root (risks accidental elevation)
Distant from inferior dental nerve	Adjacent to inferior dental nerve
Large dental follicle	Narrow dental follicle or ankylosis
Good access	Poor access (e.g. due to trismus)
Not impacted or soft tissue impacted	Impacted against bone or root of second molar
	History of complex or difficult extraction

This is a matter of judgement. You must judge your own ability and experience against the likely difficulty and also consider your ability to manage any complications. In general the following factors should be considered. The most important of these factors may be remembered using the mnemonic WHARFE:

W angulation using **W**inter's lines
H **H**eight of mandible
A **A**ngle of second molar
R **R**oot form and development
F size of **F**ollicular sac
E **E**xit path of tooth to be extracted

What are 'Winter's lines' and how might they help assess difficulty?

To apply Winter's lines, three imaginary lines are drawn on the radiographic image (Fig. 25.2). For descriptive purposes the lines are assigned colours. The white line runs along the occlusal plane, and the amber line runs along the upper bone surface through the interdental bone crests and along the bone surface behind the third molar (not up the external oblique ridge). The red line passes vertically, at right angles to the white line to the application point for an elevator. In mesioangular impactions the point of elevation lies at the mesial end of the amelocemental junction, and for distoangular impactions it lies at the distal end of the amelocemental junction.

The angle of impaction is judged against the white line. The amber line gives an indication of the amount of tooth which will be visible when the periosteal flap is raised and the amount of bone removal required over the crown. The red line gives an indication of the depth of bone removal required to gain a point of application for an elevator. If the red line is more than 5 mm in length the extraction is likely to merit general anaesthetic. If it is greater than 9 mm, it is likely that extensive bone removal will be required.

What are the deficiencies of the Winter's lines technique?

Winter's lines are useful for mesioangular impactions but the length of the red line is almost meaningless in distoangular impactions, which are always relatively difficult. The technique also ignores the possibility of sectioning the tooth which makes the extraction easier, changing the point of application of elevators and the path of removal. Winter's lines should be applied to a periapical radiograph, preferably a geometrically accurate projection obtained by a paralleling technique. The method can be used on oblique laterals or panoramic tomographs but then provides a less accurate estimate of difficulty. In addition, a correction must be made for magnification in the panoral film, which ranges from × 1.2 to × 1.4 depending on the equipment used. Winter's lines would not provide useful information in the present case, but they do provide a way of systematically examining a radiograph to ensure that no information is missed.

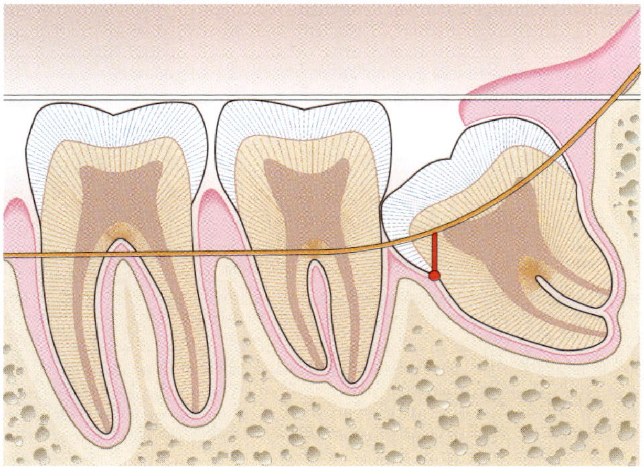

Fig. 25.2 Example of the application of Winter's lines.

How difficult are this patient's extractions likely to be?

Both lower third molars are slightly distoangularly inclined and the external oblique ridge overlies them. Though not very deeply placed these are moderately difficult extractions which should not be tackled under local anaesthetic other than by an experienced or specialized surgeon. Extraction of these teeth is not appropriate in the general practice setting.

The majority of lower third molars which meet the criteria for extraction (listed above) will be relatively difficult. This is because the commonest indication is pericoronitis which affects mostly vertically and distoangularly impacted teeth.

Prior to surgery you must warn the patient about the complications of removal. List the possible complications and give an indication of their frequency.

The complications are shown in Table 25.3. The top four are relatively common and should be discussed with patients as a matter of routine.

What warnings would you give to the patient about extraction?

Deciding exactly which complications to warn patients about can be difficult. The decision must be made for each case. The patient must be provided with sufficient information to give informed consent and the clinician must answer all the patient's questions correctly. It is generally considered mandatory to warn the patient about both sequelae and the significant complications. Sequelae may be induced by surgery or anaesthetic and should be differentiated. Surgical sequelae include swelling (for 48 hours), pain (for approximately 48 hours), bleeding (for about 2 hours), sore temporomandibular joint and trismus, sensitivity of the adjacent teeth, and remodelling of the sockets for approximately 10–12 weeks. Complications which must be described are the risk of dry socket (5%) and the risk of temporary (2%) and permanent (0.5%) damage to lingual and inferior dental nerves. Warnings concerning damage to adjacent teeth or restorations, or displacement of teeth into the antrum, are usually reserved for patients who are at particular risk.

Does the patient require antibiotic cover before surgery to prevent infection of the bone plate in his arm?

No, this is not necessary.

Would you prescribe postoperative antibiotics for these extractions?

There are no universally agreed criteria for providing antibiotics postoperatively. Antibiotics do not significantly affect the incidence of dry socket and should not be given without reason. They would be indicated if there were an increased risk of infection, as in a diabetic or immunosuppressed patient, or if infection were present at the time of operation. However, in normal individuals, antibiotics are probably less important than local measures for preventing infection. A chlorhexidine mouthrinse before operation and/or debridement of the teeth and below the operculum are highly effective in reducing the incidence of postoperative infection and bacteraemia.

In some centres antibiotics are given routinely whenever bone removal is required. In others no antibiotics are given and their value is disputed. If antibiotics are provided, patients having extractions under local anaesthesia usually receive an oral course of amoxicillin or metronidazole. When general anaesthesia is used, a suitable regimen would be a single intravenous bolus dose of 750 mg cefuroxime.

Osteomyelitis is a particular problem because it can be difficult to treat effectively. All those at increased risk should receive antibiotics. Examples are patients in whom bone is sclerotic or has a reduced blood supply, for instance after

Table 25.3 Possible complications of removal of mandibular impacted third molars

Complication	Frequency
Postsurgical pain, haemorrhage, trismus, swelling and ecchymosis	These affect all patients to some degree and in a proportion of cases may be prolonged. Inability to eat and enjoy food is considered a significant complication by patients.
Alveolar osteitis (dry socket)	Affects 1–35% lower third molar extractions, depending on difficulty and technique. An average for surgical extractions is 5%.
Sensory nerve damage, paraesthesia or anaesthesia	Affects 10–20% of cases though almost all recover spontaneously. A degree of permanent damage of inferior dental or lingual nerves affects 0.5% of cases. Temporary lingual nerve effects are seen in 2%.
Acute temporomandibular joint pain/dysfunction (myofascial pain syndrome)	About 4% of cases, higher in patients with pre-existing symptoms and those whose teeth are removed under general anaesthesia. A mild degree of muscle and joint discomfort is probably much commoner.
Iatrogenic fracture	Fracture of the mandible is fortunately rare, occurring in 1 per 10 000 cases. If minor fractures of the alveolar or lingual plates or tuberosity are included, the incidence is 2–4% of cases, but apart from tuberosity fracture these are mostly of little consequence.
Incorrect or incomplete extraction	Less than 1%.
Acute/chronic postoperative infection including osteonecrosis	Rare, affecting 2–3 per 100 000 cases.
Injury to adjacent structures including teeth and periodontium	Not uncommon; occurs in 3 per 1000 cases.
Oroantral fistula	Rare.
Introduction of tooth or fragment into another tissue space (antrum, tissue space, inhaled into lung or swallowed)	Rare.
Systemic medical/surgical complications related to surgery and/or anaesthetic	Sore throat, adverse reaction, etc. Patients must not drive or operate machinery for 48 hours after sedation or general anaesthesia.
Death under outpatient general anaesthetic	1–2 per 400 000. Increased risk in children. May be related to halothane-induced cardiac arrhythmias.

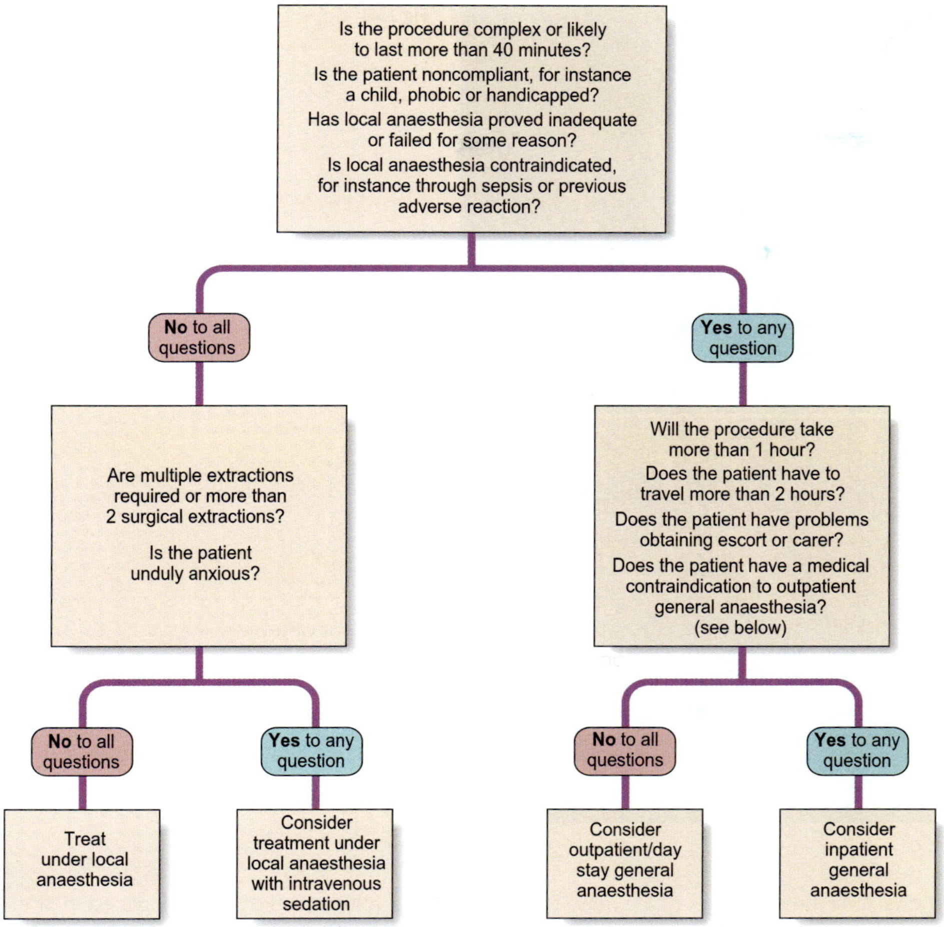

Medical constraints to outpatient general anaesthesia are:	
Cardiovascular	Myocardial infarct, angina, hypertension, anaemia, deep vein thrombosis, stroke
Respiratory	Severe asthma, chronic obstructive airway disease
Gastrointestinal	Hiatus hernia, hepatitis, obesity
Genitourinary	Renal failure
Endocrine	Diabetes, thyroid disease
Medication	Antihypertensives, anticoagulants, corticosteroids
and pregnancy or a family history of adverse reactions to a general anaesthetic	

Fig. 25.3 Flow chart for selection of patients for general anaesthesia.

radiotherapy involving the jaws or when large periosteal flaps are raised in the very elderly. Larger doses and longer courses than normal may be provided.

Is a general anaesthetic required or desirable?

The choice of anaesthetic will depend on the indications for treatment, the assessment of difficulty and the anaesthetic risk assessment for the particular patient.

This patient requires extraction of all four third molars. The indications for removal do not in themselves require a general anaesthetic. However, the surgery is likely to take longer than 20 minutes on each side under local anaesthetic. Arguably this procedure could be performed under local anaesthesia in two visits by an experienced clinician but many patients find this unacceptable. The patient's gag reflex is one factor suggesting that general anaesthesia or sedation would be appropriate, and the patient appears to have no medical contraindication. The patient must be fully informed of the risks of sedation or anaesthesia before making a decision. The risks of general anaesthesia are such that it is never the anaesthetic of choice for routine or straightforward extractions. The flow chart (Fig. 25.3) illustrates some factors in selecting a suitable anaesthetic.

What surgical technique should be used to remove the lower third molars?

There is much debate about the best method for removal of lower third molars. Some authorities suggest that the buccal technique should become the accepted method. In this system no lingual flap is raised and no lingual nerve retraction is performed so that this method carries a minimal risk of permanent lingual nerve damage. Although this is the

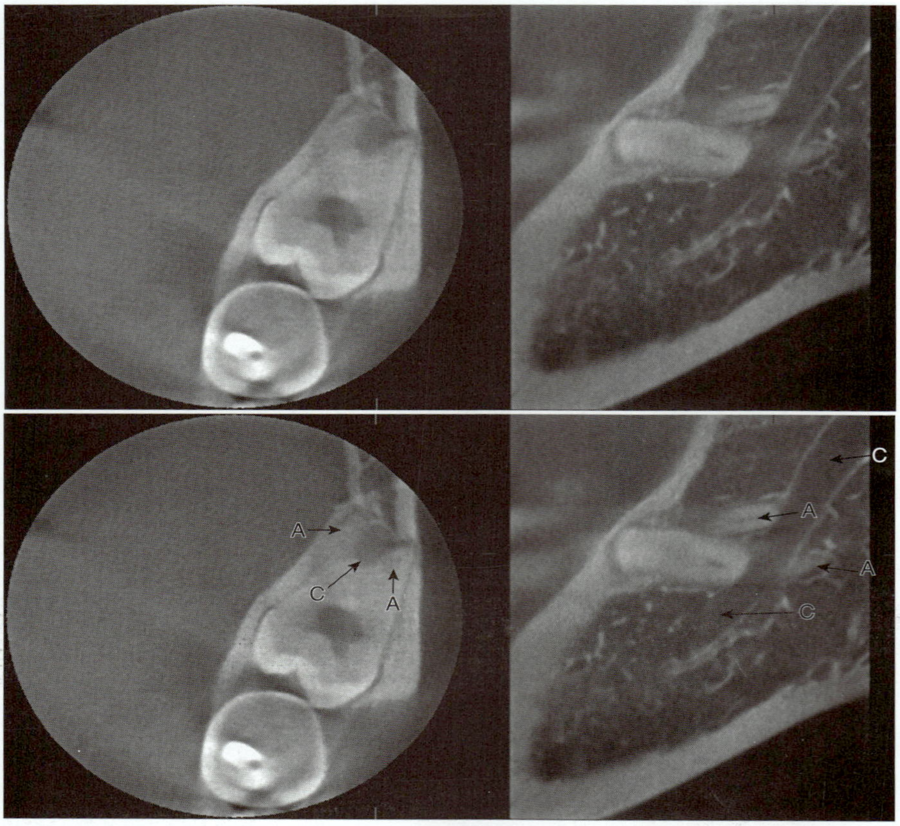

Fig 25.4 Cone beam CT images.

standard method used in Europe and the USA, in the UK it has been traditional to raise lingual and buccal flaps. Under local anaesthetic it is usual to remove bone buccally with a bur, while under general anaesthetic the lingual plate is fractured with a chisel using the lingual split technique.

Another case

■ ***What do you see in the cone beam CT images in figure 25.4?***

These images from another case demonstrate the value of this more complex imaging technique. They are selected views from the imaged volume, which is manipulated in 3D on a computer monitor. On the left is an axial slice (almost occlusal view) through a horizontally impacted lower third molar. The image is round because this system images a vertical cylinder of tissue that is being seen end-on. Unlike medical CT, cone beam images are conventionally viewed from the top, so that the patient's right is on the left of the figure. On the right is a sagittal slice. The inferior dental canal (C) can be seen clearly, outlined by thin cortical bone as it passes in contact with and between the apices of two roots (A). There is no cortex visible where the canal contacts parts of the tooth, so that the roots probably penetrate the wall of the canal.

Case 26

A phone call from school

SUMMARY

An 11-year-old schoolboy has avulsed a permanent incisor tooth. What would you do?

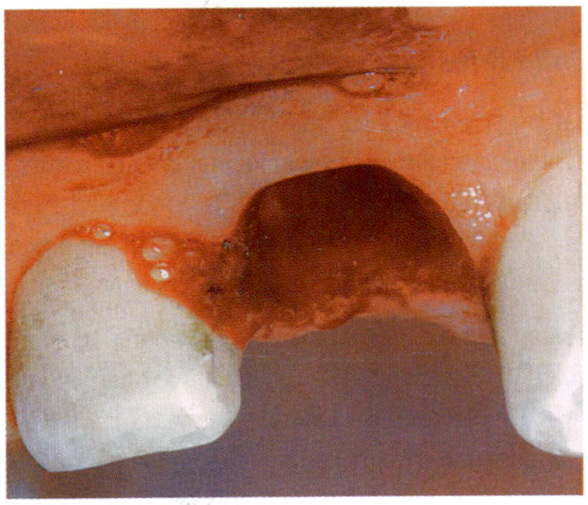

Fig. 26.1 The patient on presentation.

History

Complaint

The school nurse from a nearby primary school telephones your general dental practice to ask for advice. A child has slipped in the school playground and knocked out a front tooth. The accident happened less than 5 minutes ago, the tooth has been found and it is wrapped in a tissue.

■ ***What information would you want from the school nurse?***

Are there any other injuries? It should be established whether there has been any loss of consciousness or signs of concussion. Disorientation and impaired response to simple questions may indicate a brain injury that would require immediate hospital assessment. Limb extremity injuries are common in playground accidents, and the school nurse should be asked to establish whether there is any suspicion of limb fracture or lacerations that require suturing. Dealing with these might be a higher priority than the avulsed tooth.

Is there any relevant medical history? Reimplantation of an avulsed tooth is contraindicated in a child predisposed to infective endocarditis. Any known clotting defect could result in problematic bleeding from a tooth socket.

Has the child an up-to-date tetanus immunization? The school should have a record of immunization status, with particular reference to antitetanus immunization.

Have the parents been informed? Ideally the parents should be notified of the injury and of any intended treatment prior to it being carried out. If at all possible, a parent or legal guardian should be encouraged to either accompany the child or to meet at your practice (or hospital if indicated by other injuries).

What age is the child? The age will determine whether the tooth is primary or permanent and, if permanent, the likely stage of root development.

Is the tooth intact? This is difficult for a lay person to ascertain, but you should ask the caller to carefully examine the tooth, ideally without touching it, or at least without touching the root. A crown fracture would be easier to describe than a root fracture, but if a tapering root of approximately 2 cm in length is present, the tooth is probably intact.

Is the root contaminated with dirt or debris? The root surface must be visibly clean prior to any attempt at reimplantation. Dirt on the root must be cleaned off though any asphalt or gravel 'tattoo' on the incisal edge is not relevant at this stage.

You are told that the child is healthy and that their only other injuries are minor grazes on knees and palms of both hands. These are no signs of head injury.

■ ***What advice can you safely give over the telephone?***

Keep the tooth wet. The first advice should be to place the tooth in a cup of cold fresh milk. Storage in tap water is undesirable, as its hypotonicity reduces viability of the periodontal ligament cells adhering to the root.

Clean off visible contaminants. Rinse the root gently under cold running water for a maximum of 10 seconds to remove dirt from the root surface. The tooth will be slippery to hold but it should be held by the crown only, and under no circumstances should the root surface be scrubbed or scraped. Debris that does not rinse off may be carefully dabbed off with a clean, ideally sterile, cotton-wool bud.

If you can, reimplant the tooth straight away. The speed with which the tooth is replanted is the most important factor in determining a favourable outcome following replantation. A responsible adult should reimplant the tooth without further delay. It should be emphasised to the caller that it is relatively simple to reimplant the tooth and that they should be encouraged to try. The tooth should be placed back in the socket with firm gentle pressure until it is at the same level as the adjacent incisor and orientated labiopalatally. Reasons for failure are likely to be insufficient confidence, a distressed uncooperative child or a fracture of the socket wall. If the tooth cannot be reimplanted, you should advise that the child be escorted to a dentist as soon as possible.

Go to a dentist as soon as possible, even if the tooth is reimplanted. Deal with the other injuries and then the child should attend a dentist as soon as possible, accompanied by an adult. The child should support the tooth in the socket by gentle finger pressure on the way (biting on it may be ineffective in retaining it if there is no incisor occlusion).

You are told that the child is aged 11 years and has lost a permanent tooth. The school is unable to contact the parents and the school staff are unwilling to replant the tooth. They wish to bring the child to see you in your surgery and are setting off now.

How should the tooth be transported and why?

A successful outcome requires that the remnants of the periodontal ligament adhering to the root remain viable because after replantation the healed ligament will prevent replacement resorption and ankylosis. An appropriate transport medium is essential and the key parameter is its osmotic pressure. It has been shown that the periodontal ligament will survive if stored for only a few minutes in water, for up to 30 minutes in saliva, and up to 60 minutes in cold milk. Saliva is thus useful but it is inadvisable to ask an injured child to hold an avulsed tooth in their mouth for any period because of the risk of it being swallowed or inhaled. Storing dry or using water is to be avoided.

Examination

The child is brought to your practice within an hour of the accident, accompanied by a teacher. The parents still cannot be contacted. Before you can examine or treat the child you must obtain consent.

Is the child competent to give consent?

The legal age of consent is 16 and so the consent of a parent or legal guardian needs to be obtained. This is the preferred course of action and every effort must be made to contact the parent without wasting time as this could compromise treatment.

Individuals below the age of 16 years can give consent for medical treatment provided that they have a clear understanding of the issues involved. This is known as Gillick consent following a legal case in 1985. The principle enshrined in the case is that:

> *the parental right to determine whether or not their minor child below the age of 16 years will have medical treatment terminates if and when the child achieves a sufficient understanding and intelligence to enable him or her to fully understand what is proposed.*

It is therefore possible that this 11-year-old could give a valid consent but it would depend on your ability to explain to them and your assessment of their understanding. Detailed notes of explanations given to the child would be necessary. If the child cannot understand, they cannot be informed and so cannot be competent to give consent. A Gillick consent for dentistry is only advisable for emergency treatment.

Can the parent give consent by telephone?

Yes, a verbal consent would be perfectly valid provided it is informed. Good contemporaneous notes of the telephone conversation should be made and you should ensure, as far as possible, that you are speaking to the parent or guardian.

Can the teacher give consent?

No (unless by chance the teacher happens to be the parent or legal guardian). The teacher has a duty of care to bring the child for treatment but cannot become further involved.

Can the dentist give consent?

No, the same applies. But this does not mean that you cannot carry out treatment. You can carry out emergency treatment that is in the best interests of the child and that would be considered reasonable by the 'general body of prudent dentists'. Although the dental injury is not life threatening, delay in reimplantation will significantly reduce the chance of a successful outcome. This makes the situation a relative emergency and would be a reason to proceed without parental consent. You have a duty of care to the injured child and must use your clinical judgement to decide what course of action is reasonable. This is a difficult area. The treatment you are offering is the same as the treatment you would have performed with consent, and so you should not be criticised. If you are in doubt about consent, always check with your professional indemnity provider.

Can the child refuse treatment?

Yes, refusal by the child to any treatment must be respected (though under certain circumstances the parent's consent might override the child's wishes). To proceed further against the child's wishes might constitute assault and could be in breach of General Dental Council guidance.

You decide that reimplantation is in the child's best interests and is clinically indicated. It is still not possible to contact the parents. The patient is keen to try to put the tooth back in position after you have explained the situation.

What will you look for in the clinical examination?

The oral soft tissues	Check for mucosal and gingival tears that may require suturing and remove foreign material embedded in the soft tissues. Full examination will not be possible without cleansing the mouth with gauze soaked in saline to remove blood and debris. Avulsion is often accompanied by copious bleeding but this soon stops, leaving a dramatic and often distressing picture. Cleaning will improve patient comfort and will often reveal the injuries to be less extensive than at first thought.
The dentition	Check the adjacent teeth and those in the opposing arch. Any other injuries will have to be managed following reimplantation.
The socket	Irrigate the socket with sterile isotonic saline to remove blood clot and allow examination of the bony socket wall for comminuted fractures. If a fracture is detected, gently reduce it by pressing the fragment back into place using an instrument such as a flat plastic or a straight Warwick James elevator.

The avulsed tooth	The tooth should be examined and cleaned as outlined above, using isotonic saline as the irrigant and taking great care not to handle the root surface. The opportunity should be taken to measure the incisal–apical length (useful for later endodontic treatment) and assess the diameter and condition of the apical foramen. Any soft tissues adhering to apex should be left, as they may contain Hertwig's sheath remnants with potential for continued apical maturation.

In this case the tooth has a closed apex, as would be expected from his age.

■ ***What is the significance of the state of the apex?***

The pulp can only remain vital if it revascularizes and this is determined by the length of the pulp, the diameter of the apical foramen, the storage medium used and the speed of replantation. If the pulp in an immature tooth is less than 17mm in length and has an open apex with a diameter greater than 1 mm, revascularization may be possible provided storage of the avulsed tooth has been favourable and it is replanted within 1 hour.

In this case the apex is closed and the pulp will certainly undergo necrosis. After replantation the pulp remnants will have to be extirpated and the tooth root filled.

Treatment

■ ***You have cleaned the tooth as described above. How will you go about replanting it?***

Give local analgesia. The aim is painless replantation but local analgesia may not be required. The injured tissues may be relatively insensitive in the period immediately following trauma, and the reimplantation procedure is sufficiently rapid that local analgesia is not always required. Its use may be dictated by the presence of other soft tissue injuries or the previous dental experiences of the child. Concerns that vasoconstriction might compromise success by reducing socket vascularity are spurious.

Replant the tooth. Holding the crown either in fingers or forceps, rinse the root surface with sterile saline then swiftly and gently replace the tooth in the socket, applying sufficient pressure in an apical direction to position the tooth as near to its original position as can be estimated. The child should then bite firmly on a carefully positioned gauze roll to hold it in position. If using forceps, ensure they do not grip and thus damage the root surface.

Splint the tooth. The most practical type of splint is a short length of stainless steel wire cemented on to the labial surface of the replanted tooth and adjacent incisors with blobs of acid-etch retained composite. A paper clip will often suffice. If an orthodontic wire is used, it must be passive and flexible to avoid exerting orthodontic forces. It is important to keep the splint well away from the gingival margin to allow access for oral hygiene because bacterial ingress into the wounded periodontal ligament can significantly compromise healing. The splint should be left in place for 7–10 days. Rigid splinting for longer periods increases the chances of ankylosis.

Prescribe antibiotics. A 7-day course of oral systemic antibiotics should be prescribed to cover the immediate postimplantation period. The benefit of oral antibiotics has not been proven in human studies but in animal studies they have proved beneficial.

Prescribe chlorhexidine mouthrinse (0.1%) twice daily during the splinting period to help to keep the area clean and reduce the bacterial flora around the injured periodontal ligament.

Give dietary advice. A soft diet should be recommended during the splinting period, avoiding foods that require incising.

■ ***You replant the tooth without difficulty. What would you do next?***

The patient needs to be reviewed 7–10 days later to remove the splint. Because the apex is closed and revascularization is not expected, root treatment should be commenced by removing the pulp within 10 days. Delayed extirpation risks external resorption and discolouration of the crown.

Endodontic treatment should be commenced before the splint is removed. The necrotic pulp tissue is extirpated, the root canal cleaned and irrigated with sodium hypochlorite and a nonsetting calcium hydroxide paste is placed in the canal and sealed appropriately. A definitive gutta percha root canal filling is usually delayed for 6–12 months.

■ ***Why not extirpate the pulp and root fill the tooth while it is avulsed?***

Even if pulp extirpation is required, it should never be carried out extraorally as the need to manipulate the tooth would almost certainly cause more damage to the periodontal ligament and any delay reduces the chances of a successful outcome.

■ ***What are the main complications of replantation of an avulsed permanent tooth? How are they managed?***

See the table at the top of p. 122.

Follow up

■ ***What are the aims of treatment and chances of success?***

The aim of replantation is to maintain the tooth in the child patient thus avoiding the need for prosthetic replacement for as long as possible. While there is no frank sepsis or overt discomfort to the patient, the original tooth is the ideal space maintainer.

A failing tooth should be preserved until the patient has reached skeletal maturity, when they could be assessed for an osseointegrated implant. However, in the case of severe resorption or infraocclusion, extraction and immediate replacement with a space maintainer are required.

In one large prospective study of 400 replanted teeth followed up for 5 years, 30% were eventually lost. Immature teeth have a worse prognosis than mature teeth. The chances

necrosis (tenderness to palpation, increased tooth mobility and grey discolouration of the tooth). Sensitivity tests using ethyl chloride and electric pulp testing should be carried out but are difficult to interpret. Radiographs would have been taken at 4 weeks and at monthly intervals for 4–6 months thereafter to detect external resorption. Any signs of loss of vitality or resorption would have triggered immediate endodontic treatment with calcium hydroxide. These dressings would have been replaced every month for 3 months and then 3–6 monthly, until there was radiographic evidence of a calcific barrier across the open apex. A definitive root filling would then have been placed in the root canal.

An alternative strategy would be to place mineral trioxide aggregate (MTA) to create the apical barrier. To use MTA the tooth must be free of infection and have no evidence of progressing root resorption. Once the material has set hard at the apex, which takes a minimum of 4 hours, a conventional root filling would be placed in the canal.

■ *How would your treatment have differed if the avulsed tooth had been a primary incisor?*

No attempt should be made to replant an avulsed primary incisor. Parents should be reassured and warned of possible damage to the permanent successor. Follow up should be arranged to monitor normal development and eruption of the permanent successor.

Case 27

Discoloured anterior teeth

SUMMARY

A 22-year-old woman presents at your general dental practice surgery complaining of the poor appearance of her teeth. What is the cause and what treatment is appropriate?

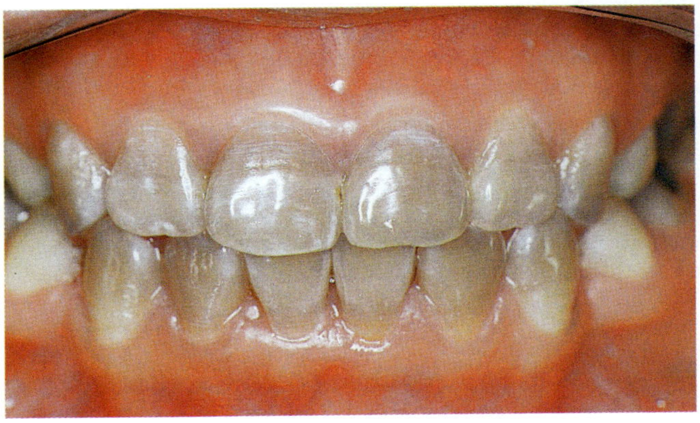

Fig. 27.1 The appearance of the teeth.

History

Complaint

She is unhappy with the colour of the teeth which she feels are becoming darker. She is very conscious of them and realizes that she is reluctant to smile because of their appearance.

History of complaint

The teeth looked slightly grey on eruption but they have slowly darkened.

Dental history

The patient has had very little dental treatment but received regular preventive care from your practice until the age of 16. Your notes record that she was given oral fluoride supplementation as a child. This was provided as fluoride drops at a dose of 0.25mg daily from birth to 2 years and 0.5 mg daily as tablets from 2 to 4 years, rising to 1 mg daily from 4 to 12 years of age.

Medical history

The patient is fit and healthy with no relevant medical conditions noted on her medical history questionnaire.

■ ***What are the possible causes of discolouration of teeth? What features of each cause aid differential diagnosis?***

The possible causes and relevant features are presented in Table 27.1.

■ ***What specific questions would you ask this patient? Explain why.***

Did she suffer any illness between birth and 6 years? This might account directly for the discolouration or could have been the reason for antibiotic treatment with tetracyclines. Further information on chronological hypoplasia will be found in Case 56.

What toothpaste was used during fluoride supplementation? The fluoride supplementation regimen provided for this patient was recommended during her childhood, but the doses would now be considered too high. On these doses, a small proportion of patients would be expected to show mild fluorosis. More severe fluorosis would be associated with a second source of fluoride. The most probable additional source would be ingestion of adult-formula fluoride toothpaste, though living in an area with fluoridated water should also be excluded.

Is there a family history of tooth discolouration or tooth loss? A positive family history aids diagnosis of inherited defects and is essential for diagnosis of some types of amelogenesis imperfecta.

In response to your questioning the patient tells you that she remembers taking many courses of antibiotics as a child for chest infections. She cannot remember what toothpaste she used before the age of 6, but for as long as she can remember she has used an adult paste. She has no family history of similar defects.

Examination

Intraoral examination

On examination the oral mucosa is healthy and oral hygiene is good. The dentition is unrestored.

■ ***The appearance of the anterior teeth is shown in Figure 27.1. What do you see? How do you interpret the appearance?***

The morphology of the tooth crowns is normal and the incisors, canines and premolars are a grey-brown colour. There are some areas which appear less affected and others which appear opaque white. Small flecks of white are

Table 27.1 Possible causes of discolouration

Causes	Features
Extrinsic staining	
Dietary stains such as tea, coffee, cigarette smoke, betel quid Chlorhexidine mouthwash Pigments produced by the normal oral flora, usually the subgingival flora	Usually worse around gingival margin and in less well cleaned areas because these agents stain pellicle and plaque rather than enamel.
Turner tooth	Infection of the deciduous predecessor causes enamel hypoplasia in a permanent tooth and the porous enamel absorbs extrinsic stains. Tooth shape abnormal.
Intrinsic staining	
Dental caries	Associated with softening. Characteristic distribution of lesions. Slowly progressing and dentine caries are the types most frequently stained.
Blood pigments	Seen most frequently in nonvital teeth (as a result of pulp necrosis). Rarely may affect all teeth in conditions including rhesus incompatibility (in the deciduous teeth only), porphyria and hyperbilirubinaemia. Colour ranges from dull red through brown to grey or black.
Tetracycline staining	Caused by administration of tetracyclines during tooth formation. When severe, this is a generalized green, brown or yellow colour, darkening with time. The teeth may fluoresce under ultraviolet light in the early stages but this reduces as the colour darkens. When mild there may be a chronological banding pattern with horizontal lines of discoloured enamel corresponding to individual courses of tetracycline. Tooth shape is normal.
Fluorosis	Varies from mild flecks of opaque white enamel to severely hypoplastic patches which take up extrinsic stain. The latter is only seen in areas where fluorosis is endemic. The mildest effects are impossible to tell from the opaque flecks seen when water fluoride concentration is very low. Affects all teeth. Moderately affected cases of endemic fluorosis may have an apparent chronological pattern of fine white lines associated with periods of exposure to higher doses. Tooth shape normal unless condition is severe.
Amelogenesis imperfecta	Numerous types. Affects all teeth, though some forms are much milder in the deciduous dentition. Colour change varies and is secondary to either hypoplasia (thin hard translucent enamel through which dentine is visible), hypocalcification (chalky white opaque soft enamel) and hypomaturation (patchy distribution of white opacities). Affected areas may also take up extrinsic stain. Tooth shape may be normal and some types have a vertical banding, pitting or ridging pattern. Family history will be positive in many cases. Mild types are difficult to distinguish from fluorosis.
Dentinogenesis imperfecta	All teeth are an even grey-brown colour with altered translucency. The shape of the tooth crowns is normal but the roots are thin and taper sharply. There is gradual pulpal obliteration by dentine. There may be a family history and, in some cases, osteogenesis imperfecta is associated. Enamel fractures from the dentine and severe wear follow shortly after eruption.
Regional odontodysplasia	Affects a group of adjacent deciduous and permanent teeth on one side of midline. Enamel hypoplasia leads to uptake of extrinsic stain and yellow cementum may be present over the crown. Characteristic defects on radiography include thin enamel and dentine, large pulps. Affected teeth often fail to erupt.
Chronological hypoplasia	Horizontal band(s) of enamel hypoplasia, each associated with a specific insult, usually a severe illness or metabolic upset including severe attacks of the common viral diseases of childhood. Affected bands are abnormal enamel which may be pitted, hypoplastic, rough, opaque or completely absent, and also take up extrinsic stain.
Age change	Teeth become yellower and slightly darker with age. This is an even colour change and it is usually mild.

scattered on the labial enamel. There are several prominent horizontal lines on the teeth, most clearly seen in the enamel of the gingival third of the crowns of both upper central incisors.

The teeth are evenly discoloured and this has the appearance of an intrinsic stain. The distribution of the affected enamel is in a chronological pattern and affects all enamel formed from birth to approximately 6 years of age. The even distribution suggests that the cause was present throughout development or that there were frequent or prolonged exposures. The fine lines in the central incisors suggest that a series of repeated exposures is the more likely cause. The grey-brown colour is typical of tetracycline staining.

The small white flecks are more difficult to explain. They are not consistent with tetracycline staining and could be either mild fluorosis or a normal feature made more prominent by the dark enamel.

Investigation

■ ***What further examinations would you carry out? Explain why?***

The teeth should be examined after drying. This makes porous defects more opaque and more visible and aids the detection of fine chronological bands and enamel flecks. The teeth could also be examined under an ultraviolet (UV) light or near UV light to see whether they fluoresce green/yellow because this would indicate tetracycline staining. The fluorescence is not bright and cannot be seen unless the room is dark and the illuminating lamp has a very low visible light output.

Though not necessary for diagnosis in this case, it is always prudent to test the vitality of discoloured teeth in case loss of vitality is the cause. The vitality of the affected teeth would determine the treatment options available.

Radiography is not a useful investigation in the present case. Periapical radiographs would be indicated if teeth were nonvital or affected by periodontitis. They would also be helpful in a younger patient to determine whether unerupted teeth were normal or if dentinogenesis imperfecta were considered a likely cause.

In this case no fluorescence could be detected in the surgery and all teeth were vital.

Differential diagnosis

What is your diagnosis?

The dark colour of the teeth is typical of intrinsic staining caused by tetracycline. The history of yellow teeth becoming darker over a period of years is also characteristic.

An enquiry to the patient's medical practitioner confirms that as a child she received repeated and sometimes prolonged courses of tetracycline for chest infection, confirming the diagnosis.

Why is fluorosis not the cause?

Fluorosis cannot account for the generalized discolouration. The appearances are quite different, with mottled brown and white patches. The scattered white flecks could be caused by mild fluorosis and the fact that the patient used a fluoride toothpaste as well as a fluoride supplement for many years makes this a possibility. However, no definitive diagnosis can be reached because there is no accepted diagnostic test for mild degrees of fluorosis. Small numbers of such small white flecks are found in normal enamel.

Treatment

How would you decide which teeth should be treated?

The patient's main concern is her appearance. Only those teeth which are affected and visible need be treated. The factors that should be taken into account are the following.

The smile line. Observe the patient relaxed, talking and smiling naturally. Note the level of the lip line, which teeth and how much of each crown is visible. This will dictate which teeth need treatment and, if restorations are necessary, where the cervical margin should be placed. In this case all upper teeth from first molar to first molar are visible during smiling but second premolars and molars lie in shadow and the staining is not obvious. The upper lip line runs along the gingival margin of all upper incisors and canines, exposing the interdental papillae.

The occlusion. Indirect porcelain or composite veneers are difficult to make where the teeth are imbricated because the teeth on the die model cannot be separated in the laboratory. Alternative methods of treatment must be used. If there is wear on the incisal edge then porcelain veneers, which are inherently brittle, may fracture and direct composite veneers may be preferable.

Occupation. A patient whose occupation depends on their appearance may require both a greater degree of correction of the tooth shade and treatment of a larger number of tooth surfaces. Performers and others who work in bright, even artificial, light may also require restorations to look natural under demanding lighting conditions. Fortunately, these more unusual constraints do not apply to this patient.

What treatment options are available? What are their advantages and disadvantages?

The treatment options are presented in Table 27.2.

Which treatment is appropriate for this patient? Explain why.

The selection of appropriate treatment is outlined in the flow chart (Figure 27.3 p.129).

A conservative approach using carbamide peroxide bleaching agents would be appropriate, and was tried initially. However, in this case the patient's lip line leaves the cervical enamel of the incisors and canines exposed and the effectiveness of the result is not predictable. Dark stain remained cervically after bleaching and the patient requested porcelain veneers to mask the discolouration.

Prognosis

The completed porcelain veneers are shown in Figure 27.2. The appearance is not ideal and the disadvantage of having to use opaque veneers is well shown. However, the patient was very happy with this result.

What is the long-term prognosis for these veneers?

The veneers on the upper right canine and lateral incisor are in crossbite with the lower canine and almost edge to edge on the lateral incisor. On the upper left the same teeth are edge to edge. There is a risk of chipping the incisal edges and debonding.

Prevention

Tetracycline should no longer be prescribed to those below the age of 12. Presumably tetracycline staining should no longer be seen?

This is true, but unfortunately courses of tetracycline are still occasionally prescribed for children. There are some specific indications, such as cystic fibrosis, for which prolonged tetracycline treatment is still provided to children. Tetracyclines are available as over-the-counter drugs in some countries.

Tetracyclines such as minocycline, which are well absorbed and reach high blood levels, are the drugs of choice to prevent infection in acne. They are frequently prescribed to adolescents and young adults and may stain dental tissues forming at this time, such as the roots of third molars. However, minocycline may also stain bone and fully formed teeth. The drug becomes incorporated into the pulpal surface of the dentine and staining is darkest in teeth where there is active secondary dentine formation. Because this stain lies deep in the tooth, it cannot be bleached by external bleaching agents.

Table 27.2 Treatment options

Option	Advantages	Disadvantages
Vital bleaching agents using carbamide (or urea) peroxide	Work best with extrinsic stains and quite well for many intrinsic stains. Easily applied in custom trays, nondestructive and easily repeated if necessary. Does not alter the underlying tooth shade or translucency. If sufficient and even lightening of the shade is achieved, bleaching produces the best appearance of all options. Can also be used to mask severe staining before a veneer is placed. This prevents the dark enamel showing through and allows a more translucent veneer to be used, improving the final appearance.	Unpredictable effectiveness with tetracycline staining, often leaving a dark zone cervically where the stained root shows through the thin cervical enamel. However, almost always some improvement and this may satisfy the patient. Only appropriate when there are minimal or no restorations in the teeth. Restorations are not bleached and there is a theoretical concern that bleaching agents might track to the pulp along the margins of restorations. Some over-the-counter formulations are acidic and others may cause local soft tissue irritation, and should not be encouraged. Licensing regulations vary between countries.
Nonvital bleach	Allows bleaching of deeper dentine than a vital bleach, producing greater effect.	Only possible in nonvital teeth and so usually inappropriate for multiple teeth. To bleach dentine below the cervical enamel the bleaching agent must be applied to the cervical part of the root canal as well as the pulp chamber.
Direct composite, indirect composite or porcelain veneers	Good appearance possible, can be as good as crowns but much less destructive.	Some tooth preparation is required, the amount varying slightly between types. The 'emergence profile' or contour at the gingival margin must be maintained by removing cervical enamel, to avoid a plaque trap. When placed over darkly stained teeth, veneer and cement must be opaque. This reduces translucency and produces a 'flat' artificial colour to the finished restoration.
Crowns	Strong and retentive, a variety of bonded or reinforced crowns are available if the occlusion is a problem. Very darkly stained teeth are best crowned. The porcelain is thicker than veneers so that opaque materials are not required. If necessary, metal-bonded crowns completely mask the underlying colour. Usually the best alternative if the teeth contain extensive restorations. Appearance can be excellent.	Destructive of tooth tissue. Margins may compromise periodontal health. Expensive.

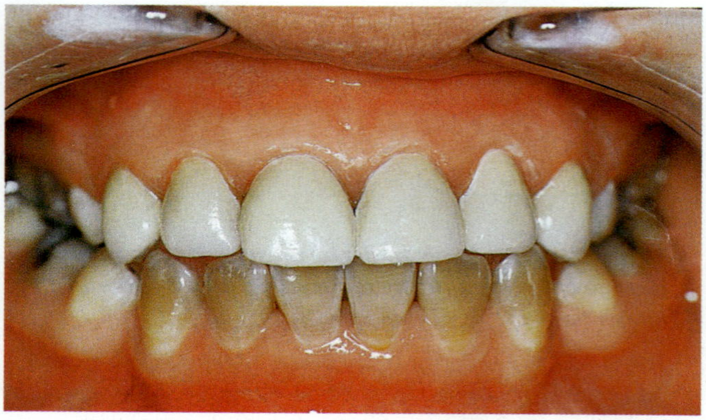

Fig. 27.2 The completed porcelain veneers immediately after cementation.

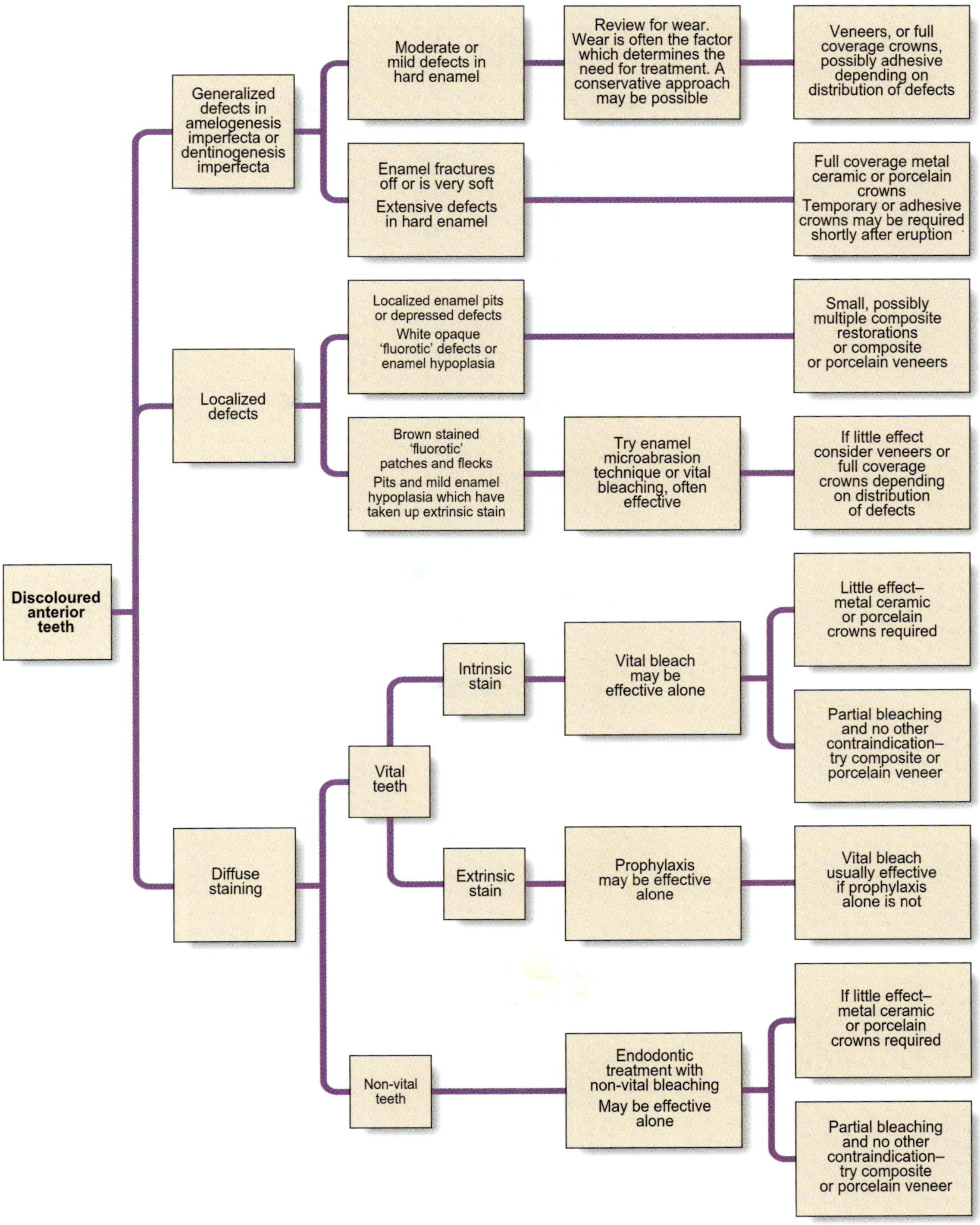

Fig. 27.3 Selection of appropriate treatment.

Case 28

A very painful mouth

SUMMARY

A 20-year-old man presents to you in your general dental practice, feeling ill and with a very sore mouth.

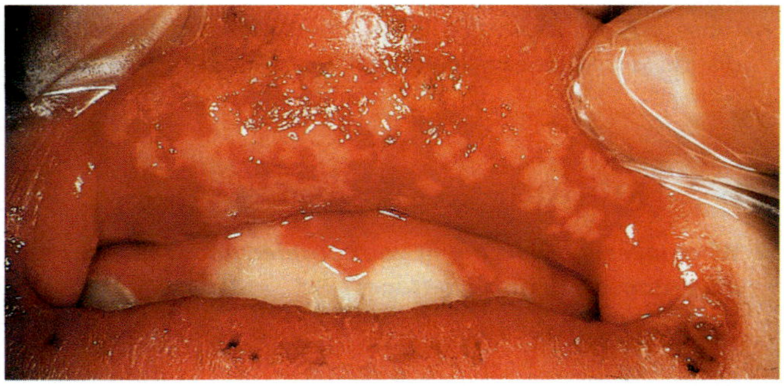

Fig. 28.1 Appearance of the patient's mouth.

History

Complaint

The patient complains of pain which is preventing eating and hampering drinking. He also feels unwell.

History of complaint

He first noticed feeling unwell 4 days previously and thought he had 'flu. He was slightly feverish and developed a headache. His mouth was sore but it was not until about 1 day later that it became very painful. Because he felt unable to take time off work, he took the remains of a course of an unknown oral antibiotic which had been prescribed for his brother who had an infected cut on his arm. This did not appear to have led to any improvement. He has had no similar attacks before.

Medical history

The patient is otherwise fit and well.

Examination

Extraoral examination

The patient has enlarged cervical lymph nodes that are slightly tender, mobile but soft or firm rather than hard. Apart from this finding no abnormalities are found in a routine examination of the head, neck and hands.

Intraoral examination

■ ***What do you see in Figure 28.1?***

There are numerous ulcers on the labial mucosa which have the following characteristics:

Site	Labial mucosa and attached gingiva
Size	A few millimetres in diameter
Shape	Well defined, rounded, sometimes coalescing to form larger irregular ulcers
Colour	Covered by a yellow-grey fibrin ulcer slough, no well-defined rim of periulcer erythema
Background	The surrounding mucosa appears uniformly inflamed

In addition, one large ulcer lies at the commissure and there are small bloodstained crusts around the lips.

If you were able to examine the patient you would discover that more ulcers affect much of the oral mucosa, including the gingivae, palate and tongue, and that they extend back into the oropharynx.

■ ***Give a differential diagnosis on the basis of the information you have so far.***

- Primary herpetic gingivostomatitis
- Erythema multiforme.

■ ***Justify this differential diagnosis.***

Primary herpetic gingivostomatitis and other oral viral infections typically cause multiple round small ulcers of acute onset, sometimes coalescing, on a background of inflamed mucosa. The patient feels unwell and has enlarged tender lymph nodes suggesting infection. Primary *Herpes simplex* infection usually affects much of the mucosa and has a predilection for the keratinized masticatory mucosa of the gingiva. The patient is older than is normally expected for a primary infection. However, the average age of patients with this infection has increased over the last few decades because improved living conditions have resulted in fewer individuals coming into contact with the virus during their childhood.

Erythema multiforme (Stevens–Johnson syndrome) is possible. The acute onset and bloody crusts on the lips suggest this diagnosis and the age of the patient is compatible. However, the distribution of ulcers is not particularly suggestive of this condition. Erythema multiforme affects primarily the lips and nonkeratinized lining mucosa of the anterior mouth, and the ulcers have ragged margins, whereas the irregular ulcers in the picture seem to be formed by coalescence of small round ulcers. A trigger for erythema multiforme is sometimes identified and antibiotics, particularly sulphonamides, are sometimes the cause. This patient has had recent antibiotics, but only after the symptoms appeared. Erythema multiforme is typically recurrent and the history of previous attacks and their periodicity is important in making the diagnosis. However, in a first attack the features may be milder and, as in this case, there is no history of similar attacks.

■ ***What diagnoses have you discounted and why?***

Other oral viral infections do not produce a clinical picture of this severity. Herpangina and hand, foot and mouth disease are milder and usually affect the soft palate of children. *Varicella zoster* would be expected to cause chicken pox in this age group though children are the age group more typically affected; oral zoster usually affects elderly patients and is unilateral.

Herpetiform aphthous stomatitis should be considered but is readily excluded. The ulcers may be numerous, small and coalescing and may have an erythematous background. However they are usually limited to the anterior or posterior of the mouth, do not affect keratinized mucosa and are not accompanied by systemic illness. Attacks are recurrent.

In a mild primary attack of *Herpes simplex* infection in an adult, the ulcers may be limited to the gingiva, raising the possibility of acute necrotizing ulcerative gingivitis. However, in this case the ulceration is too extensive for necrotizing gingivitis to be considered and in any case it is usually clinically characteristic.

■ ***What further questions would you ask and what further examinations would you perform and why?***

Do you suffer from 'cold sores'? If the patient has had recurrent *Herpes simplex* infection, usually in the form of herpes labialis, then the present ulcers cannot be due to a primary herpetic infection. Recurrent herpetic infection is sometimes a trigger for attacks of erythema multiforme and a cold sore 1–2 weeks before onset would raise this possibility.

In answer to this question, the patient indicates that he does not suffer from cold sores.

Have you been in contact with anyone with cold sores? Identification of a possible source of *Herpes simplex* 1–2 weeks before the ulcers would give further credibility to this diagnosis. Contact with *Herpes zoster* is not significant in this case but in less clear-cut cases it would be prudent to ask about both chicken pox and shingles contacts.

The patient has no known contact with any viral disease.

Did you notice small blisters in your mouth before the ulcers appeared? This would suggest herpes virus infection, each ulcer being preceded by a small round vesicle. Larger vesicles and blisters are also found in erythema multiforme but these are irregular and usually limited to the vermilion border of the lips and floor of mouth.

Have you taken any drugs or medicines in the last 3 weeks? This will clarify the possibility that medication has triggered an attack of erythema multiforme.

The patient has taken no medication apart from the antibiotic noted in the history.

Have you any rash anywhere on your body? Erythema multiforme is associated with a variety of rashes (hence its name) and the patient should have a skin examination. The presence of typical target lesions indicates erythema multiforme but other less characteristic rashes should also be noted, together with their time of onset.

No rash is present.

Take the patient's temperature. This simple investigation is easily forgotten, but often valuable. A raised temperature in the early stages indicates infection. The temperature is not raised in erythema multiforme even when severe (unless there is infection of skin lesions).

His temperature is 38°C.

Diagnosis

This differential diagnosis sometimes poses problems. If the patient has erythema multiforme he should be treated with a moderately high dose of systemic steroids, but this should be avoided if he has a viral infection. A period of time must elapse before the results of investigations will be available.

■ ***Can you make a diagnosis and commence treatment?***

Yes. In this case there is sufficient evidence to make a working diagnosis of primary *Herpes simplex* infection. Investigations should be performed to confirm the diagnosis but need not delay treatment. Investigations are probably only available to those in hospital practice. Practitioners confident in the diagnosis may well instigate treatment without confirmatory tests.

Investigations

■ ***What investigations might you consider, and what are their advantages and disadvantages?***

See Table 28.1.

In the current case, a smear for light microscopy and viral antibody titre against *Herpes simplex* were requested.

Treatment

■ ***What treatment would you provide?***

The patient should be reassured that he has a common viral infection which, while unpleasant, has no significant implications. It will run its course in a further 10 days or so but it is unlikely to worsen significantly now that it is in its fifth day. Some adult patients may confuse this diagnosis with genital herpes and require some additional explanation.

While unwell the patient should rest and maintain a good fluid intake. This is especially important in children who refuse fluids and become dehydrated rapidly. A sedative antihistamine such as promethazine is sometimes suggested for very small and fractious children who cannot sleep during the acute phase. It also has the advantage of drying the reflex salivation.

The patient should be warned about infectivity. The virus is transmitted only by close contact but while there are vesicles or ulcers in the mouth, the saliva is infectious. Care should be taken to avoid close contact with other individuals, especially

Table 28.1 Investigations to be considered

Test	Advantages and disadvantages
Smear for light microscopy	Simple and rapid. Characteristic viral changes may indicate herpes virus infection provided epithelial cells from the ulcer margin are present in the smear. Most hospitals should be able to give an urgent result the same day. However, a smear will only be positive for the first few days of ulceration. As a result, a positive smear indicates infection but a negative smear cannot exclude it in all cases.
Swab for viral culture	Simple but takes several days. In general terms this test has the advantage that it detects a wide range of viruses but in this differential diagnosis the broad specificity is not particularly helpful.
Swab for viral antigen screen	Simple and moderately fast. A small number of viruses may be identified from their antigens in a swab using ELISA (enzyme-linked immunosorbent assay). Results from this test may be available in 24 hours but it is only available in some centres.
Swab for polymerase chain reaction (PCR)-based viral detection	Obtaining the smear is simple but the laboratory procedure is complex. Highly specific and moderately fast. Results should be available in 24–48 hours. The test is only available in specialized centres.
Smear for electron microscopy	Very specific and relatively simple but again only available in specialized centres. The result is usually available the same day.
Serum for viral antibody level	Serum for antibody to herpes and other viruses is simple to obtain and provides a result in about 48 hours. A high titre of anti-viral IgM indicates acute infection (though it may take a day or two to rise to a detectable level) and a low stable titre of IgG denotes a previous infection. In the absence of raised IgM, two samples several days apart to demonstrate an increasing IgG level are required for confident diagnosis of primary infection. This test is widely available and frequently used.
Biopsy of ulcer	Relatively readily performed but almost never necessary in *Herpes simplex* infection (except for the unusual chronic infections found in the immunosuppressed). Will give the diagnosis of herpetic infection in almost all cases. Also diagnostic in most cases of erythema multiforme.

children. In the nonimmune patient (by definition anyone with a primary infection) other sites may also become infected and particular care should be taken not to spread saliva to the eye.

Antiviral treatment with aciclovir should be considered. Aciclovir is only effective in the earliest stage of the infection when the virus is replicating. It must be taken in the first 48 hours for best effect, while vesicles rather than ulcers are present. Aciclovir is not indicated in this case because of the delay in presentation (though it might be considered in an immunosuppressed patient). A dose of 200 mg five times daily is recommended for immunocompetent patients. Related drugs giving higher levels in the blood, such as valaciclovir, are usually reserved for *Varicella zoster* infection.

Preparations for symptomatic relief of the oral ulceration are indicated. Tetracycline mouthwash (250 mg capsule of a soluble preparation dissolved in water, used four times daily) is very useful in reducing discomfort and would be an appropriate choice in this patient who has presented too late to benefit from aciclovir. Antiseptic mouthwashes such as chlorhexidine are also effective. These presumably reduce oral discomfort by preventing bacterial infection of the ulcers. Chlorhexidine would also compensate for difficulty in carrying out oral hygiene procedures. Analgesic mouthwashes such as benzydamine are an alternative.

Prognosis

What is the risk that this patient will suffer from cold sores in the future?

Between 15 and 30% of individuals who come into contact with the virus develop recurrent infection. It is not clear whether those who suffer a symptomatic primary infection such as gingivostomatitis have an increased risk. Although this percentage seems high, many patients with recurrent herpes infection suffer only very occasional lesions.

What are the mechanisms and significance of recurrent infection?

During infection, *H. simplex* is transported back along axons of sensory nerves to their nuclei. There, neurones are infected but do not die and the virus becomes latent, that is, virus persists but no infectious virions are produced.

A viral latency gene and the cell mediated immune response contribute to a balance between latency and reactivation. If infection reactivates, virus travels down the nerve to cause a localised recurrent infection of the mucosa or skin, a cold sore. Because the virus is intracellular for most of this life cycle, antibodies of the humoral immune response are not effective in preventing recurrences. Environmental triggers for cold sores include ultraviolet light, illness and stress.

Latent infection has important consequences. Subclinical reactivation may result in infectious virus being shed from the mucosa without the individual realising they have an active infection. This may be a mechanism of spread in the population. Latent infection in the geniculate ganglion is one cause of Bell's palsy and very occasionally virus may spread along nerves to the brain causing herpetic encephalitis.

Labial recurrences are painful and unpleasant but relatively readily treated because there is often a characteristic prodromal sensation of burning or itching and vesicles are easily seen. Early treatment is therefore possible and antiviral drugs can be very effective. Topical preparations of 5% aciclovir are available without prescription.

When would you ask the patient to return?

The patient should return in about 1 week to check that healing is progressing, but earlier if symptoms worsen or new signs develop.

At some stage during treatment or follow up the patient should be warned not to take medications prescribed for others. The antibiotic prescribed for the patient's brother was apparently a harmless but inappropriate drug. Those who take others' drugs run the risk of hypersensitivity, drug interaction or other unwanted reaction. The importance of completing the prescribed dose should be emphasized to all patients receiving antibiotics, both to ensure effective treatment and because this is critically important in preventing the emergence of resistant strains in the community.

Final outcome

The next day a report on the smear for microscopy shows no evidence of viral infection (possibly because the ulcers have been present for several days), but on the following day the serum antibody result by complement fixation test shows an anti-*Herpes simplex* type 1 antibody titre of 160 (normal <10). The diagnosis of herpetic gingivostomatitis is confirmed.

Case 29

Caution – X-rays

SUMMARY

A patient does not wish to have radiographs taken. How should her concerns be answered?

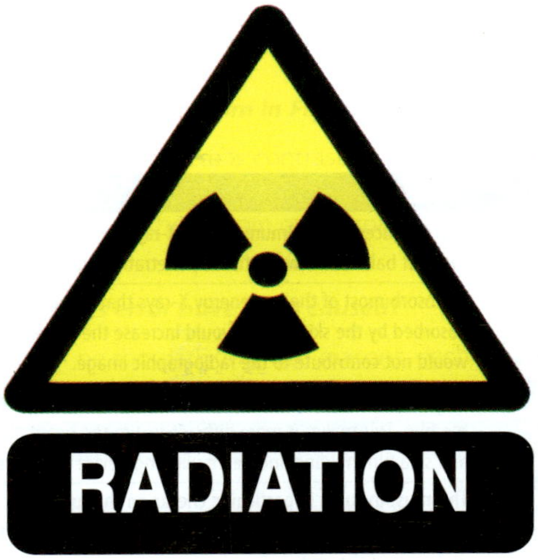

Fig. 29.1

History

Complaint

Following clinical examination, you decide that a patient attending your practice for the first time requires the following radiographs:

View	Reason
Right and left bitewings	To assess existing restorations and periodontal status
Periapical radiograph of the lower left first molar	This tooth is tender to percussion and may need extraction or root canal treatment
Panoramic radiograph	To assess partially erupted wisdom teeth

The patient is concerned about radiation and is not sure whether she wishes to have so many films taken.

■ ***What three general guiding principles must you follow in deciding whether or not to undertake any radiographic examination?***

Justification. Each radiation exposure must have a net positive benefit.

Optimization. The exposures must be at a dose which is As Low As Reasonably Practicable (ALARP), taking social and economic factors into account.

Limitation. The dose to individuals must not exceed recommended limits.

The principles are set out by the International Commission on Radiological Protection (ICRP) who also set the recommended limits.

■ ***What is the patient dose associated with these radiographs?***

Radiation dose measuring is complex. The effective dose (absorbed dose corrected to compensate for the type of radiation and susceptibility of different tissues) is usually quoted. The effective dose from an intraoral radiograph (periapical or bitewing) is in the range of 0.001–0.008 milliSieverts (mSv) and for a panoramic is in the range 0.016–0.026 mSv.

■ ***As this does not mean much to most people, how can you reassure the patient?***

The patient can be reassured that the doses are very small and equivalent to a tiny fraction of the natural background radiation to which we are all exposed every day. If the patient wants to know actual figures then she should be told that the annual dose from background radiation varies around the world, but for example the average in the UK is 2.6 mSv and in the USA is 3.5 mSv. The dose from the radiographs required equates to approximately 16 hours of background radiation for an intraoral film or 2 days for a panoramic film.

■ ***The patient accepts this but points at the hazard warning sticker on your X-ray cubicle. What exactly are the risks?***

At these low absorbed doses there is only one significant risk, that of developing a malignant neoplasm. This is a very low frequency and completely random (*stochastic*) effect induced by damage to DNA.

The risk of developing malignancy from a periapical radiograph varies between 1 in 2 million to 1 in 20 million depending on the equipment used, the speed of the image receptor and the length of the exposure time.

For a panoramic radiograph the risk varies between 0.21 and 1.9 per million, again depending on the equipment used and the type and speed of the image receptor (film/screen combination or digital).

■ ***The patient wants to know how you ensure that she will receive the minimum dose of radiation necessary. What methods limit the dose to patients and how do they work?***

Methods of dose limitation can be divided into three groups as shown in Table 29.1.

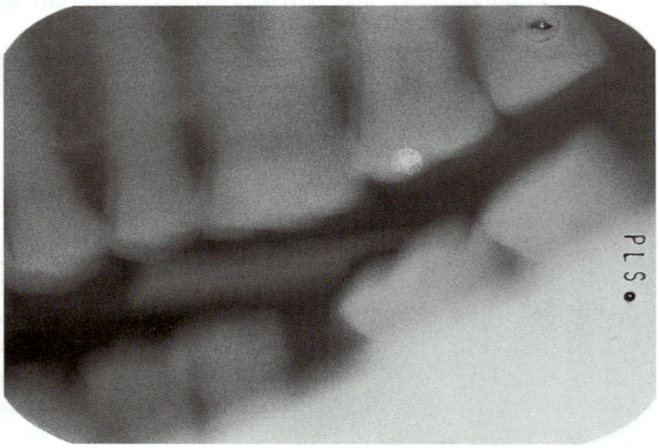

Fig. 29.4 Another bitewing film.

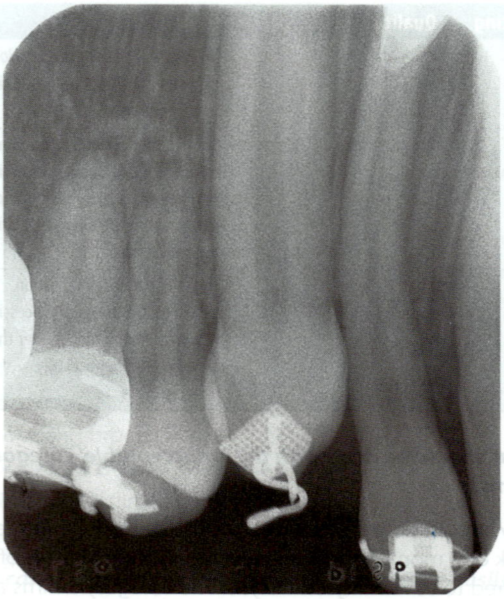

Fig. 29.5 Periapical film of upper canine.

What is wrong with the film in Figure 29.5?

The periapical image is geometrically distorted and has been elongated to such a degree that the apices of the lateral incisor and canine are not shown.

How might this error have been caused?

Error	Possible causes
Elongation	The film has been taken using the bisected angle technique and the X-ray tubehead has been positioned at too shallow an angle with respect to the teeth.
	The film could have been bent in the mouth by excessive pressure from the patient's finger supporting the film packet.

Why not use digital radiography?

The use of digital radiography has a number of advantages and one of the most important is that the sensors are much more sensitive than film, allowing a lower patient dose. Dose may be reduced by 50–90% depending on the system used. Images can also be assessed immediately for quality and may be manipulated digitally to extract useful diagnostic information from underexposed or overexposed images. Digital radiography is therefore in the patient's interest, but these advantages carry a financial cost and digital radiography is not yet universal in dentistry in the UK.

Where are the regulations governing dental radiography and radiology for UK dental practitioners published?

In the UK the 2001 *Guidance Notes for Dental Practitioners on the Safe Use of X-ray Equipment* is essential reading. This booklet brings together guidelines on good practice and the legislative requirements of the Ionising Radiations Regulations 1999 and the Ionising Radiation (Medical Exposure) Regulations 2000 (IR(ME)R 2000) as they apply to dentistry. These regulations encompass the principles of the International Commission on Radiological Protection (ICRP) of **Justification**, **Optimization** and **Limitation**.

Case 30

Whose fault this time?

SUMMARY

You seem to be having trouble communicating with the dental laboratory. How will you tackle the problems that have arisen?

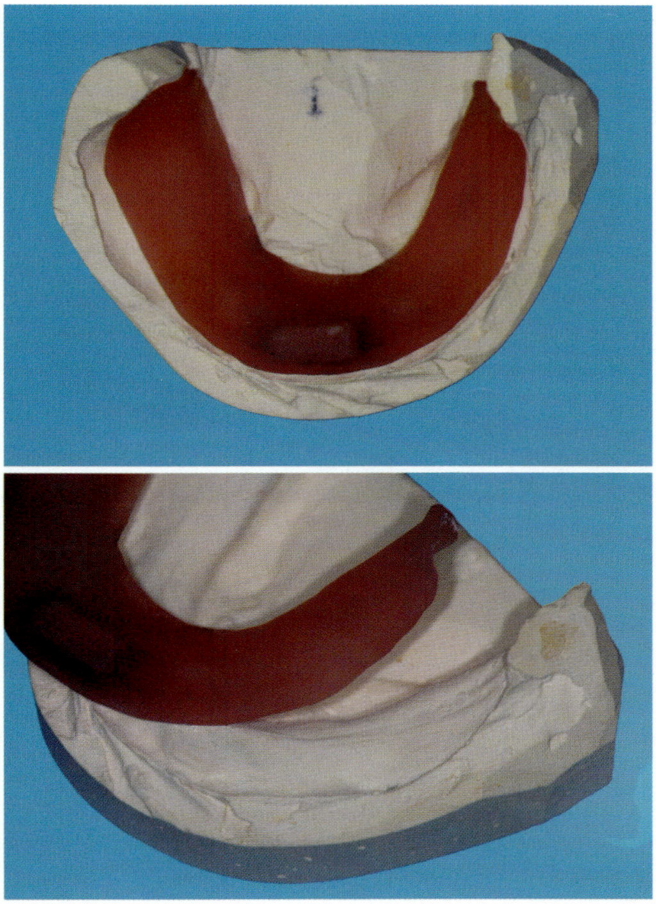

Fig. 30.1 The lower tray.

First patient

Complaint

Your nurse takes the special trays out of the laboratory package to record secondary impressions for an edentulous patient. They are not as special as you had intended.

History of complaint

You are constructing new complete dentures for a patient who has been a poor complete denture wearer. She has lost her lower denture and does not like the upper, so you have decided to make a new set from first principles rather than use a copy denture technique.

Primary impressions were recorded in stock trays adapted with silicone putty and covered with an alginate wash to record detail. You were going to take both upper and lower secondary impressions in close-fitting trays using zinc oxide and eugenol paste.

Diagnosis

- ***The lower special trays are shown in Figures 30.1 and 30.2. What is wrong?***

The tray is asymmetric: the extension on the patient's left is considerably shorter than that on the right. However, when you look at the cast you see that your impression was short in that area and the laboratory has extended the tray as much as possible. They are correct not to have extended it over the land area in this region. The result is that it is underextended on the left buccal shelf. This is important because the lower denture will need to be extended here to gain good support.

Conversely, the tray has been overextended onto the land area in the floor of mouth and this will need to be altered prior to recording a secondary impression.

- ***The upper special tray is shown in Figure 30.3. What is wrong?***

This shows a well-constructed special tray, but it has been perforated and spaced for an alginate secondary impression. The tray is properly extended but spaced trays always look slightly overextended on a primary model because it sits lower after the spacer has been removed. Your heart sinks.

You look at the laboratory request sheet to see what you prescribed and read:

'Please cast upper and lower primary impressions. Construct upper and lower special trays. N.B. lower close fitting for ZoE [zinc oxide and eugenol].'

Your diagnosis is poor communication. Many dentists and clinical dental technicians (CDTs) use alginate in a spaced tray for upper impressions. You had expected that the lab would assume that if one tray was close-fitting, then the other one would be too. You make a note to be more careful in future.

Solutions

What can you do to save the patient a further appointment and yourself the additional cost of extra trays?

Table 30.1 Upper-tray solutions

Possible solution	Disadvantages
Record the impression as planned with either zinc oxide and eugenol paste or an elastomeric material such as a medium-bodied addition-cured silicone	Will be impossible or certainly very messy to try
Record the impression with alginate	It is difficult to control the thickness of the rolled border with alginate. Unless you are using a modern 5-day-stable alginate, impressions need to be cast as soon as possible. Provided you use this material, this would be the best solution
Block perforations with composition or cold curing acrylic	Time-consuming but the tray would still have the wrong spacing for zinc oxide
Have a new tray made	Technically the best solution, but there are time and cost implications for the patient and you

What you can do about the upper tray?

There are a number of options but all have problems (Table 30.1). The only alternative would be to request a new tray.

What you can do about the lower tray?

This has one laboratory fault (overextension) and one fault resulting from your original impression (underextension). Again, you could take a new primary impression and request new special trays, but the lower tray is more easily dealt with. The best solution is to extend your tray in the buccal shelf using a material such as green or pink stick composition (pink is much easier to use as it flows at mouth temperature). The lingual overextension can be trimmed back with a bur to the correct extension, which is marked as a black line on the undersurface in the upper panel of Figure 30.2.

What else should you check before trying to adapt the trays?

The extension should be checked in the patient's mouth to ensure other areas are correct. Other common errors in tray construction relate to handle design. You need to check the handles to ensure they are properly constructed. Prosthodontists can become excited about tray handles but there are no absolute rules on what can and cannot be used. However, some tray handle designs could cause you and your patient problems.

Are these handles suitable?

From the appearances in Figures 30.1–30.3 the laboratory has provided well-made and designed handles. Faults to look for are shown in Figure 30.4. Can you identify them and the reasons why they are deficient?

The left and central images shown in Figure 30.4 show the same tray that has been poorly constructed. The handle will almost certainly get in the way of the lower lip, risking displacement during use and distortion of the sulcus. As you are aware, complete dentures develop retention from a

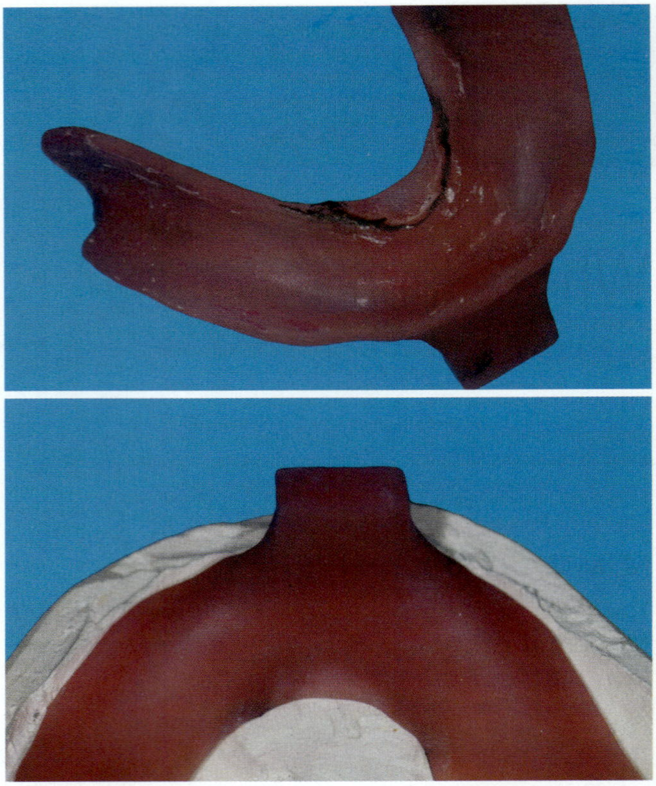

Fig. 30.2 The lower tray.

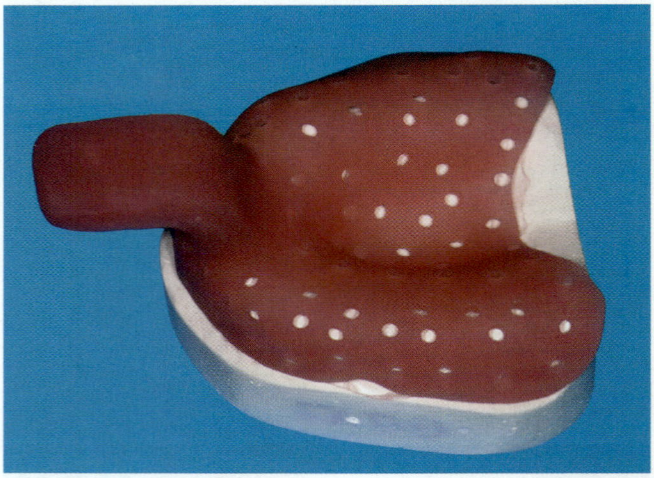

Fig. 30.3 The upper tray.

correct border seal and this might be more difficult to achieve in the master impression if the tray handle distorts the lips. This fault usually arises because the tray is left sitting on the bench before light curing, during which time the handle sags under the influence of gravity. A stub handle would be better, as seen in Figure 30.1.

The handle also deviates from the midline so that it will be very difficult for the user to centre and seat the tray without the handle as a guide. This would certainly be the case with a spaced perforated upper alginate special tray.

In the image on the right, the handle has fallen off. This is because the light-cured materials were not processed in the

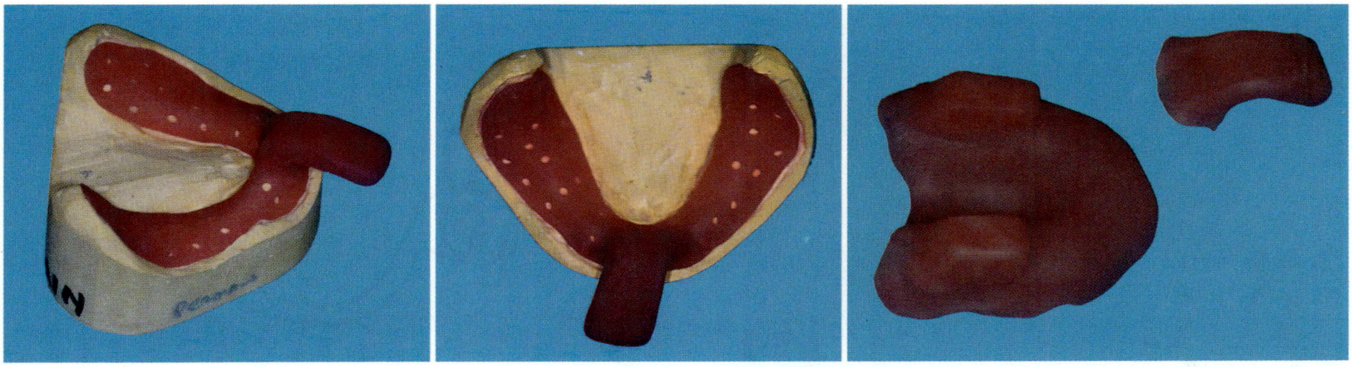

Fig. 30.4 Potential handle faults.

light box at the same time. Using this type of material a handle cannot be added at a later stage without using a special adhesive because the material has a high filler content. It is unlikely that you would have this adhesive in your surgery. This problem may only come to light when removing the impression. A well-recorded impression is normally very retentive and it can be embarrassingly difficult to remove without a strong handle.

Also the technician has placed posterior stub handles. These are not normally used on maxillary trays and have no advantage there. Their sole advantage is to help prevent the clinician's fingers from distorting the buccal sulcus when taking impressions of an edentulous lower ridge.

The next patient

SUMMARY

You are constructing a new complete denture over a lower metal-based partial denture for a 52-year-old male when things start to go wrong. How will you rectify the mistakes?

History

Complaint

The patient dislikes the worn appearance of the upper anterior teeth on his complete denture and complains that it is becoming loose.

History of complaint

The patient lost all his upper teeth due to decay in his late 20s and early 30s despite extensive dental care. He has had five dentures over a 20-year period and managed with them fairly well. The current lower metal-based partial denture was his first partial denture. He dislikes the back of the denture lifting up in function but copes reluctantly.

Examination

The upper complete denture lacks retention and no peripheral seal is evident when seated. There is some wear of the anterior teeth.

The lower partial denture has wear on the prosthetic teeth and they are no longer in occlusal contact. The patient has an inadequate posterior occlusion (posterior support).

Solution

■ *What will you prescribe?*

Both dentures must be replaced. Relining the upper denture is pointless if the teeth are worn. The lower partial denture needs replacing because it is not retentive and is worn. The posterior occlusion will have to be reconstructed with two new dentures, as neither is currently correct.

Replacing the upper denture alone might cure the cosmetic problem. However, lower natural teeth occluding against a complete denture with no lower partial or with worn teeth will accelerate alveolar bone loss and risk formation of a fibrous ridge ('flabby ridge').

You decide to construct a new metal-based partial denture for the lower arch and a new complete upper denture using a copy denture technique.

■ *In what order do you plan to provide this dental care? Why?*

It would be best to start with the metal-based partial denture first. If the copy technique for the upper denture goes to plan, five visits will be required. If the metal-based partial denture goes to plan, even ignoring the altered cast technique, it will require six visits. Some laboratories prefer 3 weeks to make a metal framework and you do not want to be recording the definitive upper impression too early in the treatment schedule.

The most efficient plan is shown in Table 30.2.

Treatment

The metal framework is shown in Figure 30.5. It looks beautiful and fits the model well. Everything seems to be going according to plan until you notice that the lab seems to have omitted the cingulum rest and minor connector for the lower left canine.

Before reaching for the phone to call the lab and complain, you look at the design that you sketched on the prescription card, shown in Figure 30.5.

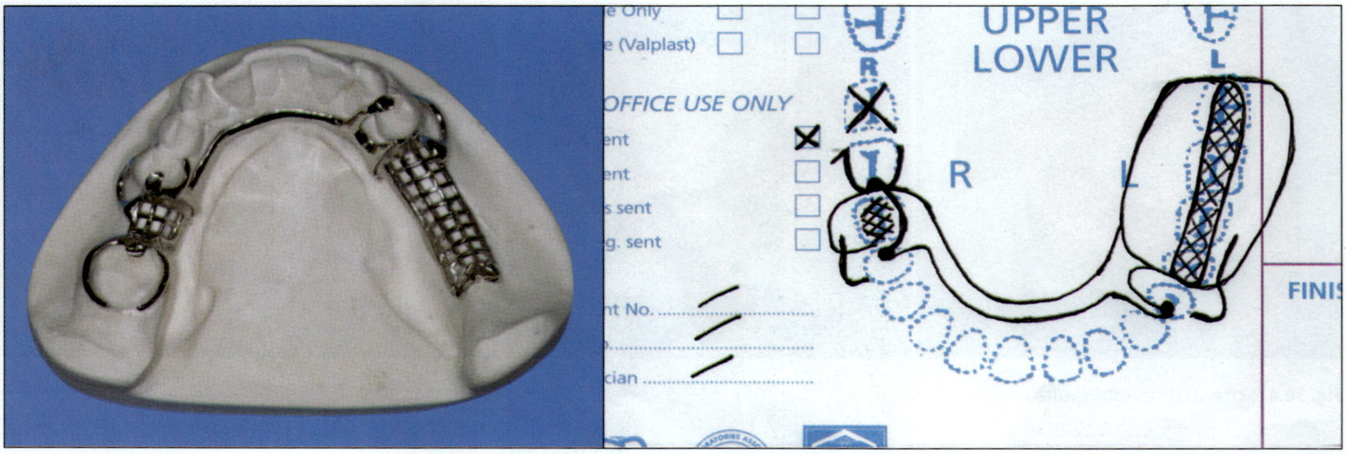

Fig. 30.5 **A** The framework back from the laboratory and **B** your original instructions.

Table 30.2 Dental care plan

Visit	Complete upper copy denture	Metal-based lower partial denture
1	Copy dentures in silicone putty and send to the laboratory	Primary impressions model and design
2		Tooth preparations and secondary impressions
3		Metal try-in and optional altered cast technique impression
4	Secondary impressions and jaw registration	Definitive jaw registration
5	Wax try-in	Wax try-in
6	Fit	Fit
7	Review	Review

■ *Is anything wrong with your prescription? If so, what?*

There are several errors:

- You have mixed up left and right, producing a mirror-image prescription – easily done if you look at an impression to help with the design.
- You have omitted to draw a cingulum rest and minor connector to the lower left canine.
- No reciprocal has been indicated for the clasp on the lower left second premolar, next to the bounded saddle. Luckily the laboratory has realised this and has put a reciprocal on the framework.

■ *Will these design faults cause problems? Why?*

Yes, probably. The patient is not keen on wearing a lower partial denture and complains of lifting of the free end (distal extension) saddle. The cingulum rest on the canine provides indirect retention (see problem 54) against this movement. As well as causing problems in function, the saddle lifting posteriorly would cause the lingual bar, which lacks support from the anterior teeth, to impinge on the soft tissues. This would cause soreness under the major connector.

■ *What can you do to rectify these errors?*

There are four options:

1. **Ignore the indirect retention** on the basis that there is good direct retention with three clasps. If the framework fits it might be possible to take a chance and go ahead. If this works you will owe the lab thanks for remembering the reciprocal because this contributes significantly to the overall retention by ensuring that the clasp is guided, reciprocated and engaged.
2. **Have a separate rest and connector cast** and ask the lab to try to laser weld that on. This is difficult, carries a cost implication and the fit might not be very satisfactory. It carries a risk of failure.
3. **Make a new framework** on the existing master cast, if it has not yet been disposed of or damaged in any way.
4. **Record a new secondary impression** and make a new framework – the optimum clinical solution, but with cost and time implications.

As the patient is already waiting, you decide at least to try-in the framework. If it does not fit, the option of adding an indirect retainer is not practical.

■ *How do you decide whether the framework fits?*

Check systematically that:

1. the rest seats are fully seated
2. there are no gaps between the soft tissues and the major connector
3. there is not an anterior–posterior or lateral rock
4. clasps and reciprocals are in close contact with the teeth
5. guide planes provide a clear single path of insertion
6. clasp tips engage in undercuts.

Bear in mind that the saddle is not supported with acrylic resin under the mesh and that if you place vertical force on the saddle at this stage the framework will lift anteriorly, even if it fits well.

When you seat the framework it seems to fit well and it appears that you may be able to adapt it. Confidently, you ask the patient how the framework feels. Unfortunately he says it is lifting at the back, and on both sides, not just the side with the distal extension saddle. Closer inspection reveals that the clasp on the lower left second molar is not providing any retention.

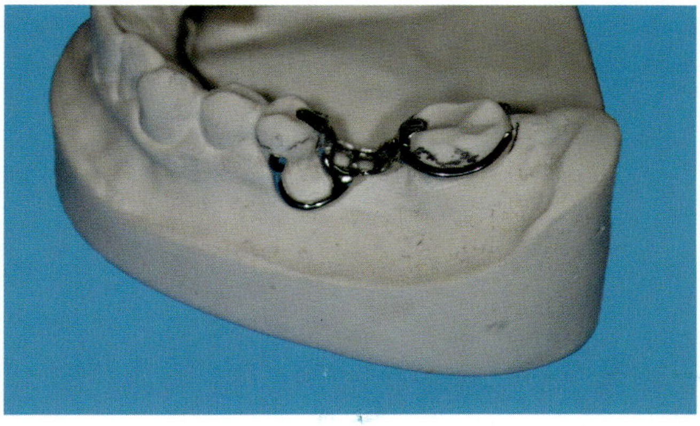

Fig. 30.6 The molar clasp.

A close-up of the clasp is shown in Figure 30.6. What is wrong?

Lack of retention indicates that the clasp tip is not in an undercut relative to the path of insertion. The fault could lie with the construction of the clasp or the lack of undercut relative to the path of insertion.

There is a design fault in the molar clasp. The clasp arm ***starts*** below the survey line and is therefore in the undercut relative to the path of insertion. The clasp tip is in contact with the tooth but above the survey line, which lies at the level of gingival margin. In such situations the clasp is usually so inflexible in the first third that it is impossible to seat the frame work in that area.

This cannot be sorted out in the surgery. You warn the patient that a new impression and framework will probably be required.

How will you take this up with the laboratory?

If you have a good dental laboratory, you cannot afford to lose its confidence or support. You will be aware that metal-based dentures have to be designed using a team approach, especially if you are not an expert (see problem 54).

You are responsible for the several prescription errors, which contribute significantly to the failure of the framework. Conversely, if the laboratory had phoned to query the design faults, they might have been rectified.

You should already have a service level agreement with the laboratory, specifying what each party expects and provides. The laboratory will expect you to provide:

- Patient identification
- An accurate legible prescription
- Identification of teeth with poor short- and long-term prognosis
- Dates that stages are required back in the surgery
- Accurate and correctly extended impressions
- Adherence to accepted infection control procedures.

In return you will expect the laboratory to contact you if they have any advice about your design or consider that it could be improved. You would expect them to contact you before changing your design and you must be happy to take calls as often as necessary for minor queries.

The agreement should include what to do in the event of errors and provides a basis for negotiating a fair solution. Errors will arise, but often both parties will need to take some responsibility for them.

Unless you have a surveyor in your practice, you would not have been able to identify that there is no undercut on the distal aspect of the tooth. The dental technician should have pointed out that a better solution would be a circumferential ring clasp, engaging the mesiolingual undercut from the distal aspect. This is exactly the sort of potential problem that is easily solved by good communication.

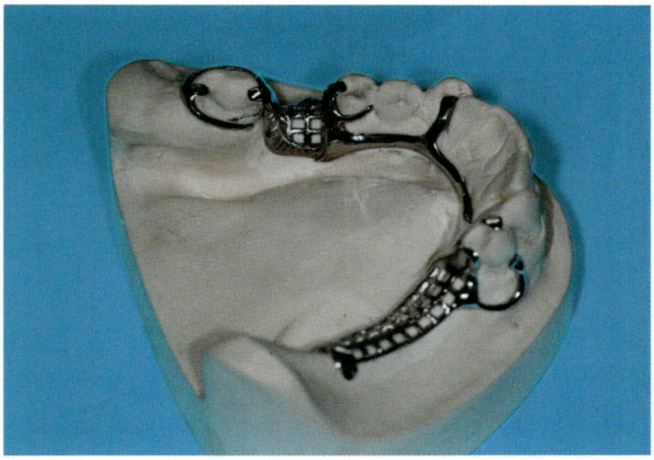

Fig. 30.7 The new framework.

What is the optimum design for this framework?

Following discussion with the laboratory, and a resolution to improve communication on both sides, the laboratory manager offers to make the framework again free of charge. This is a welcome and significant gesture of good will.

The final framework is shown in Figure 30.7.

The rest on the lower left canine provides indirect retention and the circumferential clasp of the lower left second molar now engages an undercut from above the survey line. This design is likely to be successful, though it is not necessarily the single best solution. All designs are compromises between mechanical properties, patient acceptability, reducing the damaging potential of the prosthesis and the cost.

Acknowledgement

We are grateful to PWS Direct Ltd, Bolton, for the examples of correct and incorrect laboratory work specially prepared for this problem.

Case • 31

Ouch!

SUMMARY

You sustain a substantial percutaneous injury to your foot. What should you do?

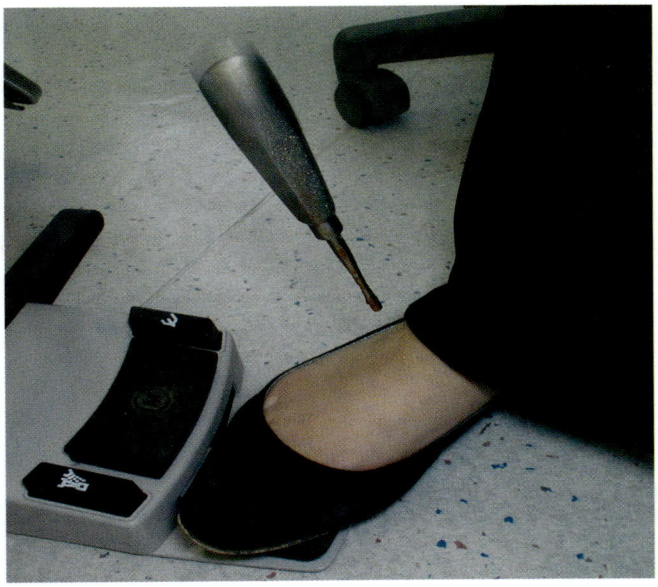

Fig. 31.1 Murphy's law in action. Nice shoes.

History

You are extracting a difficult tooth and have used a luxator to loosen the tooth prior to elevation. While transferring the luxator to the bracket table, you drop it. The luxator impales itself in your foot.

■ *What diseases of significance may be transferred by the injury?*

Most infectious diseases can be transmitted by a sharps injury but the main concerns are hepatitis B, hepatitis C and human immunodeficiency virus (HIV) infection.

■ *What would you do immediately?*

Encourage bleeding at the injury site and wash it with soap and water but without scrubbing. Antiseptics should not be used as their effects on the local defence mechanisms are unknown. Free bleeding should be encouraged.

■ *What is the most urgent priority and why?*

The most urgent priority is to assess whether there is a significant risk of transmission of HIV infection. Postexposure prophylaxis (PEP) with antiretroviral drugs can significantly reduce the chance of transmission of HIV, but for maximum effectiveness it is recommended that it is administered within 1 hour, and certainly within a few hours. The reduction in risk may be as high as 81%. There is limited evidence that some protection of transmission is still given if the administration of the PEP is delayed, even by as much as 48–72 hours.

■ *How could you obtain postexposure prophylaxis if required?*

The Health Act 2006 requires that every NHS employer has a policy on the management of exposure to blood or other bodily fluids. The policy must ensure that advice is available 24 hours a day.

PEP is only available following a formal risk assessment for each individual injury. This involves determining the severity of the injury and the risk that the patient is carrying HIV infection.

The procedure for obtaining a formal risk assessment varies with local circumstances. In hospitals, the infection control consultant(s), hospital casualty or occupational health department will perform the risk assessment and provide the appropriate medication. Those in general practice must contact their local hospital casualty department who will follow their local guidelines. Each dental practitioner should know the contact number and name/position of the appropriate person.

When you phone you will be asked details of the injury and patient. You will then be told whether or not the injury is sufficient to carry a risk of transmission and whether a risk assessment of the patient is required.

■ *What is the risk of developing HIV infection following a sharps injury?*

The average risk for transmission of HIV is estimated at 3 infections per 1000 injuries.

■ *What factors affect the risk of transmission?*

An increased risk of occupationally acquired HIV infection is associated with:

- A deep injury
- Visible blood on the device that caused the injury
- Injury with a needle that has been in a blood vessel
- A high viral load in the source patient.

The risk from a needlestick injury where the needle has been used to administer a local analgesic is therefore lower as the needle would not be expected to have been placed in a blood vessel if an aspirating syringe was used. PEP is therefore often unnecessary for a needlestick injury from a dental anaesthetic needle.

Splashes of infected blood carry a low risk. Splashes on to broken skin or mucous membranes, including the eye, carry a risk of transmission estimated at being less than 0.1%. It is considered that there is no risk of transmission from a splash of blood on to intact skin.

The viral load is a measure of the virus concentration in the blood. It is higher during the primary infection (the so-called window period), reduces with early infection but then rises with symptomatic and late-stage infection (acquired immunodeficiency syndrome: AIDS). It is reduced with effective treatment.

Your injury is a deep injury by a sharp instrument covered with blood and therefore there is a risk of transmission of HIV.

The patient has returned to the waiting room with your nurse. What will you say and do?

You should explain to the patient exactly what has happened and that there has been an accident involving a surgical instrument and that there is a practice policy, derived from national policy, that should be carried out when this happens. Introducing the HIV assessment of the patient in this way depersonalizes the incident and avoids making difficult judgements, and discriminating against perceived 'high-risk' groups for HIV infection. If the policy is written and shown to the patient then this can prevent the patient feeling discriminated against.

The patient should be asked to give informed consent for blood to be taken and tested for HIV, hepatitis B and hepatitis C and for storage of serum. If infection is transmitted, it will be necessary to compare the patient's sample and the sample of your blood for industrial injury benefit or insurance purposes.

Lengthy pretest counselling is now no longer a requirement prior to testing for HIV. It is only necessary to provide it if the patient requests it or needs it. The benefits of testing to both the dentist and the patient should be stressed. If the patient has an undiagnosed HIV infection then an earlier diagnosis is more likely to lead to effective treatment, and the dentist can have the most effective prophylaxis to prevent transmission. Most patients will be happy to give a sample of their blood under these circumstances. If not, then the reason for the refusal should be explored as sensitively as possible. It may be that patients have an inaccurate idea that they have in some way done something illegal or hold a false belief about the virus itself.

The general population have little knowledge of hepatitis but understand that it is a serious disease and may be aware that it can be transmitted sexually. As a minimum, blood should be obtained to store the serum in case testing is required at a later date.

The dentist will most likely not have the facilities to take the blood and the patient can be asked to go to his or her general medical practitioner with a request or to attend the local Accident and Emergency department. If the dentist does carry out the test then the patient should collect the results from the general medical practitioner.

The possibility that the patient might be HIV-positive will have to be addressed in order to assess the risk of transmission. This must be done in a sensitive manner, preferably in a quiet room and with reassurance about the confidentiality of any answers given. The questions should not be asked by the recipient of the needlestick injury because it is difficult to be objective if you are feeling anxious or distressed. However, in dental practice there may be no other person to handle this issue and you may have to ask the questions yourself. As an alternative you could consider asking the patient to speak on the phone to the local casualty officer responsible for the PEP, sexual health clinic medical staff, a sexual health counsellor or other experienced person.

You should remember that it is not the risk factor that denotes the risk of transmission but how the activity takes place which dictates the relative risk (Table 31.1).

Table 31.1 Risk factors for human immunodeficiency virus (HIV) infection

Type of risk	Risk factor	Relative risk
Parental infection	Transfusion	There is a small risk of infection to recipients of blood transfusion given between the middle 1970s and 1987. Most of those exposed will already have developed the infection and there is a very small risk for those who are not positive. Donor screening since 1987 has reduced this risk to a minimal level
	Haemophilia	Recipients of factor VIII-containing blood products before 1985 had a high risk of infection – almost 80%. Most of those exposed will already have developed the infection and there is a very small risk for those who are not positive. All UK factor VIII sources are now screened
	Injecting drug users (IDUs)	The risk depends on whether the needle is shared and how much contamination occurs. Needle exchange programmes have reduced the incidence of HIV in IDUs. Prisoners who are IDUs without access to needle exchange programmes represent a high-risk group for acquiring HIV
	Needlestick injury	The risk is 0.3%, but depends on the type of injury, volume of blood transmitted and the infectivity of the blood
Sexually transmitted infection	Vaginal intercourse	A risk to both partners but greater for the female. Properly lubricated condoms offer good protection
	Prostitution	Unprotected intercourse with a prostitute is a high-risk practice, but the risk varies greatly in different parts of the world
	Oral sex	Transmission has been documented but the risk is considered lower than for vaginal sex
	Anal intercourse	The highest-risk sexual activity. Condoms reduce risk but failure is common. Prisoners may have consensual or coerced sex and lack of access to condoms means they represent a high-risk group for acquiring HIV

What questions would you ask?

- Are you a regular blood donor in the UK? (Blood donations are screened for hepatitis B and C, and HIV. The rate of new infections among repeat blood donors in 2007 was 1 in 100 000 in the UK.)
- Have you ever had a blood donation refused?
- Have you ever been diagnosed with hepatitis B or C, or HIV?
- Have you ever lived in HIV high-prevalence areas such as Africa or Asia?
- Have you ever had a blood transfusion or surgery abroad?
- Have you ever had an injury when you have been exposed to someone else's blood?
- Have you ever injected drugs into a vein?
- Have you ever been to prison?
- Do you have sex without using a condom?

A positive answer to any of these questions requires further questioning to understand the degree of risk of acquiring HIV through the activity. In practice, asking these questions does not usually constitute a problem as in almost all cases there will be either no risk or a very low risk. Similarly, most HIV-positive individuals will disclose the information readily in this situation.

What are the risk factors for contracting HIV infection?

In the UK, in 2007, an estimated 55% of persons with a new diagnosis of HIV infection acquired it through heterosexual contact and 41% through men who have sex with men (MSM). The number of diagnoses acquired through injecting drug use and mother-to-child transmission has remained low over the last 5 years. Of the heterosexual-acquired infections, 77% were probably infected abroad with the vast majority from contacts from sub-Saharan Africa. However, of the MSM diagnoses, 82% probably acquired their infection in the UK.

If the patient discloses that he or she is HIV-positive, what information would you like to know? What is the significance of the answers?

Answers and significance are shown in Table 31.2. The answers to these questions would be invaluable to the person making the risk assessment.

If the patient indicates that he or she is not HIV-positive but agrees to an HIV test, can you carry it out?

Yes, UK National Guidelines for HIV Testing 2008 say that it should be within the competence of any trained health care worker to obtain consent and conduct an HIV test.

If you do not have the facilities to perform the test then you can ask the patient's general medical practitioner or the local on-call health professional who has been designated to carry out risk assessments, advice and provision of PEP. The result of the test should be given back to the patent by a person qualified to answer any initial questions that the patient might have and who has knowledge of the local specialist services for a prompt referral. This is often the patient's general medical practitioner.

Table 31.2 Information from human immunodeficiency virus (HIV)-positive patients and its significance

Information	Significance
Whether patients are generally well	Patients with asymptomatic HIV infection have low viral load and lower infectivity
Their CD4 (T-helper cell) count	An indicator of immunosuppression, the stage of disease and effectiveness of treatment
Their viral load and when it was last checked	A direct measure of infectivity
The names of any medications they are taking	The same drugs would be avoided for postexposure prophylaxis if they are not being effective in the patient
Whether their medication has changed recently and why	Recent changes in medication may indicate their strain of HIV becoming drug-resistant and this must be taken into account in choosing the drugs for postexposure prophylaxis
The address of the patient's HIV clinic	To contact for further information. Obtain consent to do this and respect the patient's confidentiality

What is PEP? Why not simply take the drugs regardless of the relative risk?

PEP is preventive treatment started immediately after exposure to an agent that causes infection. The regimes for PEP following HIV infection are complex. New drugs are being developed and knowledge is continually acquired about HIV and the emergence of drug-resistant strains. This, along with the desire to reduce side-effects of PEP to increase compliance, means that the regime for PEP is constantly under review. At the time of writing (2009) the regime includes a combination of tenofovir, emtricitabine, lopinavir and ritonavir. This is continued for 4 weeks.

The side-effects of these drugs include nausea, diarrhoea, dizziness, headache, muscle weakness and skin rash. These effects can be debilitating and automatic prophylaxis for every sharps injury cannot be advocated. Pregnancy is not a contraindication for PEP but the evidence for its safe use is limited.

What if the patient indicates a risk of HIV infection to you but you cannot obtain a formal risk assessment within 1 hour?

You should not delay starting PEP while awaiting either a formal risk assessment or the testing of the patient's sample of blood. PEP is at its most effective within the first few hours, and preferably the first hour.

Do I have to give a blood sample for testing?

You will be asked to give a blood sample for storage of serum. This is because you may need to prove that infection was not present at the time of the injury. If the patient is subsequently shown to have an infection, you will be asked to provide a sample for testing 12 weeks (as a minimum) after the injury, or cessation of PEP if it was prescribed.

What is the risk of transmission of hepatitis B by this injury?

This should be minimal. All members of the dental team should be vaccinated against hepatitis B. Once they have achieved a satisfactory antibody response of 100 mIU/ml to the vaccine, a single booster is given after 5 years. Non-responders will receive anti-hepatitis B immunoglobulin on an occupational exposure. If recent evidence of the effectiveness of the recipient's vaccination is not available, the recipient should have his or her antibody titre checked.

If the recipient is not immune, the risk of transmission has been estimated at 30% if the patient is e antigen-positive. Infection can follow transmission of as little as 0.1 ml of blood. Hepatitis B is so infectious that the degree of injury is almost immaterial. In the unlikely event that a non-immunized individual receives a sharps injury, specific hepatitis B immunoglobulin provides passive immunity and can give immediate but temporary protection after accidental inoculation or contamination with hepatitis B-infected blood.

Does this mean I have to give blood even if I know that my hepatitis B vaccination is successful?

Yes. Even if the patient is of very low risk for having HIV, you must also ensure that your serum is stored, because you may need to show that hepatitis infection was not present at the time of injury.

How can you determine whether the patient is infectious for hepatitis B?

Blood must be screened for hepatitis B antigens and antibodies (Table 31.3).

What is the risk of contracting hepatitis C?

The risk of contracting hepatitis C through a needlestick injury is 3% if the donor is infected. This risk is therefore higher than for HIV infection but, as for HIV infection, is dependent on the amount of virus present in the blood. The consequences can be severe. As many as 75% of individuals who become infected will become chronic carriers. Of these, 20% will go on to develop cirrhosis, liver cancer or liver failure.

It is estimated that 4 in 1000 individuals in England in the 15–59-years age group is infected with hepatitis C. The majority remain undiagnosed. The prevalence of hepatitis C in intravenous drug users has been estimated to be between 3 and 42%.

Is prophylaxis against hepatitis C available?

No PEP is available. However, early treatment of acute hepatitis C infection may prevent chronic hepatitis C infection.

How may the risk of needlestick or sharps injury in the dental setting be minimized?

Sharps injuries do not always result from needles. Burs, hand instruments (as you have just found out) and other contaminated sharps all constitute a risk. You should:

- Ensure that all the dental team are trained in the disposal of sharps.
- Identify and dispose of needles and other sharps immediately after use.
- *Always* pass instruments with the sharp end pointing away from any person.
- Remove burs and ultrasonic tips from handpieces immediately after use.
- Pick up instruments individually.
- Retract the patient's cheek with a mirror while administering local analgesia.
- Never resheath a needle holding the sheath in a hand: use a one-handed technique (Figure 31.2) or dispose of the needle immediately.
- Never ever place your finger, or your assistant's finger, in front of a sharp instrument, such as a scalpel or luxator.
- Always use a firm finger rest while scaling.
- Dispose of sharps into a solid container (approved to BS 7320).
- Ensure that sharps are disposed of by incineration and by an authorized person registered to collect such waste.
- Use heavy-duty gloves when cleaning instruments prior to autoclaving.
- Keep your working area well organized and uncluttered with sharps in a separate area. Do not place waste material such as swabs or tissues over instruments.

Table 31.3 Hepatitis B antigens and antibodies and their significance

Antigen or antibody	When found	Significance for infectivity
HBs (surface) antigen or 'Australia' antigen	Becomes detectable in late incubation and is present during acute hepatitis. Declines over 3–6 months but persists in carriers, whether asymptomatic or with chronic active hepatitis	Indicates infectivity, though not necessarily a high infectivity
Antibody to HBs (surface) antigen	Seen in recovery, reflecting immunity against the virus. Also found in those immunized against hepatitis B	Probably indicates no risk of infection. Denotes past exposure and immunity (including by active vaccination) to the virus and a possible need for further investigation to determine infectivity
HBc (core) antigen	Only present in the liver; not used for determining infectivity	
Antibody to HBc antigen	Found in acute disease, recovery and in carriers, whether asymptomatic or with chronic active hepatitis	Indicates past infection but a high level indicates an infection risk
HBe (envelope) antigen	Becomes detectable in late incubation and is present during acute hepatitis. Persists in carriers with chronic active hepatitis but not usually in asymptomatic carriers	Indicates acute infection or a carrier state of high infectivity
Antibody to HBe antigen	Develops as Hbe disappears. Sometimes persists in chronic asymptomatic carriers	Indicates either recovery from acute infection or a carrier state of low infectivity

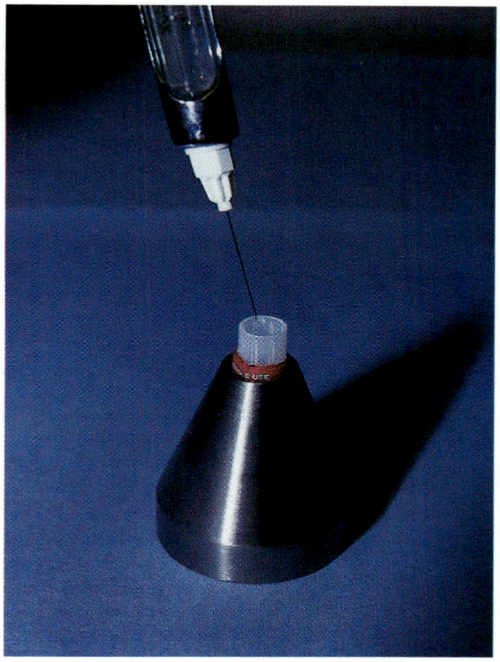

Fig. 31.2 A simple needle sheath holder. The holder is not intended to hold the syringe upright, only to hold the sheath during resheathing.

- Always wear appropriate masks, visors or protective eye protection. Modern minimalist designer glasses offer little protection.
- Footwear should cover the top of the foot. You would not have a problem today if you had worn footwear appropriate for the dental surgery.

■ ***What is your last duty before you can turn your back on this unfortunate episode?***

You must remember to fill in an incident report as required by law (the Reporting of Injuries, Disease and Dangerous Occurrences Regulations 1995) and submit it to the Health and Safety Executive. This will be important evidence for industrial injury benefit or insurance purposes, together with the records in your notes.

■ ***This injury has ruined your day. This has all proved so complex that next time you might just wash the injury and ignore it. Why not?***

The main reason is the worry that you might contract HIV infection from an unsuspected carrier. The effectiveness of PEP – reducing the risk of transmission by over 80% – cannot be ignored. Also, it would be unethical for a dentist not to follow up the possibility of developing an infection which could jeopardize the wellbeing of his or her patients. There would also be a risk of transmission to the dentist's sexual partner(s).

Case • 32

A swollen face and pericoronitis

SUMMARY

A 23-year-old woman presents in your hospital casualty department with a painful swelling of the right side of the face and neck. What is the cause and what treatment would you provide?

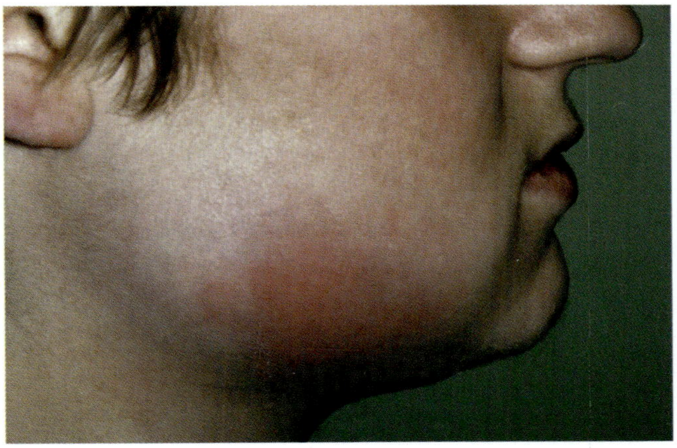

Fig. 32.1 The patient on presentation.

Further information on the diagnosis of soft tissue infection will be found in case 49.

History

History of complaint

The patient has suffered worsening pain 'from her wisdom tooth' on the lower right side for 5 days. There has been some swelling of the gum around the tooth and she has been unable to bite together for a couple of days. Yesterday she noticed pain in the floor of her mouth and found that moving her tongue was painful. Today she awoke to find the facial swelling, she feels unwell and has difficulty eating, swallowing and opening her mouth.

She had an episode of pericoronitis a few months ago and is on her local hospital waiting list to have all third molars extracted. Until the swelling developed, she thought this was just another attack of pain from her wisdom teeth. She has not had facial swelling before and has come straight to hospital.

Medical history

The patient is otherwise fit and well.

Examination

Extraoral examination

There are palpable tender lymph nodes in the upper deep cervical chain and submandibular triangle. Opening is limited to 15 mm interincisal distance.

There is swelling below and around the lower border and angle of the mandible and extending back towards the neck. The swelling is hot, tender and very firm and a dusky red colour centrally. The swelling is not pointing to the skin. There is a marked halitosis.

Intraoral examination

Trismus hampers examination. The lower right third molar can be seen to be partially erupted, the operculum is swollen and pus exudes from below it on gentle probing. The second and third molars appear caries-free.

The floor of the mouth is very tender and firm on the right side.

■ ***What additional examinations or investigations would you perform? Explain why.***

It is extremely important to take the patient's temperature to determine whether the infection is exerting systemic effects.

She has a temperature of 37.8°C (normal temperature 36.8°C) and is, therefore, pyrexic.

There is a need to confirm that pericoronitis is the cause. It would be prudent to exclude the possibility that this is infection from a nonvital molar and tests of vitality should be performed. If there were a suggestion from the examination that a lower molar was nonvital, a radiograph might be indicated, otherwise radiographs would provide little useful information for diagnosis unless another lesion were present.

Diagnosis

■ ***What do these findings tell you?***

The combination of inflammation (swelling, pain, redness and heat) together with local lymphadenitis and pus seen intraorally indicate an infection. Pericoronitis is present and this appears to be the primary source of the infection. Trismus is an important sign, indicating that the infection or inflammation has spread to involve the muscles of mastication.

The patient is pyrexic and feels unwell. These features indicate that the infection is exerting a systemic effect. Infection appears to be spreading relatively fast because the swelling has appeared overnight and there are already systemic signs.

■ ***Which type of infection is this?***

It is difficult to tell because the tissues involved are deeply sited. Pus is draining from under the operculum indicating abscess formation, but this might extend into a soft tissue space or be limited to the tissues around the unerupted tooth. The rapid spread, firmness and tenderness of the tissues ('brawny' swelling) indicate cellulitis. This might continue to spread or develop into an abscess. There is probably a mixed infection with a local pericoronal abscess and a spreading cellulitis.

To which tissue spaces may infection spread from a lower third molar? What are the boundaries of these spaces?

Pus from lower third molars may track to many spaces and spread is unpredictable, depending on many factors including the angulation of the tooth, the size of the follicle, relationship to the second molar, degree of bone loss around both teeth and the anatomical relationships between the teeth, bone and muscle attachments in the region. Pus may drain into the mouth from under an operculum, into the buccal or lingual sulcus or into one or more tissue spaces. The routes of spread to tissue spaces are shown in Figure 32.2 and are described in Table 32.1.

In what tissue spaces is the present infection tracking and why?

This swelling appears to be in the submandibular space. The main infected tissue is not visible and lies around the submandibular gland deep to the body of the mandible. The swelling just spreads round the lower border of the mandible onto the face. Moderate trismus is typical. It is relatively common for this tissue space to be involved in pericoronitis.

There may well be early sublingual space involvement. Infection readily tracks between the submandibular and sublingual spaces around the submandibular gland and posterior edge of mylohyoid. In addition infection may spread through mylohyoid which is thin, perforated by blood vessels and a poor barrier to spread of infection. There is not yet an established sublingual space infection because this would cause extensive floor of mouth swelling and deflect and limit movement of the tongue. Swelling from sublingual space infection would be readily visible in the lingual sulcus but causes considerable oedema in the loose tissues rather than the firmness and tenderness seen in this patient.

Pus from lower third molars tends to perforate the lingual plate because it is closer and thinner than the buccal plate.

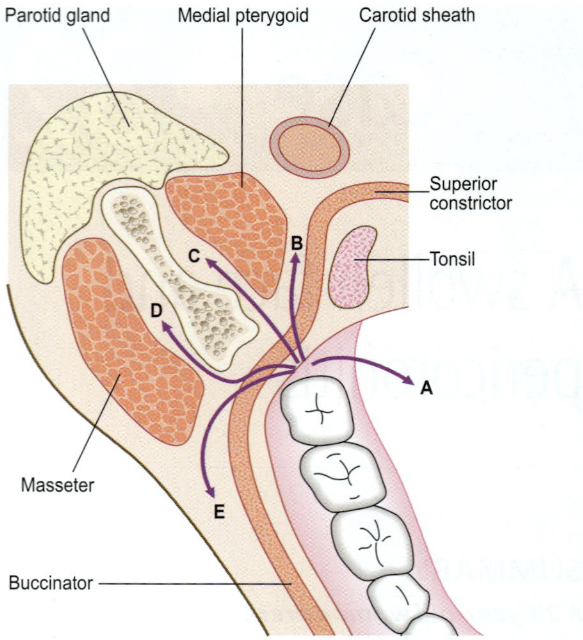

Fig. 32.2 Paths of spread of infection into tissue spaces from third molars: **A**, into the sublingual and submandibular space; **B**, into the parapharyngeal space; **C**, into the pterygomandibular space leading to the infratemporal fossa; **D**, into the submasseteric space; **E**, into the buccal space.

Infection is deflected to either the sublingual or submandibular space by the attachment of the mylohyoid muscle.

Is this a potentially life-threatening infection?

No, but it is serious. The patient's airway will be at risk if the infection continues to spread posteriorly. This would be potentially fatal and dyspnoea may develop unexpectedly and with great rapidity. Vigorous treatment of the infection must be commenced immediately.

What is Ludwig's angina? Is this a risk?

Ludwig's angina is a bilateral infection involving the submandibular and sublingual spaces. It is frequently caused

Table 32.1 Paths of spread of infection from lower third molars

Direction of spread	Tissue space	Boundaries
Medially above the attachment of mylohyoid	Sublingual space, A	Lies between the floor mouth and mylohyoid muscle with the body of the mandible laterally.
Medially below attachment of mylohyoid	Submandibular space, A	Lies between mylohyoid muscle and platysma, with the hyoid bone medially and the lower border of the mandible laterally. Contains the submandibular gland.
Posterior and medial to mandibular ramus, medial to lateral pterygoid muscle	Parapharyngeal space, B	Lies between superior constrictor muscle and the pterygoid muscles with the pterygoid plates.
Posterior and superior, between mandibular ramus and lateral pterygoid muscle	Infratemporal space via C which communicates with the cavernous sinus	Base of skull superiorly, laterally sigmoid notch of mandible and temporalis muscle, medially lateral and posterior wall of maxilla.
Posterior and medial to mandibular ramus, lateral to lateral pterygoid muscle	Pterygomandibular space, C (and potentially on into the infratemporal space)	Lies between lateral and medial pterygoid muscles and the ascending ramus of mandible. Extends up to base of skull.
Posterior and lateral to mandible ramus	Submasseteric space, D	Lies between masseter muscle and the ascending ramus of the mandible.
Posterior and superiorly, lateral to buccinator	Buccal space, E	Between the buccinator muscle and skin

by cellulitis when the classical 'brawny' (board-like) induration of the neck is seen. Spread of infection involves the epiglottis or parapharyngeal spaces rapidly and causes airway obstruction. Death may also result from septicaemia, disseminated intravascular coagulation or spread in the fascial planes of the neck to the mediastinum. Early diagnosis and prompt surgical intervention combined with definitive airway management are necessary to prevent serious morbidity or mortality.

■ ***Is there a risk that the patient might develop this condition?***

It would be possible for this patient to progress to Ludwig's angina but this is not likely to be imminent and treatment will prevent this complication. However, she could also develop airway problems from spread via other routes.

Treatment

The principles of treatment of odontogenic soft tissue infection are described in Case 49. It is necessary to drain pus, remove the cause of the infection if possible and provide antibiotics for selected cases.

■ ***Where should this patient be treated?***

Admission to hospital will be necessary for this patient because she has systemic effects of infection and there is a risk that infection might impinge on the airway.

■ ***Is pus present? If so, how will you drain it?***

It is unclear at this early stage of infection whether an accumulation of pus, as well as cellulitis, is present in the submandibular space. Incision may not be helpful. Infection at less important sites might be treated by vigorous antibiotic therapy and removal of the cause, followed by drainage, if required, 1–2 days later. However, because of the proximity of the airway, incision must be performed if there is suspicion of abscess formation. Even within a cellulitis there will be small collections of pus or necrotic tissue. Drainage is the safer option in this case.

The submandibular space must be drained through an extraoral incision, ideally 2 cm below the lower border of the mandible (to avoid damage to the mandibular branch of the facial nerve). In practice this may not be the appropriate site and a soft spot centrally in the hard swelling is the best place to incise. Distortion of the soft tissues makes the position of the mandibular branch difficult to predict. Forceps or the incision must extend up medially to the mandible to drain the submandibular space. A drain will be required.

Drainage of the sublingual space is not indicated in this case and is rarely necessary. It could be achieved via an incision in the floor of the mouth (taking care to avoid damage to the lingual nerve).

Pus should be released from the pericoronal tissue by either an intraoral incision or extraction of the tooth.

■ ***How will you remove the cause?***

A general anaesthetic will be required to drain the swelling. Fibreoptic-guided intubation may be necessary because of trismus and infection around the airway. In a more advanced case, with airway oedema or infection, intubation of a conscious patient may be required because paralysis for intubation prevents the patient from keeping their airway open voluntarily. Perforation of the pharynx during intubation is possible if it is oedematous or displaced and this might drain pus into the upper airway. Forcing the mouth open under anaesthetic may have the same effect.

It may well be possible to remove the third molar at the same time despite the poor access. This breaches the general surgical principle that surgery is best avoided in an infected field, but with effective antibiotic treatment postoperative complications are rare. Obviously the decision will depend on the difficulty of the extraction. Removal of the opposing third molar could also speed recovery and reduce the chances of another episode of pericoronitis. Removal of the lower third molar may have to await resolution of the infection.

■ ***Would you provide antibiotics? If so, which?***

Yes, prescription of antibiotics is required for such a case. An initial bolus of intravenous penicillin and metronidazole would be appropriate with an oral regimen for a few days afterwards. There is further discussion of antibiotics for odontogenic infections in Case 49.

Case 33

First permanent molars

SUMMARY

A 7-year-old girl has pain from a first permanent molar. What is the cause and how might it affect her dental development?

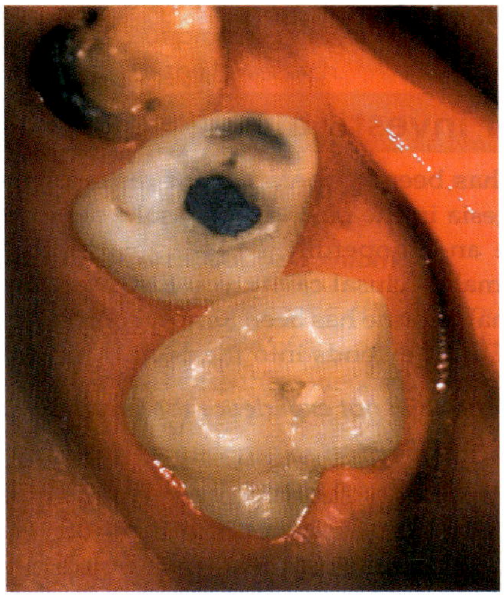

Fig. 33.1 The appearance on presentation.

History

Complaint

The patient's mother reports that the child suffers intermittent spontaneous discomfort from the upper left teeth.

History of complaint

The symptoms have been vague, no sleep has been lost and there has been no facial swelling. The patient has complained of the pain three or four times over the last month.

Medical history

The child is fit and well.

Dental history

The child has been a regular patient since the age of 3. She has required restorations in four primary molars, one requiring local analgesia. Despite intensive preventive advice and diet analysis, new carious lesions have been present at each recall visit.

Examination

You ask the child to point to the painful tooth and she points to an apparently sound upper left primary canine.

■ ***The appearance of the upper left quadrant is shown in Figure 33.1. What do you see?***

- An amalgam restoration with ditched or raised margins on the palatal aspect of the first primary molar.
- An apparently sound amalgam restoration in the second primary molar.
- Possible caries in an occlusal pit on the second primary molar.
- An erupting first permanent molar with the occlusal surface not fully through the mucosa.
- A small occlusal cavity in the confluence of the mesial fissures of the permanent molar.
- Plaque or food debris in the fissures.

■ ***How do you interpret the information so far and what are the likely diagnoses?***

The child is probably pointing at the wrong tooth. The canine appears intact and children are often poor historians. They often have difficulty in localizing the source of pain if the pain is not present at the time of examination.

Pulpitis appears likely because the pain appears poorly localized and is relatively intermittent. A history of hot or cold or sweet exacerbating factors would point to this diagnosis. The likely causes are caries beneath a restoration or carious or traumatic pulpal exposure in one of the primary molars. Any primary molar with an unrestored carious cavity or even a clinically sound restoration should be examined closely for signs of pulpal necrosis.

■ ***What features might suggest a necrotic pulp?***

- Extension of caries or fracture into the pulp
- Discolouration of the crown
- Swelling or tenderness in the buccal sulcus adjacent to the tooth
- Pus draining from a sinus in the mucosa, usually buccally but occasionally lingually or palatally
- Pus draining from the gingival margin
- Facial swelling
- Well-localized pain

None of these symptoms and signs is present. Pulpitis seems likely.

Investigations

■ ***What investigations are indicated? Why?***

- Bitewing radiographs to check the proximity of restorations to the pulps, the extent of the occlusal caries

Further information

■ ***The extracted tooth is shown in Figure 33.3 What do you see?***

Part of the crown has been removed to expose the carious cavity. On the left you can see a small periapical granuloma at the apex of the palatal root. The pulp was therefore nonvital despite the lack of symptoms. On the right you can see a large defect extending from the enamel to the pulp. The central occlusal enamel is completely unsupported but has not fractured. The carious dentine is hardly discoloured because it is progressing rapidly.

Case 34

A sore mouth

SUMMARY

A 55-year-old gentleman presents to you in general practice complaining of a sore mouth. You must make a diagnosis and institute treatment.

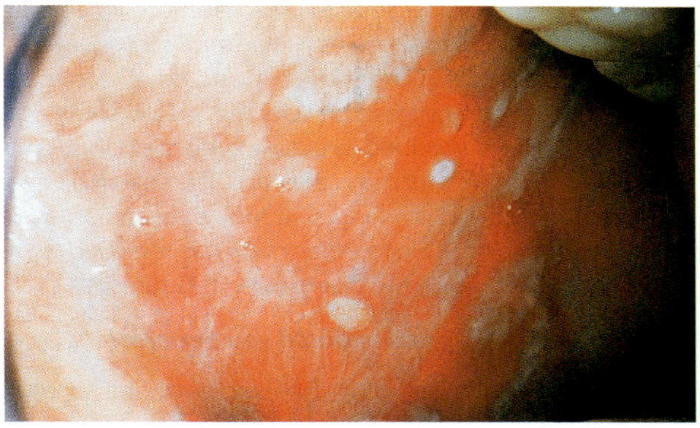

a

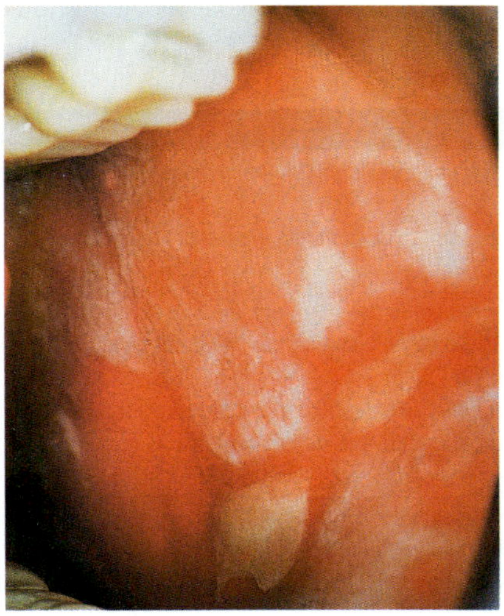

b

Fig. 34.1 a, b The patient's right and left buccal mucosa on presentation.

History

Complaint

He complains of an extremely sore mouth and the recent appearance of white patches on his cheeks. He thinks he may be allergic to his dentures.

History of complaint

The patient was fitted with a new set of complete dentures 3 weeks ago and since then his mouth has become progressively more sore. In recent days he has noticed the appearance of white patches on his cheeks. He had not noticed these before.

Medical history

One year ago the patient was diagnosed as a non-insulin-dependent diabetic and he has a history of peptic ulceration. Current medications are metformin and ranitidine. He is otherwise fit and well.

Examination

Extraoral examination

The patient appears fit and well. No cervical lymph nodes are palpable.

Intraoral examination

The patient is edentulous and his complete dentures are stable and retentive. The appearance of the right and left buccal mucosa is shown in Figure 34.1. Despite its abnormal appearance the mucosa is freely mobile with no evidence of tethering or scarring. Other parts of the oral mucosa appear healthy and the mouth is well lubricated by saliva.

■ ***Describe what you see on the buccal mucosa.***

The buccal mucosa is affected bilaterally by poorly defined ulcerated red and white lesions. These extend from the commissural region to the retromolar area, as well as vertically into the upper and lower buccal sulci. The white areas are arranged as diffuse zones but some have reticular keratotic striae within them and around their borders. Irregularly shaped erythematous zones lie around the white areas and some have ulcers centrally. There are two large oval/linear ulcers approximately a centimetre in length on the left and one smaller ulcer on the right. The ulcers have yellow fibrinous sloughs on their surfaces and appear relatively superficial and flat rather than deep or punched out. No bleeding is evident.

■ ***Suggest a differential diagnosis.***

1. Lichen planus
2. Lichenoid drug reaction
3. Lupus erythematosus.

■ ***Justify this differential diagnosis.***

The combination of white, red and ulcerated areas alone is highly suggestive of one of these three conditions, though it could also be seen in a number of other mucosal diseases including vesiculobullous diseases. However, the presence of white striae as well is almost conclusive evidence that the patient is suffering from one of this group of lichen planus-like conditions. The lesions cannot be differentiated by their clinical appearance alone.

Lichen planus. From the clinical appearance alone, lichen planus seems the most likely diagnosis. Lichen planus is a chronic condition that predominantly affects middle-aged or elderly patients and is the commonest of the three possible diagnoses. The appearances are typical of the atrophic ('erosive') form of the disease in which there are keratotic white areas associated with erythema and shallow ulceration. If this were lichen planus it would be slightly unusual. The lesions are usually less extensive and more prominent on the posterior buccal mucosa. Nevertheless, this could be a more severely affected individual.

Lichenoid drug reaction. Lichenoid drug reactions are side-effects of a number of drugs including the oral hypoglycaemic drug taken by the patient. Lichenoid reactions may be local (e.g. in response restorations) or systemic, in which case they are usually caused by medication. Some features which point to a lichenoid drug reaction rather than lichen planus include acute onset, extensive ulceration, asymmetrical distribution and severe involvement of the dorsum of the tongue. Lesions may also affect sites such as the floor of mouth which are less commonly affected by lichen planus. Lichenoid reactions may be clinically indistinguishable from lichen planus and the appearances of the buccal mucosa are consistent with a lichenoid reaction.

Lupus erythematosus. The mouth may be involved in discoid and systemic lupus erythematosus (SLE) and the oral manifestations of both types are indistinguishable. The clinical features resemble those of lichen planus and lichenoid reactions but some features may help in diagnosis. Lesions in lupus erythematosus often have a central ulcer or erythematous area around which the striae tend to radiate rather than follow the random pattern of lichen planus. Lesions are also typically asymmetrical and affect the hard and soft palate, which are rarely involved by lichen planus or lichenoid reactions. Lupus erythematosus is much rarer than either of the other two possibilities and is unlikely as a new finding in a 55-year-old male.

■ ***What further questions and examinations are appropriate? Explain why.***

See Table 34.1.

Investigations

■ ***Is a biopsy indicated? Why?***

Yes. Ideally biopsy should be performed in all cases of lichen planus. In practice asymptomatic lesions composed of striae alone are often not sampled because they can be diagnosed clinically and no treatment is required. However, when there is extensive ulceration or atrophy or when the clinical diagnosis is less clear, other conditions need to be excluded by biopsy. When a lichenoid lesion is suspected but cannot be proved clinically, the biopsy may provide evidence to implicate a drug and this can be helpful when deciding whether or not to stop or adjust the dose of an important medication. Though not present in this case, lichen planus can form plaque-type lesions and these must be sampled to exclude dysplasia. Patients with high alcohol or tobacco consumption should have a biopsy to exclude dysplasia because lichen planus has a very low risk of malignant transformation. For this patient, an incisional biopsy is indicated.

■ ***Which part of the lesion would you remove for biopsy?***

The centre of ulcers must be avoided because inflammation may mask histological features. However a sample of the ulcer margin may be useful and a piece including ulcer margin and red and white areas should be selected. Ideally some normal mucosa is always included in biopsy specimens, but in this case almost all the mucosa is affected. The specimen should be elliptical, about 1 cm long, 5–6 mm wide and an even 3–4 mm in depth. A biopsy specimen was removed from the left buccal mucosa and is shown later in Figure 34.3.

■ ***What other investigations would you perform?***

Microbiological tests. When lichen planus or a lichenoid reaction become symptomatic or extensively ulcerated the possibility of additional candidal infection should be

Table 34.1 Further questions

Subject	Questions and reasons
About the medication	Date started, dose and any recent dose changes. Previous drug history for the last 5 years. Lichenoid reactions are sometimes dose dependent and may be first noticed as a result of an increase in dosage. A close temporal relationship between starting a drug and developing lesions is good, though circumstantial, evidence of a causal link. Sometimes lichenoid reactions persist for years after the drug was administered.
About skin lesions	Are skin lesions present? Ask about and examine the flexor surface of the wrist and extensor surface of the shins. These are common sites for skin lesions of lichen planus and lichenoid reactions. The typical skin lesions are purplish polygonal papules with faint striae (Wickham's striae). They are usually very itchy. Severe lichenoid reactions may be accompanied by an extensive erythematous rash. Only a minority of cases with oral lichen planus or lichenoid reaction will have skin lesions on presentation. This is because the skin lesions often resolve spontaneously after a few years or with topical steroid treatment. In contrast, oral lesions may persist for many years and are often resistant to treatment. The skin lesions of lupus erythematosus are distinctive in distribution and appearance.
About the signs and symptoms of lupus erythematosus	Although this is an unlikely diagnosis the patient should be asked some questions to elicit evidence of lupus erythematosus. Questioning and examination should be more thorough if the oral lesions suggest lupus erythematosus by virtue of their appearance, distribution or the young age of the patient. Lupus erythematosus may be confined to the skin and/or oral mucosa (discoid lupus erythematosus). Lesions are well demarcated, round or oval red scaly plaques. The common sites are face, scalp and hands. There may be scarring and sometimes the typical 'butterfly' rash on the malar regions. Systemic lupus erythematosus has numerous signs and symptoms including those of discoid skin lesions (above), photosensitivity and hair loss. Vasculitis can affect most organs. There may be glomerulonephritis, arthritis, anaemia and CNS involvement causing infarction and/or psychiatric manifestations.

considered. The thick keratotic epithelium is more prone than normal epithelium to infection. The patient is further predisposed to candidal infection by non-insulin-dependent diabetes. A smear from the surface of the lesions on each side is an ideal investigation. Saliva sampling for candidal counts may also be helpful. This has the advantage that the organism is cultured for complete identification and sensitivity testing to antifungal agents. The disadvantage is that it does not specifically sample the lesion. In this case the patient is a complete denture wearer and is therefore likely to have an elevated salivary candida count. A smear is the better choice in this case and one was taken from the left buccal mucosa. It is shown in Figure 34.2.

Autoantibody screen. If lupus erythematosus is a possibility, an autoantibody screen may provide evidence to support the diagnosis. A serum sample should be sent for antinuclear antibody (ANA) determination. Four-fifths of patients with systemic disease are ANA-positive, often having high titres. A high titre of anti-double-stranded DNA (dsDNA) antibody is almost exclusive to SLE but is positive in only 50% of cases. In discoid lupus erythematosus this is less helpful in diagnosis because only a quarter of patients have antinuclear antibodies. Individuals with lichen planus or lichenoid reaction should have no antinuclear antibody. In this case the autoantibody screen was negative.

■ ***The smear is shown in Figure 34.2. What do you see and how do you interpret the features?***

The smear is stained with periodic acid–Schiff (PAS), which stains the carbohydrate in fungal cell walls a magenta colour. Gram stain may also be used to detect fungi; Candida stains strongly Gram-positive. A sheet of pale pink-stained buccal epithelial cells is present, together with a few dispersed cells. Numerous dark pink branching fungal hyphae are growing in and around the epithelial cells. There are also several small round blastospores budding from the hyphae. The fungus is dimorphic and branching, and the size and appearance are typical of Candida sp. The patient has candidosis.

■ ***The biopsy is shown in Figure 34.3. What do you see?***

The low power view shows mucosa with underlying fat. The surface epithelium is slightly thinner than normal buccal epithelium and has a surface layer of keratin. There is a well demarcated inflammatory infiltrate in a band immediately below the epithelium in the superficial connective tissue. The band is denser towards each side of the picture. (At this magnification the cells cannot be definitely identified as inflammatory cells but this is the most likely explanation for the very cellular zone.) There are also several foci of inflammatory cells in the deeper tissues, one particularly large one associated with a vessel near the bottom of the picture. The basement membrane is prominent.

The higher power view shows the interface between the epithelium and connective tissue. The very cellular layer can be seen to be composed of lymphocytes. Lymphocytes have infiltrated into the basal and suprabasal layers of the

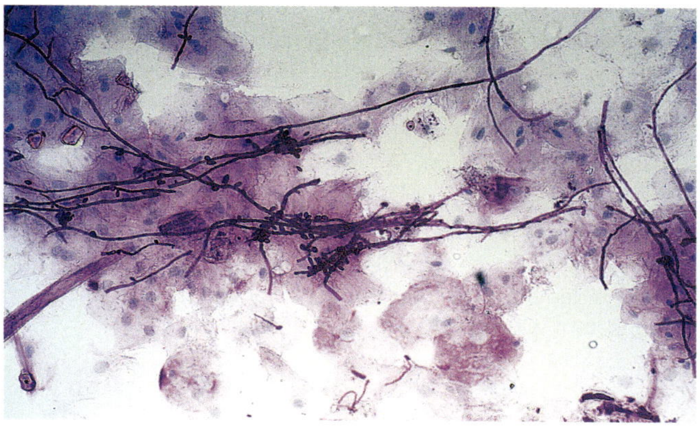

Fig. 34.2 Periodic acid–Schiff (PAS) stained smear from buccal mucosa.

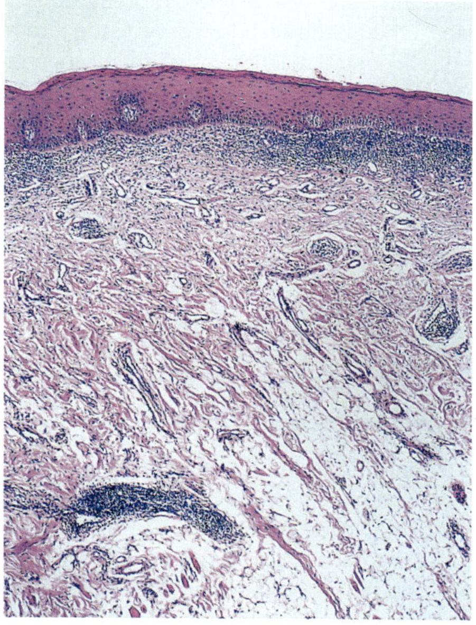

a

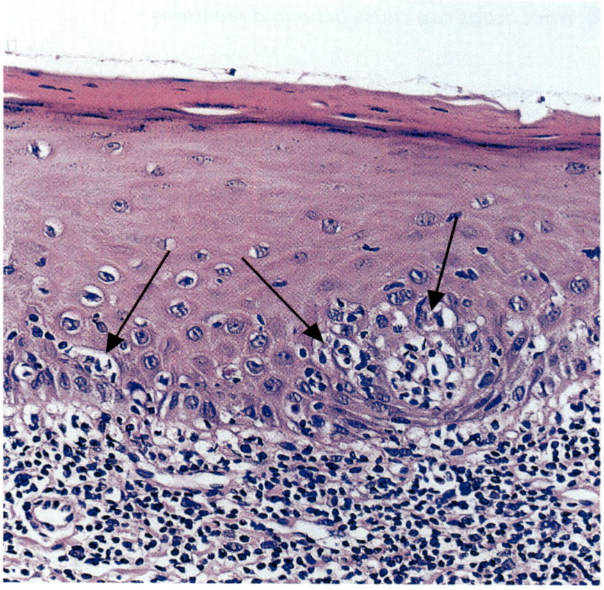

b

Fig. 34.3 Buccal biopsy; haematoxylin and eosin. **a,** Low power view; **b,** higher power view.

epithelium and caused the basal epithelial cells to undergo apoptosis. Apoptotic cells are visible as shrunken very pink cells with nuclear remnants (arrowed). There is no remaining clearly defined basal layer of small darkly stained cells and the cells lying at the basement membrane have the appearance of prickle cells. The surface is parakeratinized. Buccal epithelium is normally nonkeratinized, though a thinner layer than this may be present along the occlusal line as a result of friction.

How do you interpret the histological findings?

The dense band-like infiltrate of lymphocytes and lymphocytic infiltration of the basal cells with focal basal cell degeneration, apoptosis, loss of basal cells and a thickened basement membrane are typical of lichen planus. The deeper infiltrates of inflammatory cells around blood vessels suggest that this is the result of a systemic process rather than one localized to the epithelial–connective tissue interface. This suggests a lichenoid reaction rather than lichen planus as a cause. However, it is not usually possible to differentiate lichen planus and lichenoid reactions on histological grounds alone. For this reason the biopsy diagnosis is 'consistent with lichen planus or a lichenoid reaction'. The dentist must ensure that this histological diagnosis is compatible with the clinical features and results of any other investigations before finalizing the diagnosis.

Diagnosis

What is your final diagnosis? Explain why.

Lichenoid drug reaction with superimposed candidosis. The clinical presentation is typical of a lichenoid reaction or a severe atrophic lichen planus, the diagnosis is supported by biopsy and the patient is taking a drug known to cause such reactions. The clinical appearance does not suggest lupus erythematosus and the autoantibody screen was negative.

What drugs can cause lichenoid reactions?

A very large number of drugs may be associated with the development of a lichenoid reaction. Reactions to gold injection may be particularly severe and prolonged. Drugs of the following types cause lichenoid reactions:

- allopurinol
- captopril
- chloroquine antimalarials
- gold
- beta blockers
- methyldopa and related antihypertensives
- nonsteroidal anti-inflammatory drugs
- oral hypoglycaemic agents
- penicillamine
- some antidepressants
- occasionally other drugs.

What treatment or advice would you recommend?

Firstly the candidal infection must be treated. Denture hygiene must be checked and night wear ceased if appropriate. In view of the mucosal inflammation and ulceration, an antifungal agent should be prescribed and amphotericin or nystatin would be appropriate. Subsequently, intermittent chlorhexidine mouthwashes may help prevent repeated episodes of candidosis.

Corticosteroid preparations would be helpful for the underlying lichenoid reaction. The mode of corticosteroid delivery is determined by the extent of the lesions, a mouthrinse being more appropriate than a spray or pellets when such a large area of mucosa is affected. The potency of the steroid must be matched to the signs and symptoms. These lesions are not suitable for treatment by the low potency steroids available to dental practitioners in the UK and either the patient's medical practitioner or a hospital unit will have to prescribe a more potent steroid such as betamethasone or beclomethasone. More potent or systemic steroids may be indicated if these prove ineffective. Continued follow up for candidal infection will be required because topical steroid use would be a further predisposing factor to infection.

Would you change the patient's oral hypoglycaemic drug?

Yes, if possible. First find out whether the causative drug can be withdrawn or reduced in dose. This must be undertaken by the patient's medical practitioner who will require details of the severity of the reaction and how distressing the patient finds the symptoms. As antifungal treatment may improve the symptoms, this discussion should take place after treatment and a period to assess the reduction in symptoms. Unfortunately changing one medication for another of the same drug family may not prove effective. If the drug is changed it is important to realize that resolution may take place over a period of weeks or months and sometimes years.

The patient complained of being allergic to his dentures. Is this a possible explanation?

Such reactions are possible but statistically the likelihood is very low indeed. The oral mucosa does not generally exhibit contact sensitivity reactions. Two features suggest that this is not an allergic response. First the mucosa would usually be evenly red and sometimes oedematous. Ulceration is possible but striae and keratosis are not features. Second, the palate and alveolar ridges in contact with the denture are not involved. In this case there is no reason to investigate the possibility further, but cutaneous patch tests with the constituents of denture acrylic, in particular methylmethacrylate are possible. Tests should be carried out in a specialist centre because these unpolymerized compounds are irritant and readily give false-positive results.

The patient had had a new denture fitted 3 weeks previously. One possibility which might be considered is that it has been inadequately polymerized and contains excess monomer. However, as in true hypersensitivity, the mucosa would be red and oedematous. Neither the signs nor investigations are consistent with this diagnosis.

Case 35

A failed bridge

SUMMARY

A 40-year-old man has a missing upper incisor replaced by a spring cantilever bridge. This has become decemented and you must assess options for replacement.

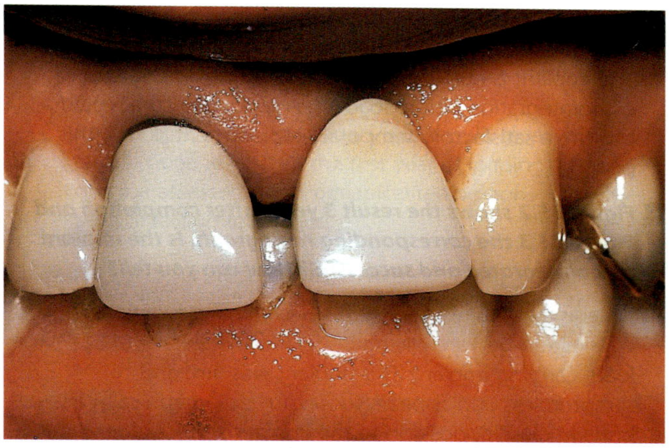

Fig. 35.1 The patient at presentation with the bridge which replaced the upper left central incisor reinserted.

History

Complaint

The patient complains that his anterior bridge has become detached. He would like it recemented or replaced.

History of complaint

The bridge had been satisfactory for many years but detached about 2 years ago. It was recemented and had been firm until yesterday when it fell off the teeth without warning.

Dental history

The upper left central incisor had been lost as a result of a bicycle accident when the patient was aged 16. It was completely avulsed and the adjacent upper right central incisor was fractured. The missing central incisor was initially replaced with a simple spoon denture and then a few years later by a spring cantilever bridge attached to full coverage crowns on the left first and second premolars. The other upper central incisor was root treated and a post crown fitted. The present bridge is a replacement made about 8 years ago after the cantilever spring fractured. The patient has never had an upper left lateral incisor.

Examination

Intraoral examination

The dentition is in good condition with few carious lesions and a small number of restorations. The upper left premolars are the abutment teeth and have relatively conservative crown preparations. There is superficial caries over much of the surface of the first premolar crown and a larger cavity at the distal gingival margin. The mesial surface of the second premolar is also slightly carious. Both abutment teeth are vital. The gingival condition is good except for bleeding on probing between the abutment premolars. Here the probing depth is 4mm. The bridge can be replaced and the appearance with it fully seated is shown in Figure 35.1. The caries in the first premolar is exposed below the crown margin.

■ ***What is the prognosis for this bridge? Why?***

Hopeless. Figure 35.1 shows that the cosmetic result is not good. The bridge pontic has moved buccally and upwards, probably a combined result of alveolar ridge resorption and distortion of the spring cantilever. It also appears to have moved distally increasing the median diastema. The abutment teeth will both require re-restoration and the first premolar appears to be very carious. In the long term, both abutment teeth are compromised by the risk of further caries and periodontitis.

■ ***Why was this method of replacing the central incisor chosen originally?***

Although a well-designed partial denture should not compromise the health of the remaining dentition, most patients prefer a fixed prosthesis without palatal coverage for a single tooth replacement.

The spring cantilever design was considered suitable for this case for the following reasons.

- It allows diastemas between adjacent crowns. Diastemas would have been present because the lateral incisor on that side was developmentally absent. A replacement crown which filled the available space would be too wide.
- The upper right central incisor was not a suitable abutment tooth for conventional fixed bridgework, having been traumatized, root-filled and post-crowned using a prefabricated post.

■ ***What replacement restorations would you consider? Explain your choices.***

A new spring cantilever bridge. For the reasons noted above, the spring cantilever design remains a good choice

Case • 36

Skateboarding accident?

SUMMARY

A 6-year-old boy with a facial injury attends late one afternoon without an appointment. Assess the child and decide what treatment he needs.

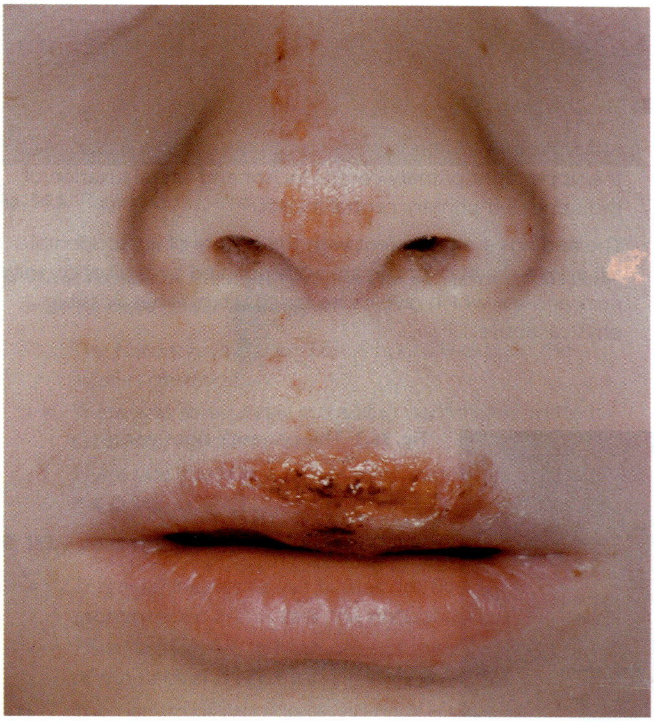

Fig. 36.1 The patient's face on presentation.

History

Complaint

The child complains of loose front teeth and that his mouth is sore and it hurts to eat.

History of complaint

The child's mother says that he fell off his skateboard and banged his teeth. The injury occurred yesterday evening when he was playing at a friend's house.

Dental history

The family attend your practice occasionally. The patient had some primary molars extracted under general anaesthesia 6 months ago and has since missed two appointments for review.

Medical history

The patient is otherwise fit and well.

■ ***What do you need to know about the accident?***

Further details, including the exact time, whether it was witnessed by others and who was responsible for looking after him at the time. Was he knocked out when he fell?

What type of surface did he fall on? Were the abrasions or mouth contaminated with soil or other dirty material? Is the patient's antitetanus immunization up-to-date?

Examination

Extraoral examination

The child looks anxious and withdrawn. Abrasions are present on the tip of the nose and the upper lip, as shown in Figure 36.1. These have a parallel vertical pattern consistent with scraping on a pavement but are not visibly contaminated with debris. When asked if he has injuries elsewhere, he does not respond at first then shows abrasions on his knees and elbows.

On examining his face, you notice faint parallel lines of petechial bruising running horizontally across the left side of his neck (Figure 36.2) and bruising on both the outer and inner surface of the right ear (Figure 36.3). No other injuries are visible on those parts of his arms and legs which are not covered by clothing.

Intraoral examination

The patient's upper anterior teeth and lip are shown in Figure 36.4.

■ ***What do you see?***

He is in the early mixed dentition, has poor oral hygiene and no obvious caries. There are abrasions on the vermilion border and inner surface of the upper lip. The upper labial frenum is torn and bruised. The upper left primary central incisor has bleeding around the gingival margin and is displaced palatally.

If you were to examine the patient you would find that both upper primary central incisors are slightly mobile and tender to pressure. The displaced incisor is not causing occlusal interference.

- Requiring repeated general anaesthesia for dental extractions.

Preschool children are particularly vulnerable and, in such cases, it is recommended that you should contact the child's health visitor to discuss how you might work together to support the family to ensure that the child's needs are met. This contributes to 'safeguarding' children, namely, not only protecting children from abuse and neglect, but taking a wider range of measures to promote their health and development and minimize risks of harm. In the vast majority of cases, lack of knowledge and difficulty accessing care account for the apparent neglect. However, if a child is already suffering significant harm from untreated dental disease, it will be necessary to make a child protection referral without delay.

Case 37

An adverse reaction

SUMMARY

A 38-year-old lady becomes unwell during routine dental treatment in your general dental practice. What would you do? What is the cause?

History

Complaint

The patient is to have a crown preparation performed on her lower second molar and a very small amalgam placed in an upper premolar on the same side. You have given an infiltration of 1.0 ml lidocaine (lignocaine) 2% with adrenaline (epinephrine) 1:80 000 (12.5µg/ml) and used a further 2-ml cartridge to give an inferior dental and lingual nerve block. Having finished injecting you turn away to prepare some instruments.

Almost immediately the patient says she feels ill. She is clearly apprehensive and is holding her chest complaining of palpitations.

Dental treatment history

The patient is in the middle of her first course of treatment for many years. She has been scared about visiting a dentist for some years. You have started a course of treatment and carried out several simple restorative procedures. You saw her only 2 days ago to insert several amalgams, using three cartridges of local anaesthetic. These restorations and one extraction have all been carried out under local anaesthesia using lidocaine (lignocaine) 2% with adrenaline (epinephrine) 1:80 000.

Medical history

The patient is apparently fit and well. The medical history records no allergies.

■ ***What would you do?***

- Reassure the patient; encourage regular breathing
- Lie her supine or slightly head down
- Feel skin and take pulse
- Prepare oxygen in case it is needed.

This applies unless the patient were pregnant or obese, in which case lying flat on her side would be more appropriate.

■ ***One minute later the patient feels no improvement. What would you do?***

- Take blood pressure and monitor pulse
- Check for pallor
- Check for rash or urticaria
- Wait and observe for dyspnoea while considering possible causes.

■ ***What causes would you consider?***

The local anaesthetic appears to be the most likely cause of her symptoms because they started immediately after the inferior dental block. However, vasovagal attacks are very common and a medical problem unrelated to dentistry cannot be excluded. Thus, possible causes include:

- vasovagal attack
- adverse reaction to local anaesthetic
- hypersensitivity reaction
- myocardial infarct or anginal attack.

■ ***Is this a vasovagal attack? Explain why?***

The features of a vasovagal attack are pallor, apprehension, restlessness, nausea, bradycardia, weak slow pulse and loss of consciousness (faint). The loss of consciousness may be immediate. In more severe attacks there may be clonic muscle contractions or rigidity as a result of cerebral hypoxia. None of these symptoms is seen in this patient. In addition, vasovagal attacks are usually caused by fear or anxiety and so may precede injection. Patients will usually be able to explain that they feel faint, either before or after the attack.

■ ***Is this is myocardial infarct?***

No. The symptoms and signs of myocardial infarct are crushing central chest pain, sometimes radiating to arm or neck, dyspnoea and possibly vomiting which may be followed by cardiac arrest. There is usually, though not always, a history of angina, coronary artery disease or hypertension. Further information on cardiac arrest will be found in Case 13.

■ ***What are the unwanted effects of local anaesthesia with lidocaine (lignocaine) and adrenaline (epinephrine)? What are their causes and signs and symptoms?***

See Table 37.1.

While these possibilities run through your mind, the patient remains conscious but nervous and agitated. She gradually calms and says that the palpitations are reducing. She takes a few breaths of oxygen but refuses more after a few minutes and says that she feels better. Her pulse is 105 beats/min and her blood pressure is 140/90.

Differential diagnosis

■ ***What is your differential diagnosis and why?***

Intravascular injection is the most likely diagnosis, the patient's symptoms being caused by the vasoconstrictor

Table 37.1 Unwanted effects of local anaesthesia

Type of reaction	Unwanted effect	Signs and symptoms
Immediate	Neuralgic pain from needle penetrating nerve.	Electric shock pain on injection, sometimes followed by prolonged anaesthesia.
	Vasomotor effect of intravascular injection of vasoconstrictor.	Tachycardia without hypertension, in overdose arrhythmias. Occasionally, skin blanching on face or neck in the event of arterial injection.
	Facial paralysis from intraparotid injection.	Paralysis of one or more branches of facial nerve; may mimic Bell's palsy.
	Anaphylaxis due to hypersensitivity to anaesthetic solution.	Anaphylactic shock, local or systemic oedema, urticaria, asthma, hypotension, pulmonary oedema, tachycardia, breathlessness and circulatory collapse.
	Drug interaction.	Though theoretically many are possible none is a practical possibility at normal dosage.
	Central nervous system stimulation or depression caused by overdose of lidocaine (lignocaine).	Only seen in **large** overdose. Sometimes initial apprehension, excitability or confusion or muscle spasm followed by respiratory and cardiac depression.
	Rare complications such as needle breakage or infection.	
Delayed	Trismus or local trauma from injection, haematoma formation or damage to analgesic tissue caused by the patient.	Vary with effect.
	Transmission of infection.	Vary with infection.

component of the local anaesthetic. The solution contains 1:80 000 adrenaline (epinephrine) which causes tachycardia felt by the patient as palpitations. Intravascular injection is most common after inferior dental blocks and posterior superior dental blocks because of the high vascularity of the injection site.

Anxiety can itself produce a significant level of adrenaline but levels rise more slowly and the patient would have to be very nervous, positively phobic, to generate endogenous adrenaline to the levels found in intravascular injection of local anaesthetic. This patient is nervous but has recently accepted routine dental treatment without problems. A vasovagal attack would be a much more likely effect of marked anxiety.

■ ***Could the local anaesthetic given 2 days ago contribute to this reaction?***

No, the adrenaline (epinephrine) will have been rapidly removed into the circulation from the site of injection in spite of its intrinsic vasoconstrictor effect. Its action is then terminated quickly by reuptake into noradrenergic fibres and other cells and tissues. Metabolism takes place within these at various sites throughout the body by the action of the enzyme catechol-O-methyl transferase and to a much lesser degree by monoamine oxidase in the liver before undergoing renal excretion.

As far as the local anaesthetic component is concerned, the symptoms experienced by this patient are not typical of an overdose and, in any event, the half-life of lidocaine (lignocaine) is only of the order of 90 minutes. We can therefore safely rule out any question of this event being related to either the local anaesthetic or vasoconstrictor given at the previous appointment.

■ ***Is an overdose possible? What are the maximum recommended doses of local anaesthetic solutions used in dentistry?***

Although theoretically possible, it is actually quite difficult to administer an overdose of local anaesthetic in dentistry. The nature of the cartridge syringe and needle system used means that doses can be accurately counted and monitored and the need to change a cartridge affords 'thinking time' for the operator. This is in contrast to the other areas of the body where large volumes of drug can be administered into body spaces more easily.

However, we cannot be complacent. In recent years the recommendations for maximum safe doses of local anaesthetics in the head and neck area have been reviewed. Because of the vascularity of the region and recognition that vasoconstrictors do not hold the drug in place for as long as was previously thought, the recommendations have been rationalized and maximum recommended doses reduced.

It is important to realize that advice based on a recommended number of cartridges or fixed dose does not take into account different formulations. Some cartridges contain only 1.8 ml solution whilst others contain 2.2 ml and therefore 22% more drug. Thus four cartridges of the larger volume will contain almost the same dose of local anaesthetic and vasoconstrictor as five of the 1.8 ml cartridges. The concentration of drug also varies from preparation to preparation. Importantly, patients come in different shapes and sizes and fixed dose recommendations are based on the safety limit for the elusive 'fit 70-kg man'!

Another way to consider the safe total dose is to relate it to body weight and the amount in a dental local anaesthetic cartridge (which varies between drugs).

Thus, 2% lidocaine in a 2.2 ml cartridge is equivalent to 44 mg of drug. With a maximum safe dose of 4.4 mg/kg, a single cartridge could be administered for every 10 kg of body weight. A 70 kg male would have a maximum safe dose of 7 cartridges and a 20 kg child a maximum safe dose of 2 catridges.

Current recommendations are expressed in the form of the maximum safe dose per body weight given over a period of treatment of 1 hour. Thus the maximum recommended doses are as shown in Table 37.2.

These limits apply to all preparations of local anaesthetic irrespective of the presence of or type of vasoconstrictor. It is no longer considered that larger doses can be given in one treatment session if the preparation contains vasoconstrictor.

Table 37.2 Maximum recommended doses

Drug	Maximum dose	Equivalent cartridges for a 70 kg male
Lidocaine (lignocaine) and mepivacaine	4.4 mg/kg	For 2% solutions about **eight** 1.8-ml or **six-and-a-half** 2.2-ml cartridges For 3% mepivacaine **five-and-a-half** 1.8-ml or **four-and-a-half** 2.2-ml cartridges
Prilocaine	6 mg/kg	For 3% prilocaine about **seven** 1.8-ml or **six** 2.2-ml cartridges For 4% prilocaine about **five-and-a-half** 1.8-ml and **four-and-a-half** 2.2-ml cartridges
Articaine	7 mg/kg	For 4% articaine about **six-and-a-half** 1.7-ml and **five-and-a-half** 2.2-ml cartridges

■ ***Immediately after calming down, the patient claims that she must be allergic to the local anaesthetic. Is this possible?***

It is possible but is excessively rare. Only a handful of cases of genuine lidocaine (lignocaine) hypersensitivity are recorded. A minority of older patients give a convincing history of local anaesthetic allergy, in some cases backed up by hospital investigations. This is because older preparations contained preservatives such as benzoates to which hypersensitivity was possible. The worst offending preservatives are no longer used, though very occasionally a reaction to sodium metabisulphite preservative is recorded. Patients can be tested for hypersensitivity to anaesthetic agents but this is only worthwhile when a typical allergic reaction is suspected.

Hypersensitivity is unlikely to follow repeated administration of lidocaine (lignocaine) for dental anaesthesia. A much more potent cause is repeated application of lidocaine (lignocaine) creams to the skin. Local anaesthetic pastes and solutions should be handled with care; the dentist is more at risk than the patient.

■ ***Would a switch to prilocaine with felypressin in future be prudent?***

No, lidocaine (lignocaine) with adrenaline (epinephrine) has been used successfully in the past for this patient and there is no evidence of an idiosyncratic or allergic response to the preparation itself. Prilocaine produces a shorter period of analgesia and the patient should not suffer suboptimal pain relief because of the remote possibility of another intravascular injection. There is no evidence that prilocaine, with or without felypressin, is safer.

Such a switch would reinforce the patient's perception that she is allergic to local anaesthetic. A spurious history of allergy might compromise the patient's general health. Lidocaine (lignocaine) is used in the emergency treatment of myocardial infarct and in many other medical situations.

■ ***How can the risk of intravascular injection be minimized?***

Good injection technique is the key to reducing the risk of intravascular injection because it ensures that the minimum amount of anaesthetic solution is used. The solution should be injected slowly, reducing the risk of a bolus injection into a vessel. An aspirating technique should always be used even though it does not always guarantee success; the narrow needle diameters used in dentistry aspirate relatively poorly.

It is impossible to completely avoid the tip of the needle entering a vessel. Indeed, in some very vascular areas penetration of a vessel is not the cause because the solution can be absorbed into the blood almost as rapidly as it can be injected. Nothing can guarantee the prevention of intravascular injection.

Another possibility

■ ***If the patient had had a genuine anaphylaxis, what causative agents would you consider?***

Anaphylaxis to other agents is considerably commoner than hypersensitivity to local anaesthetics. A number of other agents in the dental surgery should be suspected before the local anaesthetic.

Latex hypersensitivity is increasing in prevalence and is commoner in atopic patients and those who have come into contact with latex repeatedly, such as health care workers, those with spina bifida or those who are subjected to multiple surgical procedures. Rubber dam, gloves and even traces of rubber from local anaesthetic cartridges or drug vials can trigger reactions. Other less obvious items in the dental surgery which may contain latex are face masks with elastic components, amalgam carriers, plastic syringes, aspirator tubes, orthodontic elastics and emergency equipment such as ventilating bags and sphygmomanometer cuffs. These usually cause type 1 reactions such as urticaria, asthma or anaphylactic shock. Glove powder is a particularly potent method of disseminating latex allergen into the atmosphere and powdered gloves should no longer be used to reduce the risk of allergy developing among the dental team.

In addition to latex, staff and more rarely patients may develop hypersensitivity to acrylics, composite resins, dentine bonding agents, eugenol, cleaning and disinfection solutions and metal alloys. Almost all materials may be allergenic to some individuals. The worst offending agents usually have their formulations changed and the most notorious examples, particularly some synthetic impression materials and self-curing acrylics are no longer available in their original form. It is worth remembering that many of these agents are irritant as well as allergenic and rashes may not be true hypersensitivity reactions.

Case • 38

Advanced periodontitis

SUMMARY

A 56-year-old man has severe periodontitis. Diagnose and plan treatment for his condition.

History

Complaint

The patient complains of loose back teeth, particularly the last tooth on the lower right.

History of complaint

He has recently moved to your area and has been a regular dental attender. His previous dental practitioner diagnosed periodontal disease several years ago and organized repeated courses of oral hygiene instruction and scaling. Despite this, several teeth are loose though he has suffered no pain.

Three years ago the remaining upper right molar teeth became very loose and were extracted when abscesses developed. Subsequently two implant fixtures were placed because he could not tolerate partial dentures. An implant-retained bridge was planned but the implants remain unused.

Medical history

The patient is fit and well and no illness is revealed by his medical history questionnaire.

■ ***What questions will you ask the patient? Explain why.***

Ask about his tooth cleaning regime, because it is clearly failing. The patient tells you that he cleans his teeth three times a day using a modified Bass technique and changes his toothbrush at monthly intervals. He uses floss on his anterior teeth every day and occasionally on his molars and premolars where access is difficult.

Whether he smokes. Smoking is a risk factor for periodontitis.

Whether he is diabetic or has any other susceptibility to infection. This is relatively severe periodontitis and there is a history of multiple abscesses. These features do not necessarily indicate an underlying condition but it would be worthwhile to exclude diabetes. Other features which might suggest diabetes are a period of rapid tooth destruction in middle age, suggesting late-onset diabetes.

Examination

Extraoral examination

No cervical lymphadenopathy is present. The temporomandibular joint and mandibular movements appear normal.

Intraoral examination

The mucosa and soft tissues of the mouth are normal. The teeth present are:

4321	1234 78
7654321	1234567

Most molars contain small- to medium-sized amalgam restorations. No caries is detected.

The patient's oral hygiene is fair but the lower second molar teeth and upper left molars are mobile. The plaque control around the anterior teeth is good with minimal deposits of plaque or calculus. There is bleeding on probing around most posterior teeth and increased probing depths of 7–8 mm around the molars. No recession is present.

■ ***How will you assess the patient's periodontal health and oral hygiene?***

They will be assessed by a combination of measurements and indices.

The measurements are:

- recession
- probing depths
- attachment loss.

Recession and probing depth measurements are made at six points around the circumference of a tooth: mesially, at the midpoint and distally on the buccal and palatal surfaces. The distance from the cementoenamel junction to the gingival margin records the amount of recession. Probing depths are measured from the gingival margin to the base of the periodontal pocket. The sum of recession and probing depth gives the length of attachment loss.

The indices are described in Table 38.1.

The results of these examinations are shown in Figure 38.1. The lower right second molar is mobile to grade 3. All other molars are mobile to grade 2 and there is bleeding on probing from most pockets. The anterior teeth have only 2–3 mm probing depths and no bleeding on probing or gross attachment loss.

Investigations

■ ***What further examinations or investigations would you perform?***

Vitality tests are indicated for all teeth with marked attachment loss or furcation involvement. This would include all molars.

Table 38.1 Indices of oral health and periodontal hygiene

	Index score	Significance of score
Oral hygiene		
Degree 0	No plaque or debris	Reflection of effectiveness of cleaning.
Degree 1	Looks clean but material can be removed from the gingival third with a probe.	
Degree 2	Visible plaque	
Degree 3	Tooth surface covered with abundant plaque.	
Bleeding on probing		
Degree 0	None	Healthy or inactive disease.
Degree 1	Bleeding	Active disease. N.B. in smokers bleeding may be less than expected for the disease activity.
Tooth mobility		
Degree 1	Movement of the crown of the tooth between 0.2–1 mm in a horizontal direction.	Minor movement, possibly physiological. If periodontal disease present, treat conservatively.
Degree 2	Movement of the crown of the tooth exceeding 1 mm in a horizontal direction.	Caused by loss of attachment. The degree of mobility depends on remaining periodontal support and the shape of the roots. Conical roots on molars are more likely to develop mobility than divergent roots on teeth with a similar degree of attachment loss.
Degree 3	Movement of the crown of the tooth in a vertical and horizontal direction.	Indicates bone loss below the apex and little or no bony support. Usually indicates a need for extraction.
Furcation involvement		
Degree 1	Horizontal loss of supporting tissues not exceeding 1/3 of the width of the tooth.	Early furcation involvement, can be treated conservatively; predisposes to further and more rapid attachment loss if untreated.
Degree 2	Horizontal loss of supporting tissue exceeding 1/3 but not a 'through and through' lesion	Much more difficult to keep clean. Unlikely to respond to conservative treatment.
Degree 3	A 'through and through' lesion	May be easier to clean depending on soft tissue contour. The prognosis for the tooth would depend upon the remaining amount of periodontal attachment and the length and shape of the roots. Indicates susceptibility to furcation caries and risk of loss of vitality.

Mobility					1	1	1	1	1	1	1	1			2	2
Attachment loss – Buccal	X	X	X	X	5 4 3	3 2 3	3 2 3	3 2 2	2 3 3	2 2 3	3 3 3	3 3 4	X	X	6 7 7	8 7 7
Attachment loss – Palatal	X	X	X	X	5 4 3	3 2 3	3 2 3	3 2 2	2 3 3	2 2 3	3 3 3	3 3 4	X	X	6 7 8	8 8 8
Tooth	8	7	6	5	4	3	2	1	1	2	3	4	5	6	7	8
Tooth	8	7	6	5	4	3	2	1	1	2	3	4	5	6	7	8
Attachment loss – Lingual	X	9 9 8	7 8 7	4 4 3	3 3 3	3 4 4	3 3 3	3 3 2	2 3 3	3 3 3	2 3 2	3 4 4	3 4 5	6 7 8	8 9 9	X
Attachment loss – Buccal	X	9 9 9	8 9 8	4 3 4	4 3 3	3 3 3	3 3 3	3 3 2	3 3 3	3 3 2	2 3 3	3 4 4	4 4 5	6 7 7	9 9 9	X
Mobility		3	2	1	1	1	1	1	1	1	1	1	1	2	2	

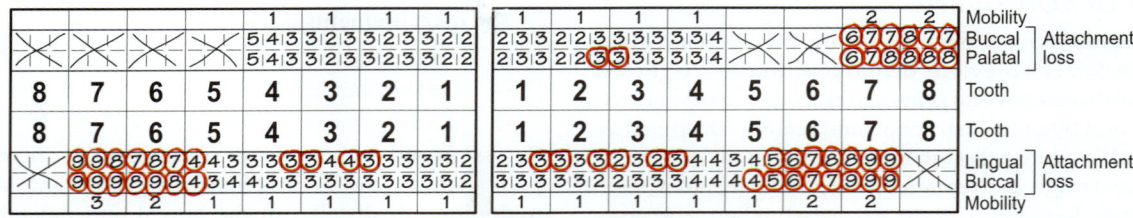

Fig. 38.1 The probing depths (in mm) at six points, bleeding sites (ringed) and mobility (grade), recorded for each tooth. No recession is present.

■ ***What radiographs would you take? Why?***

See Table 38.2.

■ ***The dental panoramic radiograph is shown in Figure 38.2. What do you see?***

The panoramic film is of poor quality. The patient's head was not correctly positioned and this has produced a number of distortions. The lower border of the mandible appears bowed down and the lower anterior teeth are foreshortened. Spinal shadows are also accentuated by poor positioning and the teeth in the midline appear out of focus because of superimposition. The head was also twisted, enlarging one side of the film. This can be seen most easily by looking at the molar crowns which are wider on the right than on the left. The patient's postoperative film in Figure 38.3 (p. 179) shows what the film should have looked like.

The radiograph shows extensive bone loss around the lower right and left second molars. The lower left second molar has bone loss and caries in the furcation. Furcation involvement was also evident on both lower first molars which were not as mobile.

■ ***Where are the implants? How might you localize them more accurately?***

The panoramic view is insufficient to localize the implants accurately. They appear in focus but the focal trough in the molar region is quite wide so that this gives no clue as to their buccolingual position. Their position and angulation will be critical in determining whether they can be used to support restorations.

If the end of the implant cannot be identified in the mouth, the implants could only be accurately localized using a tomographic technique, either CT scanning or multidirectional tomography. Conventional CT scanning is expensive and requires special software to prevent 'star artefact' shadows on the film. Multidirectional (spiral or

Table 38.2 Radiographic views

View	Advantages	Disadvantages
Dental panoramic radiograph (DPT)	This is the appropriate initial view for periodontal assessment; also as a general survey for a new patient and to identify the number of implants present and their approximate site.	Distortion and poor resolution make detailed assessment of periodontal bone support and caries difficult, especially around incisors.
Full mouth periapical films	Ideal for assessing bone loss if taken with a paralleling technique. Selected films, based on the panoramic view, would be ideal and still involve a lower dose than full mouth films because the panoramic provides a dose equivalent to only 4 E-speed periapical films.	Not necessary: probing depths around the upper and lower anterior teeth were normal or only slightly increased. Full mouth films cannot be justified as an initial investigation on the basis of the radiation dose.
Vertical bitewings	Ideal for molars and premolars when there is no more than moderate bone loss.	The missing upper molars would have made the positioning of the films difficult, if not impossible.

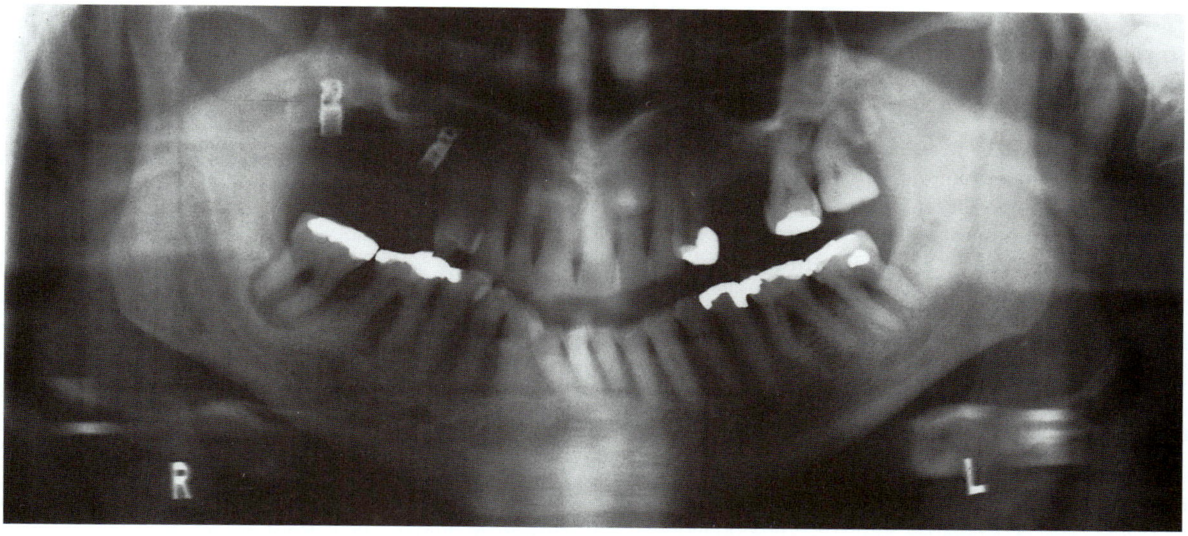

Fig. 38.2 Dental panoramic radiograph of the patient at presentation.

epicycloid) tomography performed in machines such as the Scanora or Tomax produces cross-sectional images of any part of the jaws much more easily and this or cone beam CT would be the best method. If the implants were misplaced, the film might be taken with radiopaque markers on the ridge to aid localization. Alternatively it could be assumed that the implants are in an appropriate position and a flap could be raised.

Are any other investigations necessary?

Yes, a urine glucose test to exclude diabetes would be prudent. This was negative.

Diagnosis

What is your diagnosis?

Chronic adult periodontitis, at a relatively advanced stage with considerable bone destruction around the molar teeth. There is grade 3 involvement of furcations on all lower molars and grade 2 involvement of the upper molars.

This patient has problems with furcation involvement. What are the possible sequelae?

- Devitalization of the tooth
- Further and more rapid periodontal destruction
- Periodontal abscess
- Root caries.

This patient has already had courses of periodontal treatment. Why have they failed?

Conservative periodontal treatment comprising oral hygiene instruction and scaling/root planing has been effective anteriorly. Posteriorly, where there are much deeper pockets and inacessible furcations, further intervention is required to halt progression. Oral hygiene must improve around the posterior teeth, particularly interdental cleaning. The patient is flossing too infrequently and in any case wide interdental spaces are more effectively cleaned with tape, brush floss or miniature bottle brushes.

Treatment

There is a need for immediate extraction of those teeth with a hopeless prognosis. A further period of improved cleaning and assessment is required before a definitive treatment plan can be made. There is root caries in one furcation and a caries prevention regime is also required.

Which teeth would you extract immediately?

Both lower second molars require extraction. The right molar has no bone support and is almost certainly nonvital. Bone loss around the mesial root is compromising the first molar. The left molar is less severely involved but has extensive caries in the furcation which renders the tooth unrestorable.

All the remaining molars have a poor prognosis and extraction must be considered. The upper molars have furcation involvement and the fused roots will make conservative treatment difficult. The lower first molars also have a poor prognosis and may require extraction later. However, all these molars are grade 2 mobile at maximum and are in occlusion and functional. They could be preserved in the short or medium term. The patient has shown some ability to control his disease around the anterior teeth and a definitive decision on extraction could be delayed until an attempt has been made to stabilize the periodontitis. If these extractions are carried out, the patient will either have to accept a premolar-to-premolar occlusion or a prosthesis.

The patient did not wish to lose more teeth than absolutely necessary and accepted a plan to retain a completely natural dentition for as long as possible. The remaining molars will be retained for the time being. There is a risk of excessive bone loss if abscesses develop or disease progresses. Close follow up will be required.

In the long term, what are the broad treatment options?

The broad options are presented in Table 38.3.

What is the appropriate solution for this patient?

This will depend largely on the patient, who has expressed a wish to retain a natural dentition for as long as possible making plans C and D preferable. Some recommendations can be made:

- The implants should be retained for use later. These have been placed at some expense and provide an insurance policy for the future. If a molar occlusion can be retained, they are not required in the short term.
- A premolar-to-premolar occlusion provides acceptable function, though the appearance may be unacceptable depending on the visibility of the molar spaces.
- The upper molars provide useful occlusion and, though compromised, will probably last many years with conservative treatment. If the upper molars are to be retained, the lower first molar should be preserved if at all possible.
- Preservation of the lower right first molar would provide occlusion against the upper second premolar and possibly against an implant-supported prosthesis in the longer term. However, complex treatment may be required and saving it might be regarded as a less essential element of treatment. The main reason for preserving it is that all the left molars may eventually be lost and it opposes the implants.
- Conservative treatment will take a long time and its success will depend primarily on the patient's ability to clean the teeth.

What are the treatment options for the lower first molars? Under what circumstances are these possible and practical?

See Table 38.4.

The patient quickly develops a more effective cleaning regime and root planing is performed. Over a period of 3 months the bleeding is eliminated and the mobility of all posterior teeth improves. There is still slight bleeding from the furcations of the lower first molars but the gingival condition is good. Conservative management appears to have been successful and more complex treatment options can be considered.

The following treatment is provided and the results are shown in Figure 38.3. Root resection is performed on the lower left molar and hemisection on the right. This eliminates the furcation and enables cleaning. The inflammation around the roots resolves.

Do the hemisected or root-resected teeth require restoration?

Ideally, yes. The large area of exposed dentine and risk of fracture of the overhanging crown after root resection really

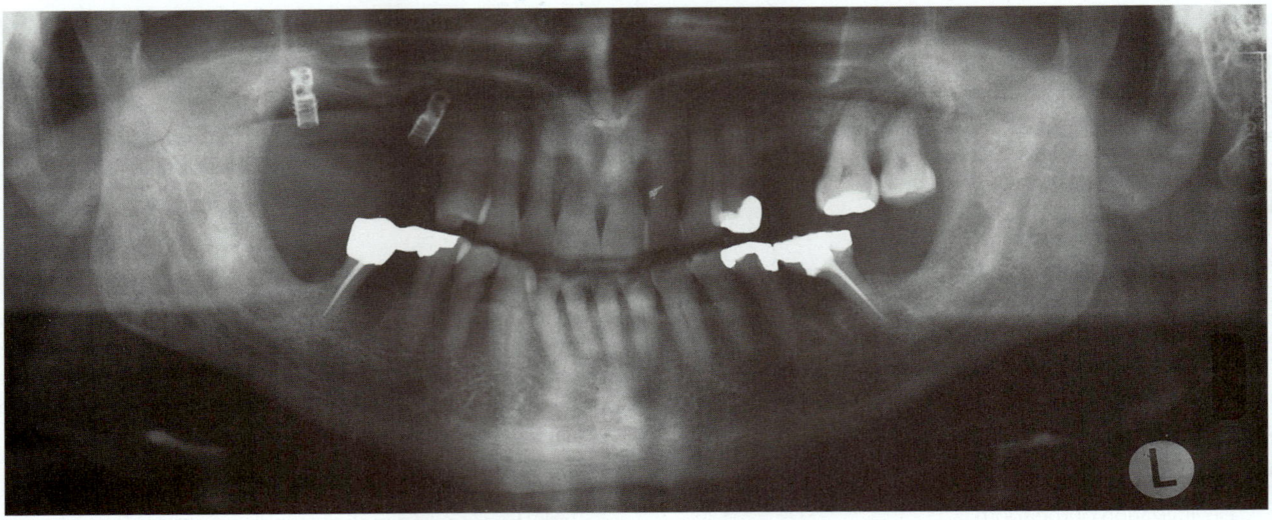

Fig. 38.3 Dental panoramic radiograph showing the result of treatment.

Table 38.3 Broad treatment options

Treatment plan	Advantages	Disadvantages
Lower arch		
Plan A. Extract all lower molar teeth and either leave or replace with an acrylic or cobalt–chrome based partial denture.	Simple approach with minimal need to treat the periodontal disease.	Transition to artificial dentition will be difficult especially with free end saddles in the mandible. Initially, acrylic dentures would be indicated in both jaws which may predispose to further deterioration of the periodontal tissues.
Plan B. Extraction of all lower molar teeth, provisional denture, and replacement of the teeth with implant-supported fixed or removable prosthesis.	The prognosis of the implants would be good and would eliminate the need for dentures.	This is a costly procedure but probably the most effective way to retain a molar occlusion.
Plan C. Conservative management with surgical investigation of the first molar teeth.	The only choice if the teeth are to be kept. The first molars are usually relatively easily cleaned and the root morphology makes preservation possible.	There is a cost implication of surgery and follow up treatment, and the procedure is uncomfortable. Oral hygiene must be excellent to embark on this course of action.
Upper arch		
Plan D. Retain the upper left molar and treat conservatively. Leave the implants buried for future use.	Retains natural dentition, inexpensive. Retains natural occlusion for lower first molar. If these teeth can be retained, no prosthesis will be necessary.	Accepting teeth with a poor prognosis means that dentures or bridges must be designed with their future loss in mind.
Plan E. Extract molars. Leave the implants buried, accepting the existing premolar-to-premolar occlusion.	A simple and inexpensive procedure.	The implants would not be used. The discomfort and expense associated with their placement would be needless.
Plan F. Extract molars. Use the implants to retain a removable partial denture replacing all the missing teeth.	The restoration would be relatively simple and have good retention and stability.	An expensive route because of the need for precision attachments within the denture. Often the attachments in the denture wear and need replacement.
Plan G. Extract molars. Maintain the edentulous space on the left side and replace the missing teeth on the right with an implant-supported bridge.	The implants would be used to retain a bridge. Eating would be easier and teeth provided on one side.	The loss of teeth on the contralateral side may become a problem. The position of the implants may mean that a bridge is not possible.

Table 38.4 Treatment options for the lower first molars

	Treatment	Indications and contraindications
Eliminate tooth	Extraction	Very mobile; poor oral hygiene or compliance; patient wishes; caries in furcation or elsewhere rendering tooth unrestorable; insufficient bone support on either root to conserve. This option has already been discussed and rejected.
Retain furcation	Root planing alone	Effective only for grade 1 involvement. Inappropriate in this case where furcations cannot be debrided without raising a flap.
	Root planing with surgery	Still difficult; possible for lower first molars only. The chances of success are improved if the furcation contour is changed ('furcoplasty').
	Tunnel prep/apically repositioned flaps	Opens furcation for cleaning but also risks caries.
Eliminate furcation	Hemisection or root resection	Difficult procedure; expensive; hemisected tooth loses contact on one side; full coverage restoration may be required. Only suitable for teeth with bone far enough below the furcation to allow surgical access.

demand full coverage restorations. However, complex and expensive treatment is often avoided because hemisected and root-resected teeth are compromised.

Hemisected or root-resected teeth which have proved themselves stable over a period of months or years are best restored. In this case the hemisected molar root was linked to the premolar with a fixed movable bridge. Care must be taken that the design of the bridge does not overload the periodontal support of the root. Both teeth remain in function and are excellent semipermanent solutions to this patient's problem.

Restoration, root treatment and surgery add up to a huge investment in time and money spent on one very compromised tooth root. If a definite need for a bridge or denture had been identified at the outset, an implant would have provided the support required at lower cost and with a better long-term prognosis.

■ *How do you assess the potential usefulness of the implants?*

The position of the implants is not favourable. Even on the panoramic view it can be seen that the fixtures are not parallel, making them unsuitable for a fixed prosthesis. The fixtures are small, of different types and partially integrated. The mesial implant would appear to have less bone supporting it, and it is unclear whether it could support significant occlusal load.

Case 39

Fractured incisors

SUMMARY

A 38-year-old man presents to you in your local hospital accident and emergency department. He has fractured his front teeth. You must manage the injury and outline a treatment plan for restoration.

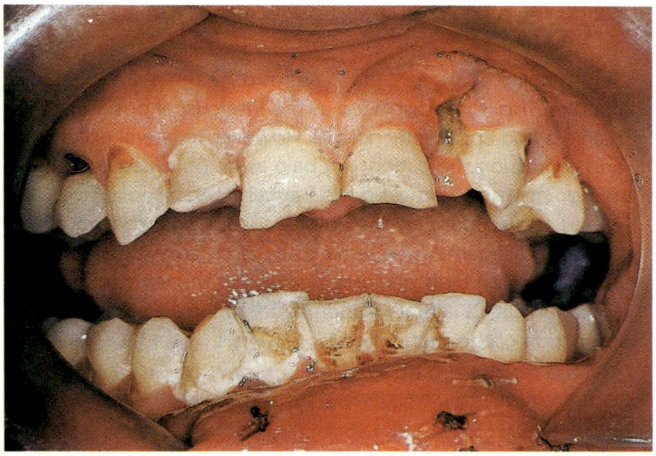

Fig. 39.1 The appearance of the anterior teeth on presentation.

History

Complaint

The patient's front teeth have been fractured and they are all loose. One tooth was knocked out and he feels pain when he bites.

History of complaint

The car accident occurred yesterday. The patient was sitting in the driver's seat when another car drove into his. He was stationary and not wearing a seat belt and was thrown forward, his lower face hitting the steering wheel. He did not lose consciousness and was taken to a local accident and emergency department where a laceration of his lower lip was sutured and no other injuries were found. At that time his teeth and jaws were not examined or radiographed and he has returned for a follow up appointment with you.

Medical history

Prior to the accident the patient was fit and healthy, with only allergy to penicillins and erythromycin noted on his medical history questionnaire.

Examination

Extraoral examination

■ ***How will you assess the possibility of a mandibular fracture?***

Fracture is suggested by:

- pain, swelling and tenderness at the fracture site
- bleeding, bruising or haematoma at fracture site
- displacement, step deformity
- change in occlusion
- mobility of fragments or of teeth
- difficulty opening the mouth or in lateral excursion
- paraesthesia or anaesthesia in the distribution of nerves involved in the fracture.

■ ***How will you assess the possibility of a fracture of the zygomatic arch or facial skeleton?***

In addition to the features noted above, fracture at these sites may produce:

- facial asymmetry and flattening of facial contour (may be masked by swelling for a few days)
- step deformity along infraorbital margin
- anaesthesia or paraesthesia of cheek, nose, upper lip and teeth
- unilateral epistaxis
- subconjunctival haemorrhage with no definable posterior limit
- restricted eye movements and diplopia.

On extraoral examination you cannot identify a mandibular or facial fracture. The lower lip is swollen and lacerated to the left of the midline. There is no restriction or pain on opening, nor swelling associated with the temporomandibular joint.

Intraoral examination

■ ***The anterior teeth are shown in Figure 39.1. What do you see?***

The swollen lower lip is just visible. The upper right lateral and both central incisors have been fractured. The upper left lateral incisor appears to be missing. The upper left canine is not fractured but has caries buccally and is mesially inclined. This inclination could predate the injury, in which case the lateral incisor may have been buccally positioned, or it could be a result of injury.

The oral hygiene is poor. This does not appear to be a result of injury because there are large accumulations of plaque,

Table 40.1 Methods of controlling anxiety

Method	Advantages and disadvantages
Behaviour modification	Simple to perform but time consuming. Methods include identifying causes of anxiety (which may be visual, auditory or olfactory), modifying anxiety using desensitization techniques and a 'tell-show-do' approach. Works well in mild or moderate anxiety and for routine dental treatment but is unlikely to be appropriate for surgical extractions.
Hypnosis	Requires trained clinician and several relatively time-consuming episodes of training prior to surgery. Can produce pain relief as well as anxiety suppression. If patient has already received hypnotherapy their suggestibility will be known and the preliminary episodes may not be necessary. No after-effects and no drugs required.
Preoperative oral anxiolytic drug	Suitable for mild anxiety and restorative procedures but unlikely to be sufficient for surgical extraction. May be used in addition to other techniques if the patient is so anxious that they may not even attend for their appointment. Unpredictable effect in children.
Inhalational sedation	Can be combined with oral anxiolytic drug. Requires trained operator and team. Suitable for routine dental treatment in mild and moderate anxiety and especially useful in anxiety-related gagging reflex. Ineffective in nasal obstruction or if patient fears mask.
Intravenous sedation	Requires trained operator and team but relatively simple in comparison with general anaesthesia and easily administered in a general practice setting. Fast and with few medical contraindications or adverse effects. Patient remains conscious throughout procedure.
General anaesthesia	Never the method of choice for minor procedures because of the risk of fatality. Though very low, this risk is sufficient to contraindicate general anaesthesia for most dental treatment in normal individuals. General Dental Council regulations require general anaesthesia to be performed in a hospital. May be required for patients with severe disabilities or more complex surgical procedures. Indications for general anaesthesia for removal of lower third molars are considered in Case 25.

The choice of anaesthesia for extraction of third molars is discussed in case 25.

The patient had originally wanted to be completely unconscious for her dental treatment. Following discussion about the risks and alternative options, she decided to try sedation.

Is epilepsy a contraindication to the use of sedation?

No. Benzodiazepines (e.g. midazolam) are the drugs of choice and have anticonvulsant properties. In any case, this patient's epilepsy is well controlled. An epileptic fit under sedation is most unlikely.

How would you assess the patient's fitness for intravenous sedation?

The American Society of Anesthesiologists (ASA) has a classification which is useful when assessing fitness for sedation or general anaesthesia:

ASA group	Definition
ASA I	Normal healthy patient
ASA II	Patient with mild systemic disease
ASA III	Patient with severe disease that is limiting but not incapacitating
ASA IV	Patient with incapacitating disease that is a constant threat to life
ASA V	Patient not expected to live more than 24 hours

Which groups would normally be considered suitable for treatment in an outpatient setting?

ASA groups I and II.

Does this mean that ASA group III-IV patients should never be treated under sedation?

No. Many ASA group III and IV patients may benefit from sedation because it reduces the patient's anxiety and, as a result, their endogenous catecholamine secretion. However, such patients should be treated in a hospital or specialist centre.

What medical investigation would you perform?

The systemic arterial blood pressure must be checked. 'Normal' blood pressure is 120/80 mmHg but small variations are common and the systolic blood pressure is often raised in anxious subjects. Hypertension which is well controlled is not a contraindication to sedation. However, patients with a diastolic blood pressure that is consistently above 110 mmHg should be investigated before sedation is given.

When you take the patient's blood pressure it is 140/90, consistent with her anxious demeanour.

Is this patient suitable for treatment under local anaesthetic with intravenous sedation?

Intravenous sedation would appear to be an ideal adjunct to local anaesthetic. The patient has practically no experience of dental procedures, has a history of failed treatment under local anaesthetic alone and is anxious about the extractions.

Treatment

What is the drug of choice for intravenous sedation?

Midazolam is a benzodiazepine well suited to dental sedation. It is soluble in water and presented in a 2-ml ampoule in a concentration of 5 mg/ml or in a 5-ml ampoule in a concentration of 2 mg/ml. Both presentations contain the same quantity of midazolam but the 5-ml (2 mg/ml) solution, being less concentrated, is easier to titrate.

Are there any contraindications to the use of midazolam?

Allergy to benzodiazepines is an absolute contraindication but is extremely rare. Some drugs interact with midazolam but careful administration of the sedative drug will minimize any difficulties. Drug abusers are notoriously difficult to sedate and treatment should only be carried out by very experienced practitioners.

■ ***What is meant by titration of the dose? Suggest a suitable titration regimen for a fit (ASA group I) adult patient being sedated with midazolam.***

Titration is administration of a drug in small quantities whilst observing the patient's response. Sedation is judged to be adequate when the patient looks relaxed, and displays a slight delay in response to questioning of commands (such as 'raise your arm'). There is often a degree of slurring of speech.

A suitable regimen would be 2 mg of midazolam injected intravenously over a period of 30 seconds followed by a pause of 90 seconds during which the patient's response is observed. If sedation is inadequate further increments of 1 mg should be administered every 30 seconds until sedation is sufficient. Local anaesthetic can then be administered and treatment carried out in the normal way.

■ ***What are the undesirable side-effects of intravenous midazolam?***

Intravenous sedation with midazolam is an extremely safe procedure when the drug is administered according to the above guidelines. However, all drugs have side-effects and the major worry with midazolam sedation is respiratory depression. There is a dose-related decrease in both respiratory rate and tidal volume which is most pronounced in the first 10 minutes of sedation.

■ ***How should a patient be protected from this potentially dangerous side-effect?***

Clinical monitoring by observing the patient must be carried out by both the dentist and a suitably trained and experienced dental nurse. The use of a pulse oximeter to monitor the arterial oxygen saturation and heart rate is mandatory for intravenous sedation.

All suitable pulse oximeters have 'alarm limits'. The minimum acceptable arterial oxygen saturation is 90%. If the alarm sounds the patient should be encouraged to take deep breaths. If this is not successful the airway must be opened (by tilting the head and lifting the chin) and the patient ventilated with the aid of a ventilator bag or mask. If breathing is still inadequate as judged by arterial oxygen saturation you should consider abandoning the dental procedure and administering the benzodiazepine antagonist flumazenil (Anexate).

■ ***Why must a 'second appropriate person' such as a dental nurse always be present during sedation and recovery?***

To help monitor the patient's condition, assist with any emergency and act as a chaperone in case the patient experiences a benzodiazepine-induced sexual fantasy which might result in charges being brought against the dentist (or another member of the dental team).

■ ***What postoperative care is required?***

At the end of the procedure, the patient is slowly returned to the upright position over a period of 3–5 minutes and helped to a supervised rest area. The patient must not be discharged until sufficiently recovered so as to be able to stand and walk without assistance.

The patient should be discharged into the care of an escort who must also be given written and verbal instructions.

■ ***What instructions would you give this patient and their escort following treatment?***

- Do not travel alone: travel home with your escort, by car if possible.
- For the next 8 hours:
  - Do not drive or ride a bicycle
  - Do not operate machinery
  - Do not drink alcohol
  - Do not return to work or sign legal documents.

■ ***Are benzodiazepine antagonists used routinely to hasten recovery after dental sedation?***

At present antagonists such as flumazenil are only recommended for emergency procedures such as countering benzodiazepine overdose and should not be used to hasten recovery. However, elective reversal of benzodiazepines may be helpful for some patients such as those who must travel some distance home on public transport. In such cases it is **imperative** that the usual postoperative instructions for intravenous sedation are given and adhered to.

Prognosis

■ ***Is the patient likely to require intravenous sedation for all future dental treatment?***

Not necessarily. Sedation will have ensured that the extractions were performed as pleasantly as possible and any existing dental phobia should not have been reinforced. The amnesic effect of benzodiazepines is likely to reduce the patient's memory of the whole procedure. During future visits for dental care anxiety-reducing methods should be used, so that eventually dental care can be provided routinely.

Case • 41

A blister on the cheek

SUMMARY

A 58-year-old lady patient of your general dental practice complains of a sore mouth with blisters. Identify the cause and outline appropriate management.

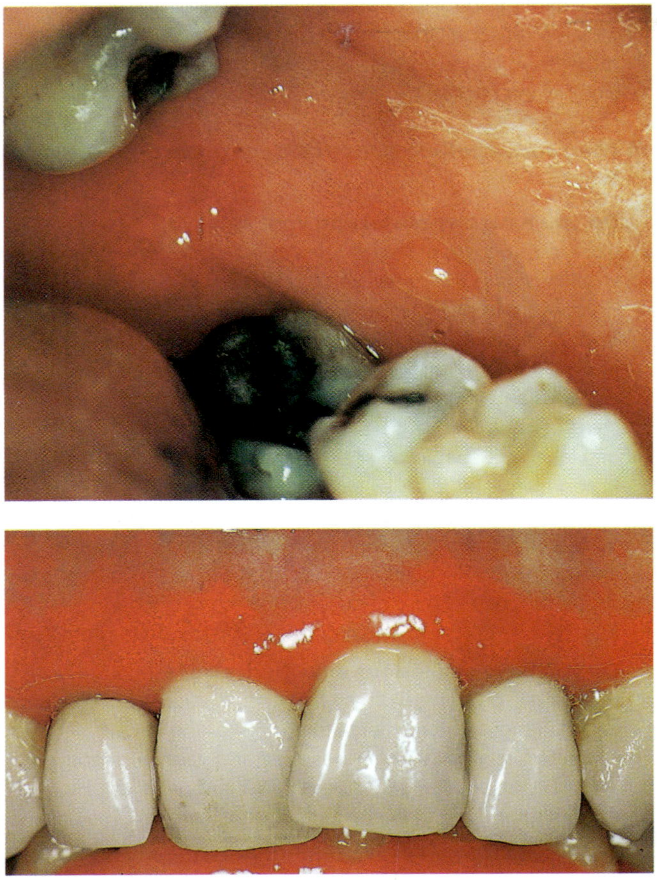

Fig. 41.1 a, b The patient on presentation.

History

Complaint

The patient complains of a very sore mouth. She describes blisters which last a few hours before bursting to release a clear fluid, or sometimes blood. The palate is particularly affected though lesions may develop anywhere in the mouth and often follow minor trauma. Each blister heals very slowly and the area is painful until healing is complete. She often finds she cannot brush her teeth.

History of complaint

The symptoms started about 1 year ago and are worsening.

Medical history

She has had hypertension for many years and her elderly medical practitioner has been treating her with methyldopa.

Examination

Extraoral examination

A fit-looking woman with a blood pressure of 140/90 when sitting. Visible skin and nails appear normal.

Intraoral examination

■ ***The appearance of the buccal mucosa and gingivae is presented in Figure 41.1. What do you see?***

The buccal mucosa has an extensive area of red atrophic mucosa posteriorly, possibly with small ulcers towards the anterior edge. The red area has an irregular margin. A small blister, a few millimetres across, lies near the centre of the buccal mucosa, just above the buccal cusp of the second premolar in the photograph.

The gingivae are also red but no blisters are present. The red area extends from the gingival margin across the mucogingival junction to involve the adjacent alveolar mucosa. The margin is poorly defined. The gingivae around all visible teeth are involved and the distribution of inflammation is not consistent with plaque accumulation as the cause.

Differential diagnosis

■ ***Which conditions cause oral blisters?***

- Mucous membrane pemphigoid
- Pemphigus vulgaris
- Lichen planus
- Erythema multiforme
- Angina bullosa haemorrhagica
- Epidermolysis bullosa
- Dermatitis herpetiformis
- Viral infections
- Trauma.

■ ***What name is given to the gingival lesions?***

A band of red atrophic or eroded mucosa affecting the attached gingiva is known as desquamative gingivitis. Unlike plaque-induced inflammation it is a dusky red colour and extends beyond the marginal gingiva, often to the full width of the attached gingiva and sometimes onto the alveolar mucosa. Some reserve the term for cases where the epithelium blisters or peels while others use it whenever the characteristic red appearance is present.

■ ***What are the main causes of desquamative gingivitis?***

- Lichen planus
- Mucous membrane pemphigoid
- Pemphigus.

■ ***Which of these conditions would you include in your initial differential diagnosis? Explain why.***

Either pemphigoid or pemphigus is the most likely diagnosis whenever there is a good history of blister formation. The most frequent cause of oral blisters is mucous membrane ('cicatricial') pemphigoid. This typically affects middle-aged and elderly women causing relatively long-lived vesicles and bullae (bullae are blisters greater than 10 mm in diameter) in areas of friction. Pemphigus vulgaris is less common and predominantly affects women in early middle age. In pemphigus it is unusual to notice long-lived vesicles or bullae, because the loss of keratinocyte adhesion which causes the disease makes the blister roof extremely fragile. Both diseases cause desquamative gingivitis. In this case, the history is more suggestive of pemphigoid than pemphigus. However, pemphigus must be specifically excluded by investigation because it can progress to extensive skin lesions and be difficult to treat.

These conditions would also need to be considered whenever a patient presents with chronic ulceration or erosion of the oral mucosa. This is because the vesicles and bullae often break down so rapidly that patients may be unaware of the blistering phase. Ragged tags of epithelium around ulcer margins would suggest that the ulcer was derived from a pre-existing bulla.

Lichen planus is the commonest condition in the differential diagnosis and also affects the middle-aged. However, it rarely produces well-defined blisters and when it does they are usually on the gingivae. Some refer to this situation as *bullous lichen planus*. However, this is not a specific form of lichen planus. Bulla formation merely reflects separation of the epithelium as a result of inflammatory destruction of its basal cells by the underlying disease process. In this case lichen planus seems an unlikely cause. Blisters are a prominent feature and no white striae are present on the buccal mucosa or the affected gingivae.

■ ***What diagnoses have you excluded? Explain why.***

Erythema multiforme is an unlikely possibility. Although erythema multiforme does cause blistering it is distinctive clinically. The pattern of recurrent episodes of acute blistering and ulceration, particularly affecting the anterior mouth and lips of young males, is characteristic. Occasionally patients, including the middle-aged, have a more chronic form of erythema multiforme and the diagnosis might be considered when other more common blistering conditions have been excluded. Erythema multiforme does not cause typical desquamative gingivitis.

Angina bullosa haemorrhagica is the name given to recurrent oral blood blisters. The blisters usually affect the palate or oropharynx and are often long lived to the extent that patients burst them for symptomatic relief. The condition is diagnosed on the basis of exclusion of other conditions and the typical presentation, particularly the constant presence of blood as the blister fluid. In this case blood was present in only a minority of the lesions and the sites involved would not be typical. Angina bullosa haemorrhagica does not cause desquamative gingivitis.

Drug reactions may occasionally lead to pemphigus and pemphigoid-like presentations, lichenoid reactions and erythema multiforme. This patient is taking methyldopa which is commonly implicated in lichenoid reactions but these are lichen planus-like rather than vesiculobullous. Of these conditions, only a lichenoid reaction might cause desquamative gingivitis.

A number of less common vesiculobullous conditions may affect the mouth, but can be effectively excluded at this stage. Dermatitis herpetiformis may be associated with coeliac disease and is usually accompanied by skin lesions and usually affects the soft palate. The various forms of epidermolysis bullosa are inherited and most are accompanied by skin lesions from a young age. Unlike the skin, direct trauma is almost never a cause of oral vesicles or bullae. Viral conditions cause acute single attacks of vesicles rather than bullae and are usually accompanied by systemic signs of infection.

■ ***What additional questions would you ask in the history? Why?***

Do you have any blisters on your skin? This is the most important question. Skin lesions, or a clear history of them, would confirm the presence of a systemic disease, may aid diagnosis and provide further lesions for investigation. Approximately half of pemphigus patients have oral lesions alone during the first year but develop skin lesions later. Lichen planus may be accompanied by a rash on the wrists, shins or back. Though the rash may resolve long before the oral lesions, it should be specifically sought in the history if lichen planus is a possibility. Erythema multiforme may be accompanied by the typical target lesions, though these usually signify typical severe oral erythema multiforme (Stevens–Johnson syndrome), which is unlike this patient's presentation. A history of onset following specific triggers (e.g. cold sore) would also suggest erythema multiforme.

Do you have any lesions anywhere else? Mucous membrane pemphigoid may be accompanied by ocular and vaginal lesions, the former leading to scarring and, if untreated, sometimes blindness. Eye and vaginal symptoms should be sought by questioning and, if appropriate, by examination.

If you were able to examine the patient you would find that she has no skin lesions and gives no history of a rash.

Table 41.1 Tests and special procedures

Test	Significance/special procedures
Nikolsky's sign	Some clinicians attempt to elicit Nikolsky's sign, in which gentle lateral pressure on apparently unaffected mucosa or skin (not rubbing the surface) raises a bulla. This is positive in vesiculobullous diseases but is somewhat unpredictable. In pemphigus the epithelium tends to disintegrate rather than form a bulla. If no lesions are present on examination it may be a useful way of demonstrating reduced epithelial adhesion, but it is often not necessary for diagnosis. Unsurprisingly, it is also unpopular with patients who are left with a large new ulcer which may take weeks to heal.
Biopsy	An incisional biopsy is indicated and it will almost certainly need to be investigated by immunofluorescence to differentiate the autoimmune blistering conditions. An incisional specimen removed from a vesicle or bulla margin or from apparently normal perilesional mucosa is best. Skin may also be sampled if involved. The biopsy must include epithelium and may be difficult to perform because the mucosa may disintegrate on slight trauma. The specimen should be either taken fresh to the laboratory immediately, frozen in liquid nitrogen at the chairside or placed in a special transport medium. Tissue fixed in formalin is useless for immunofluorescence.
Serum autoantibody determination	A sample of clotted blood should also be sent for indirect immunofluorescence to detect circulating pemphigus or pemphigoid autoantibody.

Investigations

■ ***What special tests would you perform and what is their significance? Are any special procedures required?***

See Table 41.1.

■ ***The biopsy specimen is shown in Figure 41.2. What do you see?***

The epithelium has separated cleanly from the underlying connective tissue in the plane of the basement membrane. A few erythrocytes lie in the cleft between the two. No cause for the separation is evident. The epithelium appears almost normal and there are only a few inflammatory cells in the lamina propria.

■ ***The immunofluorescence stain for complement C3 is shown in Figure 41.3. What do you see?***

The immunofluorescence staining has been carried out on a separate part of the specimen in which there is no epithelial separation. A bright line of fluorescence runs along the basement membrane, outlining the rete processes of the epithelium. Immunofluorescence for IgG gave an identical result.

■ ***How do you interpret these histological features?***

Separation of the full thickness of the epithelium at the level of the basement membrane, without epithelial damage, almost certainly signifies pemphigoid. Pemphigus is excluded by the lack of acantholysis and the level of separation. Lichen planus is excluded by the lack of basal cell degeneration and lymphocytic infiltration of the epithelium. The direct immunofluorescence indicates binding of IgG at the basement membrane and activation of complement. This indicates pemphigoid in which IgG autoantibody binds and fixes complement. Taken together, these features indicate pemphigoid.

Diagnosis

The patient has pemphigoid. There are different variants of pemphigoid but, as there is no skin involvement, mucous membrane pemphigoid is almost certainly the diagnosis. Bullous pemphigoid, linear IgA disease and epidermolysis bullosa acquisita are pemphigoid variants which very rarely affect the mouth.

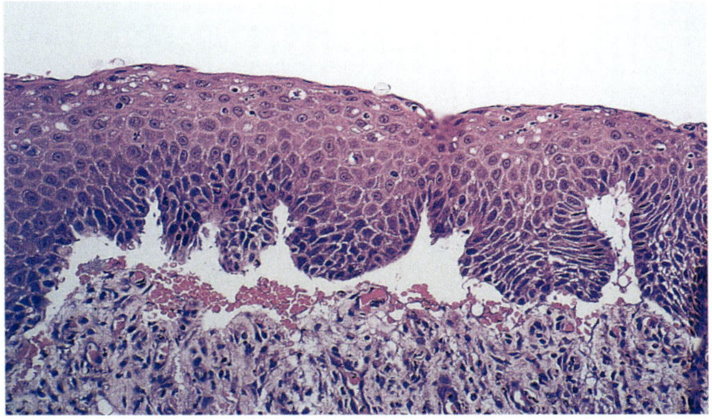

Fig. 41.2 Histological appearances of the biopsy specimen stained with haematoxylin and eosin.

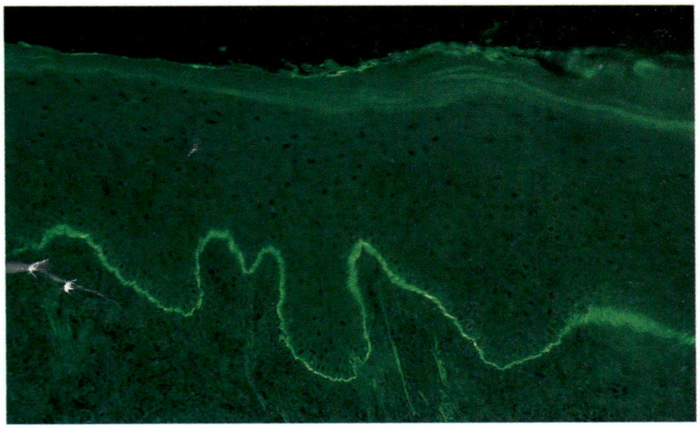

Fig. 41.3 The biopsy specimen after immunofluorescence staining for complement component C3.

Treatment

■ ***How should this patient be managed?***

The patient should preferably be treated in a hospital environment, at least initially. This will probably be necessary in order to perform the immunofluorescence tests. Treatment of pemphigoid requires more potent steroids than are usually considered appropriate in a general dental practice setting. However, there is no reason why routine dental treatment should be transferred to hospital.

The patient should be referred to an ophthalmologist to identify and manage any ocular lesions that may be present.

Lesions limited to the mouth and of relatively minor severity can be treated with topical steroids. Potent steroids are required, such as betamethasone 0.5 mg qds used as a mouthwash. Patients must be warned not to swallow such potent steroids and must be regularly checked for adverse effects. However, if oral lesions are widespread from the outset, if there are eye signs or if topical steroids fail, dapsone is the drug of choice. If this proves ineffective, systemic steroids, sometimes with azathioprine, are required. After the disease is brought under control, topical steroids may be sufficient for maintenance.

All patients using systemic or topical steroids are predisposed to oral candidal infection and this should be monitored at subsequent visits.

Case • 42

Will *you* see my son?

SUMMARY

The mother of a 6-year-old child brings him to your practice to ask for an appointment. She cannot find another dentist to see him.

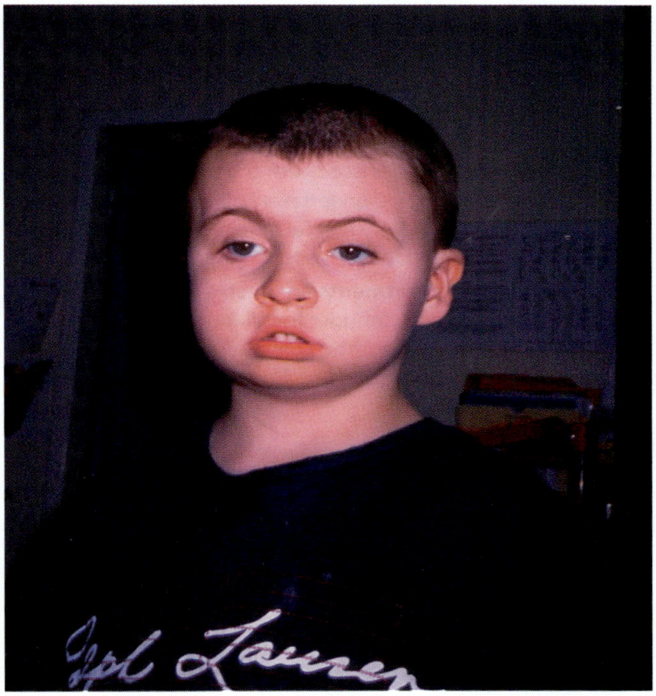

Fig. 42.1 The patient on presentation.

History

Complaint

The mother reports that she has asked several dentists to see her autistic son, but they all find reasons not to.

History of complaint

No one has ever been able to perform a proper check-up on her son. A recent attempt by another dentist ended in failure. Recently he has been putting objects into his mouth and biting his clothes. His mother is worried that he may be in pain but is unable to tell her.

Medical history

The patient was diagnosed with autism at age 3 years. He has no other medical conditions and takes melatonin to help him sleep. His mother thinks that he may be allergic to wheat and dairy produce and consequently tries to exclude these from his diet.

Examination

Extraoral examination

■ ***The patient is shown in Figure 42.1. What do you see?***

In a still photograph the patient appears essentially normal, as most children with autism do. However, he fails to make eye contact (or look at the camera) and has a relatively large head, a feature seen in some young children.

While you speak to the mother in the waiting room the child is flapping his hands and rocking backwards and forwards. He does not seem to be aware of his surroundings.

It appears that you will not be able to perform an examination easily.

■ ***What is autism?***

Autism is a developmental disorder, more accurately described as autistic spectrum disorder (ASD) because it includes a range of conditions. All are characterized by three key diagnostic features:

1. Impairment of social interaction
2. Impairment of communication
3. Repetitive, stereotypical patterns of behaviour.

Autism has a wide range of expression. Some individuals have normal or near-normal intelligence, though three-quarters have some degree of learning disability. Males are four times more frequently affected than females. The mildest form, Asperger's syndrome, is compatible with a near-normal life.

■ ***What is the cause of autism?***

Autism is considered to be primarily genetic in origin. It is not unusual for siblings to be affected, though they may not be recognized if signs are limited to subtle lack of social skills or failure of language development. Autism appears to be a complex multifactorial condition and several genes have been identified that may contribute, on both autosomes and sex chromosomes. It appears that there are changes in brain structure in autism, but these remain to be defined.

■ ***What features of autism will affect your management?***

Verbal communication is a major problem. Many children never develop functional speech and are reliant on communication aids. Some develop the ability to repeat back what is said to them (echolalia), seemingly understanding, but usually not. One positive aspect of this behaviour is that copying the sound 'ah' may allow you to see inside the mouth.

Lack of nonverbal communication may prevent you from using alternative strategies. There is a lack of eye contact, making it difficult to gain and maintain attention, and an inability to interpret nonverbal signals or emotions from facial expression or tone of voice.

Aversion to physical contact makes examination, treatment and the usual means of physical reassurance ineffective.

Hypersensitivity to sights, sounds, smells and touch may be a feature and present problems with tooth brushing and dental treatment.

Idiosyncratic behaviours, such as highly specific insistence on the colour or consistency of food, are frequent. This may make dietary control difficult.

Resistance to change. Autism is associated with a strong need for routine. Individuals will like events to be predictable and new experiences may unbalance the whole day.

Unusual diets are frequent because many parents exclude wheat, dairy products or yeast in an attempt to improve the condition. In combination with the patient's own dietary demands, this may make dietary prevention very difficult.

You may also need to consider that the parents themselves may suffer a mild form of the disorder and their communication and social interaction may appear unusual.

■ *Are other significant medical conditions associated with autism?*

Yes, the behavioural pattern of autism can have several causes and 10% of individuals will have other conditions such as Rett's syndrome, fragile X syndrome, tuberous sclerosis or phenylketonuria.

Epilepsy is a common association and, if not present in childhood, often manifests as in adolescence. Attention deficit hyperactivity disorder is sometimes present and patients may take methylphenidate (Ritalin) to help address this behaviour.

■ *Should this patient be referred for hospital or specialist care?*

Given time and careful planning you would probably be able to examine and carry out simple treatment for the patient. If you consider that there is severe pain, infection or other acute condition, then immediate referral to a specialist care centre where general anaesthesia is available would be appropriate.

However, you still need to examine him to explore alternatives. There is no reason why patients at the more able end of the spectrum cannot be treated in general practice for routine preventive and even simple restorative care.

■ *What will you do next?*

It appears that the patient may be in pain. You will wish to determine the cause quickly, but without a careful plan of action you will probably fail. Before you can proceed you will need some information from the mother.

■ *What information will help you plan treatment?*

The following information would be helpful:

- Patient's likes and dislikes – useful in establishing a rapport with the child
- Any communication aids that are used (see below)
- Possible associated behavioural conditions such as attention deficit hyperactivitiy disorder
- Possible associated medical conditions such as medication and epilepsy
- Therapies being used to help the condition
- Whether tooth brushing is managed and whether toothpaste is tolerated
- Whether the child is able to give a degree of cooperation and accept physical contact. Experiences such as having a haircut are often good indicators of this.

If you see many patients with special care requirements you would probably have a special questionnaire to collect this information, but this is an emergency situation.

■ *Might treatment for autism affect or aid dental care?*

Drug treatments include antiepileptics, methylphenidate (Ritalin), selective serotonin reuptake inhibitors, antigastric reflux drugs and melatonin. While these have some oral adverse effects, such as dry mouth, they should not compromise treatment. Some medication addresses anxiety and aggressive behaviour.

Behavioural therapy is the most effective treatment but is very labour-intensive, costly and of limited availability. Applied behavioural analysis (ABA) breaks down learning into tiny chunks, using imitation and reinforcement to encourage autistic children to communicate, then speak and follow commands, before moving on to more advanced skills. Positive responses are rewarded by reinforcers such as food, social interactions, games or toys. Given more time, visits to the dentist could be rehearsed with the patient's ABA teacher. If, as here, this cannot be undertaken, at least knowing the rewards used may be very helpful in reinforcing good behaviour at this, and future, visits.

Complementary treatments are often sought by parents. Some parents consider that fluorides, amalgam or foods worsen or cause autism. Some negotiation and compromise may be required on both sides to allow successful treatment.

■ *What is your plan to examine the child?*

As the child may be in pain, you need to make some attempt to examine the mouth. If you are not successful, you need to ensure that the visit does not become a negative experience. You will need to reinforce all positive behaviour and regard this as the first of, perhaps several, short experience visits. These may achieve little more than 'saying hello' and allowing the child to see you, your staff and the surgery and experience its smells. Autistic children are highly anxious in new situations but repeated exposure helps.

Invite the mother and child into the surgery. Reassure the mother that her child's behaviour does not worry you or your staff and try to appear confident. Make sure there is a quiet calm atmosphere, without distractions such as telephones ringing. Observe the child's behaviour and remember that the most likely cause of poor behaviour will be anxiety.

Don't expect him to sit in a dental chair. Try engaging him at a sink, playing with running water. Try a toothbrush, if acceptable. This may allow you to view the child's mouth.

How can you communicate with the patient?

There are some basic rules that will stand you in good stead. Keep the language very simple and limit yourself to a few concepts.

- Use the child's name at the beginning of every sentence to get his attention.
- Always look at the child when you are talking to him.
- Speak slowly.
- Omit unnecessary words, especially social language – 'please' and 'thank you' will only be understood by mildly affected individuals.
- Avoid idiomatic expressions. 'Take a seat' will be taken literally.
- Humour has no effect and will not be understood.
- Be patient.

Some individuals may use pictorial communication aids such as Makaton or the Pictorial Exchange Communication System (PECS). Makaton uses iconic symbols and line drawings to convey the meaning of words. The more user-friendly PECS system teaches nonspeaking children to exchange pictures of things that they want for the item, using their visual rather than verbal skills. An example is shown in Figure 42.2.

Parents or teachers can produce a series of pictures or photographs to make a 'social storyline' that will help prepare the child for the next dental visit and reduce anxiety. An example is shown in Figure 42.3. You will need to investigate the child's own communication strengths.

Try to engage the child. Knowing what he likes and dislikes is most important. Try to identify something in the surgery, perhaps moving the dental chair, playing with the light or a toy, that can be used to reinforce good behaviour.

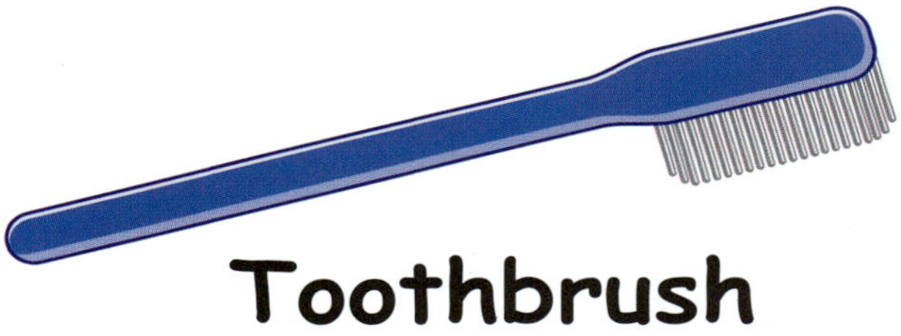

Fig. 42.2 A pictorial exchange picture.

If the patient is in pain, what causes would be likely?

Without having set up the visit in the way described above, you may only achieve a glimpse of the teeth so you will need to know likely causes in advance. For this patient, these are:

- **Caries,** especially if the diet or behavioural reinforcers are cariogenic
- **Trauma** from a nonvital deciduous incisor, because children with autism with epilepsy are prone to trauma
- **Self-mutilation** is sometimes seen: patients may pick at their gingivae causing ulceration or inflammation
- **Mobile lower incisors** resulting from physiological loss in a child aged 6 years
- **Discomfort or pericoronitis** associated with erupting first permanent molars.

The history of mouthing and chewing objects would be suggestive of either of the last two causes.

Using the strategies described above you manage to get the child to let you look at his teeth while his mother brushes them. No caries is obvious, but both lower central deciduous incisors are very mobile. These appear to be the cause of the discomfort and the mother can be reassured. No intervention is likely to be helpful or possible. This is a self-limiting problem.

If caries had been noted, there would probably have been no option but to refer the patient for treatment under general anaesthetic. This would have the benefit of allowing a complete examination and radiographs, which might otherwise take months to achieve. If the first permanent molars were erupted, fissure sealing could also be performed under anaesthetic.

You ask the mother to bring the child back for a subsequent visit. There will be time for the child to be properly prepared using pictures, as described above, and possibly one or more trips to your surgery waiting room. The mother should bring the patient's own toothbrush and paste. These form a conceptual link for the patient between visiting the dentist and his teeth and also allow you to capitalize on

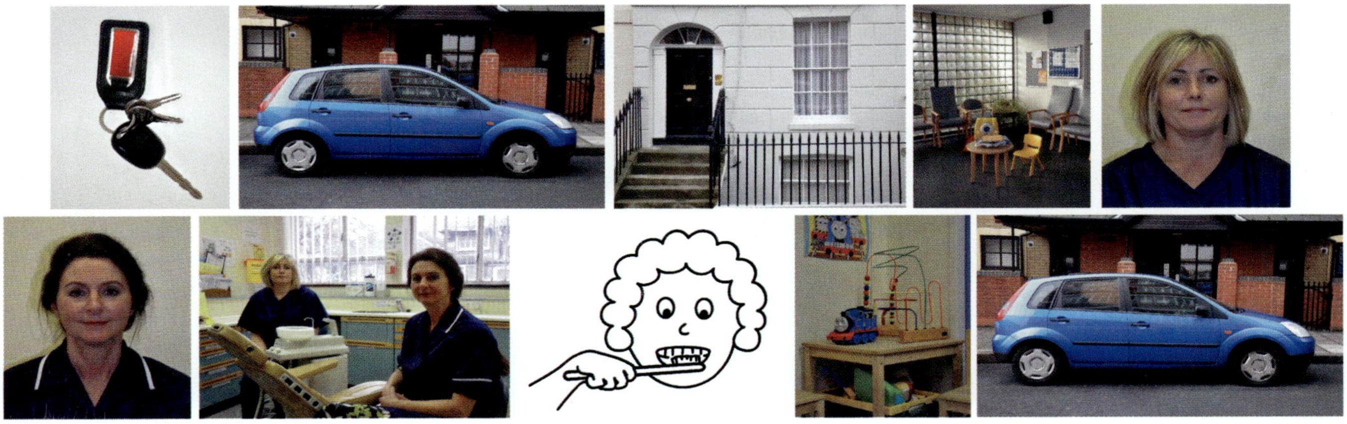

Fig. 42.3 Example of social storyline preparing for a visit to the dentist.

behaviour that is normally part of the patient's home routine. The parent should be instructed to show the mobile teeth to the child in a mirror.

■ *What is your strategy for further visits?*

Plan frequent short visits making progress in small increments, until the child accepts dental examination sitting in the dental chair. The aims are to provide an intensive preventive regime so that treatment is unnecessary and to be able to undertake examinations to ensure the regime is effective. The 'social storyline' prepared for the next visit is shown in Figure 42.3.

Dietary analysis is critical, given the unusual diets noted above. Safe reinforcers and snacks may need some imaginative thought since wheat and dairy products are unacceptable, chronic diarrhoea rules out fruit and the child will only eat food of one colour. Sugar-free confectionery may have to be considered.

Establishing toothbrushing habits is essential for autistic children. Not only does it maintain gingival health but it will also deliver fluoride toothpaste. As for other children with disability, an adult toothpaste with a high fluoride dose is appropriate given the importance of preventing caries. If toothbrushing habits are established, a toothbrush is usually the best way to entice children with learning difficulty to open their mouth.

The dental treatment of children with autism in a general practice can be a challenge. The dental visit can be a very positive experience for some families with children who are mildly affected. However, the degree of learning disability and communication in the majority of patients usually requires referral to a specialist.

Case 43

Bridge design

SUMMARY

A 28-year-old woman presents to you in your general dental practice with an edentulous premolar space on the upper left. She would like this space filled. What are the options?

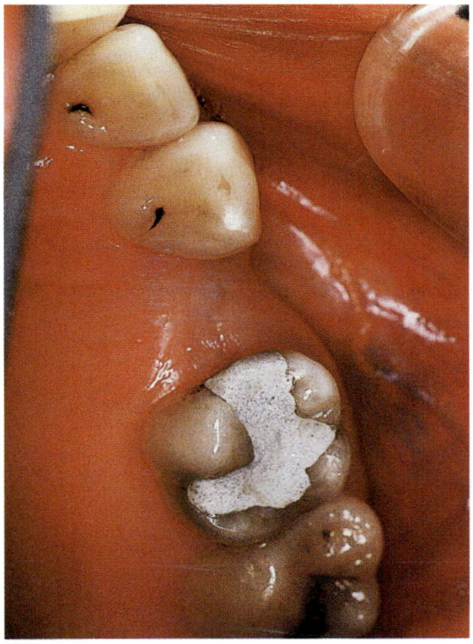

Fig. 43.1 The premolar space on presentation.

History

Complaint

Her complaint is the appearance of the gap. She would like it filled in time for her wedding in a few months time and requests a bridge.

History of complaint

The patient had all four first premolars extracted for orthodontic treatment in her early teens. After treatment with fixed appliances the premolar space was closed and the result had been stable. However, she then lost the upper left second premolar because of a combination of caries and root fracture following root canal treatment. This was about 2 years ago and she has had no replacement since.

Dental history

The patient first came to your practice 18 months ago, shortly after having had the second premolar extracted. You have made her dentally fit and instituted preventive treatment which appears to have been successful. No caries is present in any teeth and the gingival condition is good. The patient consumes a low sugar diet and has good oral hygiene.

Medical history

The patient is fit and well with no medical problems.

Examination

Extraoral examination

No abnormalities are present on extraoral examination. The premolar space is visible during speech.

Intraoral examination

The patient has an almost complete and well restored dentition with small- or medium-sized amalgam restorations. Although two premolars are missing, the gap is only a single premolar-sized unit of space because of the orthodontic treatment. This is her only missing tooth.

There is a mesio-occlusal restoration in the upper left first molar tooth. The first molar and the incisor teeth are in class I occlusion, with canine guidance in left lateral excursion. The orthodontic treatment has left the canine and molar vertically aligned and there has been no significant mesial drift of the first molar in the 2 years since extraction. The features are shown in Figure 43.1.

- ***What alternatives are there for replacing the missing tooth and what are their relative advantages and disadvantages?***

The options are shown in Table 43.1.

- ***What specific features of importance with regard to restoration would you examine? Explain why.***

The degree of bone loss of the edentulous alveolar ridge is important. If this is extensively resorbed, an elongate pontic would be necessary to hide the bone loss. This might well be unacceptable if the pontic is easily seen during talking or smiling. This problem can be overcome with ridge augmentation prior to placement of the bridge, but this would prolong the treatment and make it considerably more complex. A diagnostic wax-up may help the patient visualize the potential result if resorption is a problem or the appearance is critical.

Size of existing restorations in potential abutment tooth. This is the most important consideration for minimal

Table 43.1 Replacement options

Replacement	Advantages	Disadvantages
Removable partial denture	Removable for cleaning; cheaper than a fixed replacement; flange useful to improve appearance if significant bone loss has developed buccally; appearance can be good.	Patients rarely prefer a removable prosthesis and dislike palatal coverage. If poorly cleaned it will compromise the gingival margin around several teeth. Retention may deteriorate with time.
Minimal preparation bridge	Appearance can be excellent. No coverage of the palate required. Conservative of tooth tissue. Subsequent preparation for a conventional bridge is possible.	More expensive, significant laboratory fees. Not suitable if there is significant loss of alveolar ridge after the extraction. Must be cleaned in place. Average lifespan of restoration only about 5 years.
Conventional bridge	As for the minimal preparation bridge. Additionally, crowning adjacent teeth allows their appearance to be improved if heavily restored. Reasonable longevity approaching 10 years.	As for the minimal preparation bridge. Additionally destructive of tooth tissue.
Implant retained crown	Conservative of tooth tissue; no abutment preparation needed. Long-term survival rates are good.	Expensive. Involves surgical procedures as well as laboratory fees. Not an immediate result; may take 6–9 months to complete. Patient may require temporary prosthesis while implant integrates. Good quality bone and sufficient alveolar width and height required.

preparation bridges which require either no restorations or only small restorations in abutment teeth. Extensively restored teeth leave little natural tooth tissue to supply retention for conventional bridges. The quality of existing restorations must be known if they are to be used to prepare a core.

Inclination of the potential abutment teeth. A degree of vertical alignment is necessary to eliminate undercuts and allow the bridge to be made in the laboratory. Provided the teeth are fairly parallel this can be provided by preparation. If the teeth are not parallel, a fixed–movable design is useful because it allows the restoration on each tooth to have a different path of withdrawal.

Reduced length of clinical crown on either potential abutment tooth. Toothwear or repeated restoration may reduce the length of the clinical crown. There may be insufficient crown length to guarantee a retentive preparation. In extreme cases additional retention such as a post may need to be considered. However, post crowns do not make very good bridge retainers. They fail relatively frequently and should be avoided wherever possible.

Increased length of clinical crown on either potential abutment tooth. Recession makes crown preparation more difficult because it is difficult to prevent undercuts in long preparations. It may be necessary to place the crown margin some distance from the gingival margin and this might compromise the appearance if the margin were visible.

The width of the alveolar ridge is also important if implants are to be considered. For standard implants a minimum of 7 mm mesiodistal space between the adjacent teeth and 7 mm interocclusal space is needed. Particular attention should be given to the buccal contour of the edentulous ridge as a concavity would make implant placement difficult.

What investigations would you carry out? Explain why.

Tests of vitality of the potential abutment teeth, in this case the upper left first molar and canine.

If teeth are nonvital, any bridge design would need to take this into account. If required, endodontic treatment would have to be performed before bridge construction. The bridge should not be made until root filling is proved successful. Also, it would be a pity to have to weaken the bridge by making access to the root canals after placement.

Periapical radiographs of the potential abutment teeth are required. These are to exclude unsuspected caries, periodontal bone loss and other pathological lesions. They may also be required to assess the quality of pre-existing root fillings or for root treatment if either tooth proves to be nonvital.

Study models are useful in some cases. They can be used to make a diagnostic wax-up to show the patient the likely shape of the proposed bridges and to mould a former to make a provisional restoration. They also allow the clinician to plan treatment, including abutment preparation and pontic size outside the mouth. Articulated models mounted using a facebow could be used to analyse the occlusion.

Diagnosis

What type of replacement appears ideal?

The patient has indicated a preference for a fixed prosthesis and there seems no clinical reason to suggest any other option. A minimal preparation bridge is the most conservative option. A conventional bridge in this region would mean considerable destruction of the unrestored abutment teeth. Minimal preparation bridges carry the risk of failure sooner than conventional bridges, but a lifespan of about 5 years can be expected and a conventional bridge or implants could be considered then. There would be no advantage in providing a metal-based partial denture. The costs would be similar to those of a bridge.

The possibility of leaving the gap unfilled should also be considered. The adjacent teeth might drift into the gap or the opposing teeth might overerupt. These changes could be kept under review using study casts. However, even if the teeth did move, a prosthesis remains only advisable and not essential. This is a decision based on appearance and the final decision must rest with the patient.

What factors might make you suggest a removable prosthesis instead?

The cost is probably the most common reason for choosing a denture rather than a bridge. However a number of specific reasons might favour the removable prosthesis:

- Missing teeth requiring replacement on both sides of the arch.
- Mobility or significant periodontal bone loss or inflammation around either abutment tooth.
- If the patient is likely to lose further teeth in the short term, replacements would be more easily added to a partial denture.
- A high smile line with marked resorption of the edentulous alveolar bone. This is most satisfactorily hidden by an acrylic flange.
- Poor oral hygiene or a high caries rate would make it unwise to expensively restore the abutments and provide a fixed prosthesis which is difficult to clean. A denture could compromise a larger number of teeth, and neither replacement is ideal in this instance. However, a carefully designed partial denture is the better option.

If the patient opted for a removable prosthesis, what designs would you consider?

In this bounded saddle situation a metal-based tooth-supported design is ideal. Both abutment teeth would require a rest seat preparation and one abutment tooth would require a clasp. A palatal connector would be required but need not cover the whole palate, provided sufficient rigidity can be achieved to prevent distortion (which usually occurs out of the mouth). A second clasp on the opposite side would provide sufficient retention.

A mucosa-supported acrylic denture with minimal coverage of the palatal gingival tissues is possible. However this would be difficult to design. There are no other edentulous spaces and an Every-type design would not be possible.

Should the study models be mounted on an articulator to make the bridge?

Properly articulated models mounted with the use of a facebow are essential when a bridge:

- involves many teeth
- changes the anterior guidance
- includes occlusal surfaces involved in guidance
- increases the vertical dimension.

In general an articulator can be helpful when planning and making posterior crowns or bridges on patients who have a class II division 1 incisal relationship and anterior crowns and bridges on patients with a class II division 2 incisal relationship. The choice of articulator will depend on the clinician's preference, but in most cases with straightforward restorations a semiadjustable articulator is satisfactory. For simple crowns and bridges when the guidance is straightforward, such as the present case, either hand-held models or a simple hinge articulator are satisfactory.

What is the ideal design of minimal preparation bridge?

The ideal design of bridge varies with the site of the edentulous space. Various possibilities are shown in Figure 43.2. In the upper anterior region a simple cantilever design lasts longest. In the lower anterior region a fixed–fixed design is usually more dependable because the surface area of enamel on lower incisors is insufficient to support a simple cantilever design. In this situation, a simple cantilever using the molar as a retainer or fixed–fixed or fixed–movable designs are possible.

In this case a simple cantilever design was selected. The completed bridge is shown in Figure 43.3 and 43.4. To maximize the rigidity of the retainer and increase the surface area of enamel available for bonding, the existing amalgam restoration in the molar was removed and the cavity incorporated into the design. A minimum of 1mm retainer

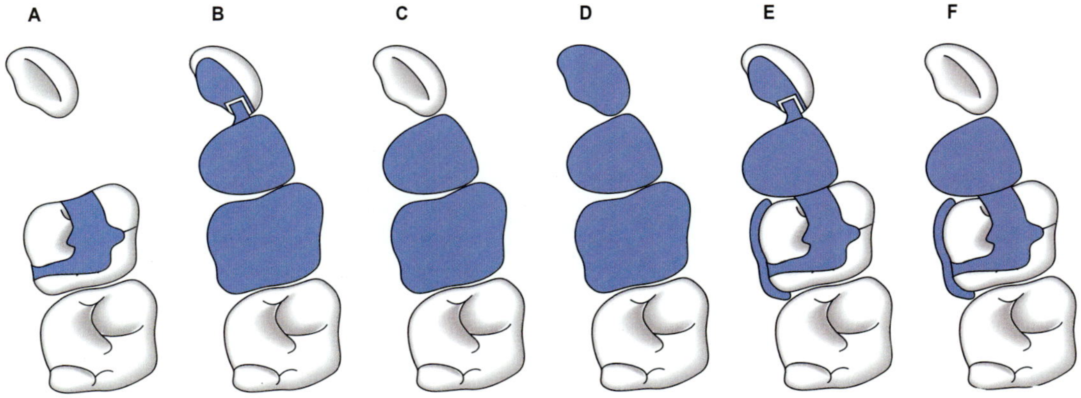

Fig. 43.2 Possible bridge designs. The gap can be left and provided overeruption of the opposing teeth does not occur, the existing situation would be stable (A). A possible fixed-movable design (B) would be a minor retainer covering part of the canine and secured to the tooth with an adhesive cement and a conventionally prepared full coverage retainer on the molar. The molar can be conventionally prepared for a full coverage restoration, either for a simple cantilever (C), or in addition the canine can be prepared producing a fixed–fixed design (D). A minimal preparation bridge is also possible. The existing restoration can be partly removed to secure the retainer, and the canine can be either included in a fixed–movable design (E) or avoided to produce a simple cantilever design (F).

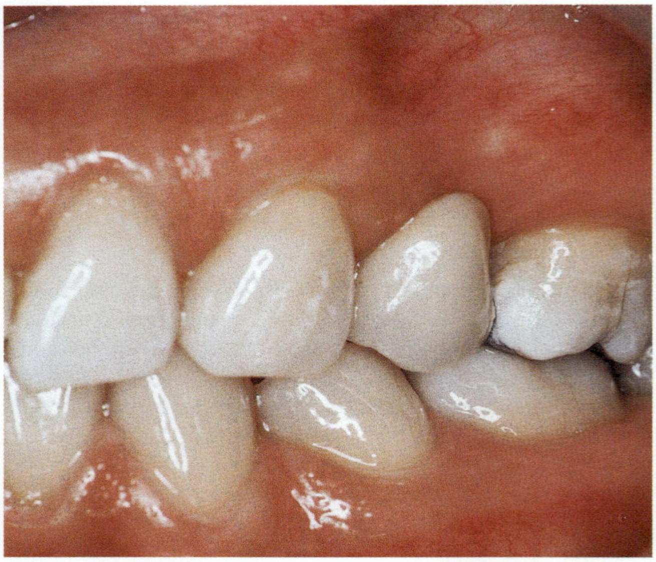

Fig. 43.3 The completed bridge.

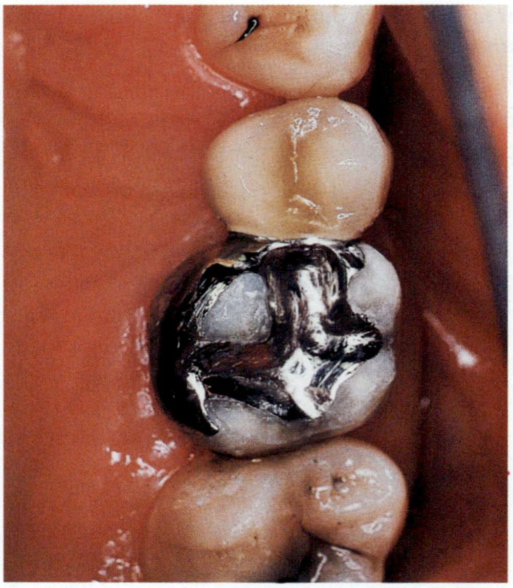

Fig. 43.4 The completed bridge showing retainer design.

thickness is required for rigidity, and including the existing cavity into the thickness provides a significant increase in rigidity, reducing flexion and reducing the risk of failure of the bond.

The retainer should cover as much tooth tissue as possible to maximize surface area for bonding. Metal should be wrapped around the abutment tooth as far as possible without encroaching on the contact point. The prepared area should be either within enamel or just into dentine. Modern luting cements bond to dentine and placing part of the preparation in dentine reduces the reliance on the enamel bond. Including the existing cavity also helps, by providing a dentine surface for bonding. The pontic is usually made of porcelain bonded to the metal.

■ *What would you do if the bridge fails through debonding?*

If the bridge decements shortly after placement, it is acceptable to recement the bridge and ensure that there is no occlusal interference. If the problem persists, a conventional bridge would then be indicated, probably using the same abutment teeth for conventional crowns.

Case 44

Management of anticoagulation

SUMMARY

A 60-year-old man presents to you in your general dental practice requiring a dental extraction. He is taking oral anticoagulants. How will you deal with his extraction?

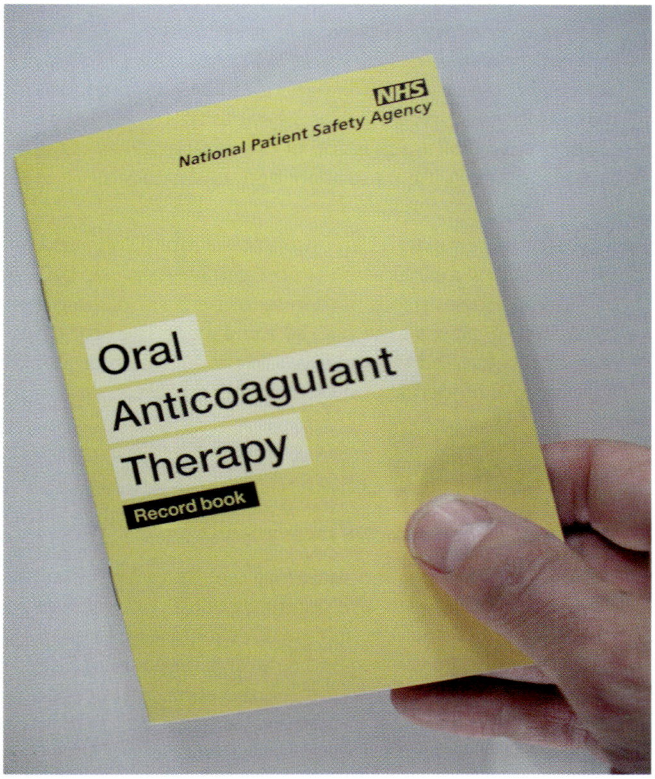

Fig. 44.1 Oral anticoagulant record book.

History

Complaint

The patient has a broken-down upper first molar that is tender on biting. The patient points directly at the tooth and requests extraction.

History of complaint

The tooth has been root-filled and crowned, but is tender to percussion. There have been several episodes of similar pain in the past year. The crown has been lost from the tooth.

Medical history

The patient reports that he had rheumatic fever as a child and as a result of cardiac valve damage he received a prosthetic heart valve 7 years ago. He is taking warfarin (9 mg daily) and co-amilofruse (amiloride/furosemide diuretic combination; 2 tablets daily). The patient carries an anticoagulation card from his local clinic showing that his international normalized ratio (INR) prothrombin time is usually between 3.5 and 4.5 (Figure 44.1). It was last checked 10 days ago, when it was 3.9.

■ ***How does warfarin work and how is anticoagulation monitored?***

Warfarin is a vitamin K antagonist. It prevents the liver from utilizing vitamin K to make clotting factors II, VII, IX and X. The patient is usually under the care of an anticoagulation clinic, although some patients are monitored by their GP. Blood tests are performed regularly and the results and drug doses are recorded in a yellow book that the patient should always carry.

■ ***What is the INR test, what is its normal therapeutic range and how should the result be interpreted?***

The INR is a standardized method of presenting the result of a prothrombin time test. The result is the ratio of the patient's prothrombin time to that of a standardized control and measures the effectiveness of the extrinsic and common pathways of blood coagulation, those most affected by warfarin. The therapeutic range for patients who have had deep-vein thrombosis or pulmonary embolism is 2.5–3.5. For patients with a prosthetic heart valve it is 3.5–4.5, depending on valve type, at the top of the therapeutic range.

In theory the INR is a standardized test using an internationally accepted standard. Unfortunately, in practice accurate standardization of the INR is often not reproducible, and small changes in the decimal places of the result cannot be relied upon to reflect small changes in anticoagulation. The test should be regarded as an estimate of anticoagulation rather than an accurate measure.

■ ***Is this patient at risk of infective endocarditis?***

Yes, all patients with the following conditions are considered at risk and a prosthetic heart valve is a relatively high risk factor that carries a very high risk of fatal outcome if endocarditis develops:

- Valve replacement
- Acquired valvular heart disease with stenosis or regurgitation
- Surgically corrected or altered congenital heart defects*
- Previous infective endocarditis
- Hypertrophic cardiomyopathy.

*excluding isolated atrial septal defect, fully repaired ventricular septal defect or fully repaired patent ductus arteriosus, and closure devices that are judged to be covered by an intact layer of endothelium.

Examination

Extraoral examination

No lymphadenopathy is present and the extraoral examination reveals no abnormalities. However, a large bruise is apparent on the patient's right forearm, consistent with the degree of anticoagulation.

Intraoral examination

The patient has a number of teeth with large restorations and several crowned teeth. His periodontal condition and oral hygiene are relatively good with only small amounts of detectable interdental plaque.

The upper first molar tooth is broken down. Root-filling material can be seen in the open pulp chamber and much of the root surface is carious. The tooth is tender to percussion. The second premolar is not tender to percussion but produces a dull percussive note. No sinus is present. The periodontal condition seems reasonable and there is no significant bone loss around the tooth on probing.

There is caries around the distal margin of a crown on the first premolar.

Investigations

■ *What investigations are required and why?*

The premolars and molars should be checked for vitality. The first premolar is vital but both second premolar and first molar do not respond to testing with an electric pulp tester. A radiograph is required in order to decide whether the molar is restorable, that is, to gauge the extent of caries and determine the success of the root filling. If extraction turns out to be required, a radiograph will be necessary to assess the difficulty of the extraction. This is particularly important in a patient who may suffer prolonged bleeding. A periapical view is the ideal view.

■ *The periapical view is shown in Figure 44.2. What does it show?*

The first permanent molar is extensively carious. A root filling is present but only one gutta percha or silver point is visible, in the palatal canal. It extends beyond the apex by approximately 2 mm. The buccal roots are not clearly visible but appear to contain no root filling. The overextended root filling lies close to the antrum and the antrum extends down between the roots of the first molar and second premolar. There is no apical radiolucency. The second premolar is also

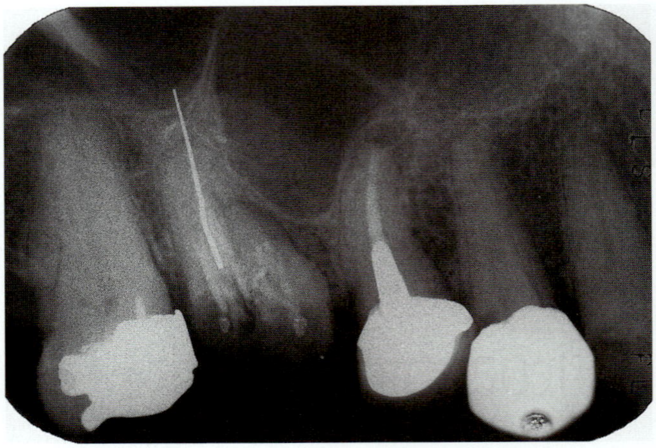

Fig. 44.2 Periapical radiograph of the upper first molar.

root-filled. The root filling appears to stop just short of the anatomical apex at an appropriate point but a small apical radiolucency is present, surrounded by the lamina dura of the tooth socket. The caries below the crown on the first premolar is visible and the second molar contains a large pinned amalgam.

Diagnosis

■ *What is your diagnosis? Explain your diagnosis.*

The patient's pain is caused by periapical periodontitis of the first permanent molar.

The patient points clearly to this tooth as the cause of his pain. This and the tenderness on percussion indicate inflammation of the periodontal ligament and the overfilled root canal provides a likely cause. No radiolucency is shown on the radiograph. However, none is required for diagnosis in the presence of typical signs and symptoms. There may be either only a small apical lesion or one on the apices of the buccal roots or in the trifurcation, both of which are superimposed on the film.

The second premolar has an unsuccessful root filling and small periapical radiolucency, almost certainly a periapical granuloma. However, it is not tender to percussion and is not felt to be the cause of the pain by the patient. The first premolar is vital and the caries would produce pain of pulpitis type without tenderness on biting or percussion.

Treatment

■ *What treatment would you recommend?*

The primary consideration should be that the patient is at risk of infective endocarditis and potential sources of infection should be eradicated. The first molar cannot be restored without another root filling and extensive preparation. The patient prefers extraction and this is the appropriate course of action. The first premolar is more problematic. It appears to be symptom-free and the apical granuloma has probably been present for some time. This lesion is a further potential source of infection and it must be eliminated, either by extraction or another root filling. The success of the new root filling must be monitored to ensure that it is successful and if not, either apicectomy or extraction will need to be considered. Treatment may be complicated by the anticoagulation, so there must be a comprehensive treatment plan that takes the rest of the dentition into account.

■ *Is the extraction of the first molar likely to be straightforward?*

No. The tooth is broken down and root-filled and there is little or no bone loss from periodontitis. It will be difficult to grasp with forceps and may be brittle. The roots extend close to the antrum and there is a risk of creating a surgical oroantral fistula.

A simple forceps extraction might turn out to be possible, but extraction may well require a mucoperiosteal flap and bone removal. A simple forceps extraction would be preferable in an anticoagulated patient because bleeding is more easily controlled when it is limited to a socket and surrounding gingiva. A surgical extraction would be less traumatic overall and separating the roots and elevating them singly would reduce the chances of creating an oroantral fistula.

■ *The patient is at risk of endocarditis. Is antibiotic cover required?*

No. Before 2008 antibiotic cover would have been routine and the patient would have been administered oral amoxicillin or an alternative antibiotic regime. Since 2008 antibiotic cover is no longer recommended for dental procedures, even for the highest-risk patients.

■ *Why have the recommendations changed so dramatically?*

In the past, antibiotic prophylaxis was based on the precautionary principle. It seemed logical because bacterial endocarditis had a high fatality rate, oral bacteria were sometimes implicated and antibiotics could prevent bacteraemia. However, much of the presumed benefit was based on animal models of the disease that could not be extrapolated to humans. There were cases where prophylaxis was correctly given but failed. More recent evidence from case control studies suggests that prophylaxis is hardly effective, and is possibly ineffective.

Although dentistry has frequently been blamed for bacterial endocarditis, there is little or no evidence to suggest that dental *procedures*, as opposed to oral bacteria, were to blame. Low-grade bacteraemias caused by eating and tooth brushing are common enough to be considered normal. There is no evidence to link the level of bacteraemia with the risk of endocarditis and these normal bacteraemias would appear to be as dangerous as those following dental procedures.

If there is little benefit from antibiotic prophylaxis, there is significant risk. Adverse effects of antibiotics range from fatal anaphylaxis to the development of resistant strains. It has been suggested that death from anaphylaxis is five times more likely than death from endocarditis. Though this is difficult to ascertain (and anaphylaxis is both avoidable and treatable) it sheds a rather different light on the value of antibiotic cover. A further factor is cost; resources spent on antibiotic prophylaxis are probably wasted and may cause harm.

■ *How should endocarditis be avoided?*

The emphasis should be on prevention and patients at risk of endocarditis must achieve a high standard of oral and dental health. They will require effective preventive regimes for caries and periodontal disease and must have infection identified and treated promptly and effectively. Patients need to be aware of the signs and symptoms of endocarditis and told to return or seek other expert advice immediately if they develop. Unnecessary medical and dental interventions should be avoided and patients need to understand infection risks from nonmedical sources as well. Chlorhexidine mouthwash or other topical agents should not be offered as prophylaxis against infective endocarditis. They are not effective.

■ *If the patient requested antibiotic prophylaxis, what would you do?*

National Institute for Health and Clinical Excellence guidance states that practitioners must be able to give clear and consistent information about endocarditis and explain the risks and benefit of antibiotic prophylaxis. However, patients have previously been told that antibiotic prophylaxis is a life-saving precaution and may be unwilling to stop. It may be helpful to note that cover is no longer recommended for many other medical interventions and that dentistry is only falling into line with other medical specialties. If a patient insists on receiving antibiotic cover, support from the patient's medical practitioner or cardiologist may assist. A disagreement over antibiotic cover cannot be allowed to delay treatment of infection in a patient at risk of endocarditis. This sudden change of guidance could place you in a difficult situation: you would be responsible if a patient developed an adverse reaction to antibiotics administered for no better reason than the patient's request. If either the patient or cardiologist consider antibiotic cover to be necessary despite national guidance, it would prudent to arrange for the cardiologist to determine the antibiotic regimen.

■ *Would you expect this patient to suffer prolonged bleeding after a dental extraction?*

Potentially yes and, if untreated, such bleeding could require hospital admission. The mouth is a vascular site and saliva has fibrinolytic activity. Untreated prolonged haemorrhage could be fatal, though the risk is low.

■ *Does the patient require reduction of the INR to enable minor oral surgery?*

Until recently it was accepted that the INR had to be reduced for procedures such as intramuscular injections, minor surgery and dental extraction. The INR was reduced to 2.5 or below for inferior dental (ID) nerve block, simple extractions and soft-tissue surgery. However, it has recently been demonstrated that the incidence of bleeding following dental extraction without reducing or stopping warfarin is less than has been thought, and that any bleeding may be relatively easily controlled. Current guidelines from the British Committee for Standards in Haematology, British Dental Association and National Patient Safety Agency recommend that oral anticoagulants should not be stopped for outpatient oral surgery, including extraction, provided the degree of anticoagulation is stable with an INR between 2 and 4. Additional procedures to reduce the risk of bleeding, such as suturing sockets with an oxidized cellulose (Surgicel) dressing and use of tranexamic acid mouthwashes, are recommended.

As these guidelines are relatively new, some patients' haematologists, cardiologists or surgeons may still request reduction of warfarin dose on the basis that a short reduction is without complication. It may be necessary to consult with the patient's physician in this interim period.

Why did these guidelines change?

For two reasons. Firstly, clinical research has shown that it is safe to extract teeth without reducing or stopping warfarin if the INR is below 4.0 and when the sockets have been packed with a haemostatic agent and sutured. Secondly, it has been realized that stopping anticoagulants places patients at risk of thrombosis, embolism or both. Clearly these complications are of major importance and potentially fatal. The risk of thromboembolism following withdrawal of anticoagulants for a day or two is debated, but it is clear that significant complications can arise when anticoagulants are stopped for a few days. To ensure patient safety, the decision has been made to maintain the level of anticoagulation if at all possible.

Suppose more extensive surgery were planned?

For more major surgery the risk of haemorrhage would rise significantly. The patient would then have to be treated in a hospital setting because he would need to be switched from warfarin to heparin. Heparin is given as a daily dose using new low-molecular-weight heparin preparations such as enoxaparin (Clexane), avoiding heparin infusion. These have a half-life of only a few hours, allowing anticoagulation to be readily reversed in an emergency using antagonist drugs. Anticoagulation with heparin is monitored by the activated partial thromboplastin time and is usually kept at 1.5–2.5 times normal.

Do you still need to check the INR? How recently should the last INR test have been done?

Yes, you still need to ensure that the INR is 4.0 or less. The more recent the test, the better. In the past it was suggested that a result less than 24 hours old was required to adjust the warfarin dose.

Now that the warfarin is not adjusted, a test result up to 72 hours old may be accepted. However, if the INR result on the patient's anticoagulation record card fluctuates without change in dose, only a test performed on the day of treatment should be accepted. If there has been no recent test, one should be requested, or alternatively the appointment may be postponed until the next test result is available.

The patient says he tests his own INR. Is that acceptable?

Coagulation testing can now be performed using small hand-held battery-operated devices, allowing coagulation testing to be performed by medical practitioners or patients (point of care testing or near-patient testing). Results from a medical practice can be considered reliable as machines are checked and calibrated regularly. Some patients now test their own INR at home and some evidence suggests their anticoagulation is managed very well. Selected patients are trained to interpret their own results and are able to adjust their own doses. Provided the patient's coagulometer is subject to a quality assurance scheme, the results can be relied on. However, patients cannot take responsibility for adjusting their dose for a medical procedure, only for routine dosing. With approximately 1 million UK patients taking warfarin, and the total rising, this type of testing is likely to be encountered more frequently.

How can warfarin anticoagulation be reversed in an emergency?

Warfarin is a vitamin K antagonist and administering vitamin K intravenously can reverse its effects (oral dosing is effective but much slower in action). Vitamin K takes some time to become effective as the liver must synthesize the necessary clotting factors. For a more rapid effect the missing clotting factors can be replaced immediately by transfusing fresh frozen plasma.

What additional precautions might you take to ensure haemostasis?

In general, warfarin is associated with oozing of blood from soft tissues rather than bleeding from bone. Following current guidelines with no reduced warfarin dose, a single interrupted or mattress suture across the mouth of the socket and an oxidized cellulose (Surgicel) pack is recommended for all extractions. Haemostasis must be achieved, usually by gentle pressure on the gingiva. Tranexamic acid is an antifibrinolytic agent that inhibits conversion of plasminogen to plasmin, stabilizing clots once formed. It can be administered as a 5% mouthwash and must be used four times a day for several days after extraction.

If there is severe periodontitis, then treating this first, even if only around a few teeth, much reduces postoperative bleeding.

In this case a further test was required and the INR had fallen slightly to 3.7. The tooth was extracted and the socket sutured. Haemostasis was achieved after a slightly prolonged period.

What postoperative instructions are necessary for the bleeding tendency?

No specific instructions are necessary. The patient should be warned not to eat or drink or rinse the mouth for a few hours after extraction. A little blood in saliva is to be expected but should vanish over a few hours. If there is bleeding from the socket or fresh blood in saliva, then biting on a damp gauze swab (provided on discharge for the purpose) should stop bleeding. Pressure must be maintained for at least 5 minutes at a time to stop bleeding. If this fails, the patient should not hesitate to contact your practice or a local hospital Accident and Emergency department. The patient may rinse with hot salt mouthwashes on the following day.

What postoperative instructions are necessary for the risk of endocarditis?

All patients at risk of endocarditis must be warned to be alert for signs and symptoms of endocarditis. Unfortunately these are relatively nonspecific in the early stages. They may be of acute onset and progress rapidly or persist for weeks or months before cardiac signs develop. Endocarditis caused by oral streptococci is usually of this latter subacute type. Patients with endocarditis of prosthetic valves progress to heart failure more rapidly. Low-grade endocarditis is often a diagnostic challenge in the early stages and patients and dentists need to have a high index of suspicion. Patients should seek advice if they develop:

- Influenza-like symptoms of malaise and fatigue
- Fever or night sweats
- Weight loss and loss of appetite
- Rash
- Vague and poorly localized pains
- Splinter haemorrhages beneath the nails
- Painful red nodules in finger tips (Osler's nodes)
- Haematuria
- Joint pains
- Signs of heart failure
- Change in heart murmur
- Transient ischaemic attacks and strokes.

Postoperative

The patient returns 3 hours later indicating that bleeding has continued throughout most of this period. Why has bleeding restarted?

Bleeding in the immediate postoperative period is stopped by platelet plugs forming in the vessels. This mechanism is unaffected by warfarin, which inhibits only coagulation. After the initial haemostasis, coagulation fails to consolidate the platelet plugs. When the vasoconstrictor in the local anaesthetic wears off, there is a period of hyperaemia as a result of inflammation and bleeding may start again.

How would you manage this postextraction bleeding?

Initially, check that the socket is only oozing as rapid bleeding would necessitate immediate measures. Then take a history and assess the degree of blood loss which, to the patient (and sometimes the dentist), always seems worse than it actually is. Examine the patient using a good light and suction to remove the old socket dressing and poorly formed blood clots and identify the bleeding area.

If only the soft tissue is bleeding, pressure and a new dressing will probably be all that is required. However, bleeding after a pack and suturing may be arising from the bone. If a bleeding point can be identified it can be crushed with a hand instrument. Electrocautery should not be used on or near bone. Bone wax should only be used if all else fails because it delays healing in the longer term. Replace the Surgicel pack, or place a Whitehead's varnish pack, resuture the socket over the pack to provide pressure to the gingival margins and to keep the pack firmly in the socket. Bleeding from the surgical incision may require additional sutures and deeper sutures to compress the sides of the incision on to the underlying tissues.

Take the blood pressure and pulse to assess whether there has been serious blood loss.

Reassure the patient, who is often very worried and well aware of the problems of the anticoagulation treatment. Observe for 15–30 minutes and reinforce normal postoperative instructions. It is emphasized that the patient must not rinse until the next day. It is unlikely that these measures will fail.

What would you do if there were tachycardia and lowered blood pressure?

This would indicate significant blood loss and, as above, the patient should be speedily admitted to hospital for intravenous fluids to prevent circulatory collapse.

What would you do if these steps did fail?

In a practice setting the patient should be transferred to a hospital casualty or specialist unit, or the anticoagulation clinic. This should be arranged speedily and the patient will require an escort. There the INR and platelet count would be checked. Antifibrinolytics, such as aprotinin and tranexamic acid, can be used in conjunction with packing and suturing. If the bleeding persists or if the INR is above the therapeutic range, the patient will need to be admitted for reversal of the anticoagulation by infusion of fresh frozen plasma or prothrombin complex concentrates (a more effective preparation of concentrated dried factors II, VII, IX and X) and vitamin K. The vitamin K injections will not reverse the action of the warfarin for 12 hours and so are not effective in such emergency situations, but aid stabilization of anticoagulation after the bleeding is stopped. A major bleed is likely to necessitate a few days in hospital.

Warfarin interacts with a variety of other drugs. Which drugs that might be prescribed in dental practice can affect warfarin anticoagulation?

In all drug interactions with warfarin there is increased anticoagulation and a risk of bleeding. Aspirin and related drugs also increase the risk of bleeding, not by interaction but through their separate antiplatelet activity. Discussion with the patient's anticoagulation clinic would be prudent if any of these drugs are required:

- Nonsteroidal anti-inflammatory drugs
- Antibiotics, including erythromycin, metronidazole, tetracyclines and penicillins
- Fluconazole, ketoconazole and miconazole (including topical preparations).

How can I keep up with all these changes in guidance?

This case demonstrates how rapidly accepted practice can change. Only a year or two ago the patient would have had antibiotic cover and adjustment of the warfarin dose before treatment. Guidance can, unfortunately, come from a wide variety of sources and it is not always clear whether it is generally accepted, recommended or mandatory. Guidelines from the National Institute for Health and Clinical Excellence apply to the NHS in England and Wales, but not in Scotland, where a separate institution, the Scottish Intercollegiate Guidelines Network, plays the equivalent role. Guidance or references to it may also be provided by Royal Colleges, the British Dental Association, the General Dental Council and professional indemnity organizations. Guidelines, evidence and other clinical best practice are available online at the NHS National Library for Heath (http://www.library.nhs.uk). Guidance on medications in the *British National Formulary* or *Dental Practitioners Formulary* is regularly updated and usually considered definitive. Almost all guidelines first appear in peer-reviewed scientific or professional journals, though it may take some time for them to become accepted and be given an official seal of approval. This demonstrates the importance of continuing professional development to ensure all dentists remain up to date. In the UK, the General Dental Councils ethics guidance *Standards for Dental Professionals* has six key principles and maintaining your professional knowledge and competence is one.

Case 45

A white patch on the tongue

SUMMARY

A 52-year-old woman has a white patch on her tongue. Make a diagnosis and decide on appropriate treatment.

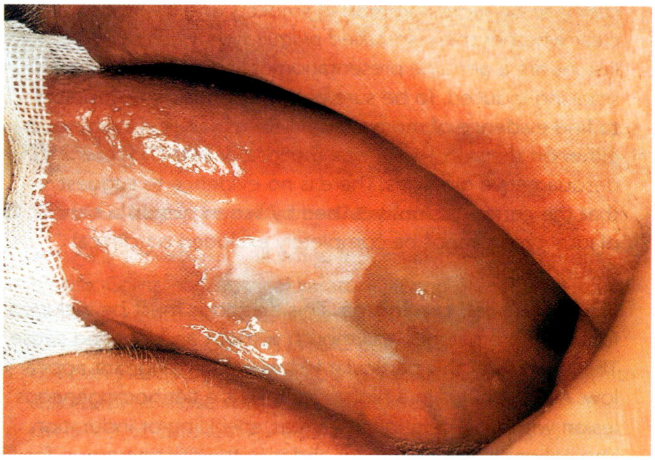

Fig. 45.1 The patient's tongue.

History

Complaint

The patient has no complaint.

History of complaint

You have just noticed the lesion in a patient attending for the first time for several years. There is no written record of the white patch in her notes. The patient had noticed the lesion but has ignored it. She thinks it has probably been there for several years.

Medical history

The patient is otherwise fit and well. She smokes 4 cigarettes a day and drinks 4–8 units of alcohol each week.

Examination

Extraoral examination

No lymph nodes are palpable in the neck and there are no abnormal findings on extraoral examination.

Intraoral examination

Apart from this lesion, the remainder of the oral mucosa is normal.

■ ***The appearance of the lesion is shown in Figure 45.1. What do you see?***

There is a flat and homogeneous white patch on the left lateral border and ventral tongue mucosa. It is well defined and varies slightly in whiteness.

If you were able to feel the lesion you would find that it is soft and feels no different from the surrounding mucosa.

Differential diagnosis

■ ***What are the common or important white patches in the mouth? How are they caused?***

Almost all oral white patches are caused by increased keratinization of the epithelium. Keratin absorbs water and appears white, brighter white where it is thicker. The exception is a chemical burn where the white surface layer is caused by necrosis or ulceration.

Type of lesion	White lesion(s)
Normal mucosal variants	Leukoedema Fordyce spots/granules
Inherited epithelial disorders	White sponge naevus Pachyonychia congenita
Traumatic lesions	Frictional keratosis Chemical burn Cheek and tongue biting
Infections	Thrush (acute hyperplastic candidosis) Chronic hyperplastic candidosis (candidal 'leukoplakia') Chronic mucocutaneous candidosis Hairy leukoplakia Syphilitic leukoplakia
Lichen planus and similar conditions	Lichen planus Lichenoid reaction (topical and systemic) Lupus erythematosus
Unknown or smoking-related	Idiopathic keratosis (*leukoplakia*), including: Homogeneous leukoplakia Verrucous/nodular leukoplakia Sublingual keratosis Smoker's keratosis Speckled leukoplakia Stomatitis nicotina (smoker's palate)
Neoplastic	Squamous cell carcinoma

Lesions with moderate or severe dysplasia may be excised, ablated by laser or treated with topical chemotherapeutic agents such as bleomycin. Occasionally patches are too large to treat in these ways and the only option is to monitor to detect malignant transformation as early as possible.

In addition it is important to remember that dysplasia probably affects all mucosa exposed to tobacco smoke and alcohol. There is a risk of carcinoma arising in the pharynx and respiratory tract and symptoms from these areas indicate a need for endoscopy.

Prognosis

■ ***What features would indicate that a white patch might become malignant over the coming years?***

See Table on p. 213.

In this case the lesion remained unchanged and the patient was reviewed at 3-monthly intervals for 1 year, 6-monthly intervals for 2 years and she continues under annual review. Four years after presentation a second biopsy was performed and the degree of dysplasia was still mild. Excision has been considered because the lesion is relatively accessible and in a high risk site for carcinoma, but has not been carried out because the dysplasia remains mild and the patient prefers not to have surgery. She keeps her patch under close observation, returning for an earlier appointment if she feels it has changed.

Case 46

Another white patch on the tongue

SUMMARY

A 39-year-old woman has a white patch on the lateral margin of her tongue. What is the cause and what are the treatment options?

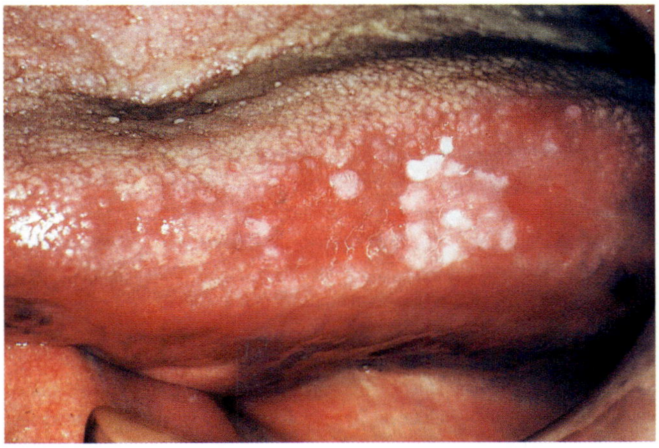

Fig. 46.1 The patient's tongue.

History

Complaint

The patient has no symptoms.

History of complaint

The patient is an infrequent dental attender and has not been to the dentist for at least 5 years. Following an oral cancer awareness week she inspected her mouth and became nervous about her tongue. She would like it checked.

Medical history

She has had cervical dysplasia treated in the previous year by cone biopsy and this has left her very worried about cancer. She is otherwise fit and well.

She has smoked 40 cigarettes daily since the age of 18 years and drinks 14 units of alcohol per week as wine.

Examination

Extraoral examination

She seems a healthy woman with no obvious skin, nail or eye lesions present on visible skin. No lymph nodes are palpable in the neck.

Intraoral examination

The oral mucosa appears normal, except for the tongue which is shown in Figure 46.1.

■ ***Describe the appearance of the tongue lesion.***

Site	Right lateral border of tongue
Size	1 × 3 cm approximately
Shape	Ill defined ellipse
Colour	Mixture of white and red components
Surface	Appears nodular or irregular

Palpation reveals the lesion to be firmer than the adjacent mucosa. The white component of the area cannot be rubbed away. The tongue is freely mobile.

Differential diagnosis

■ ***What are the causes of mixed red and white patches in the mouth?***

The causes of white patches are discussed more fully in Case 45. Several may also be associated with red areas.

Cause	Red and white lesion(s)
Trauma	Chemical burn Cheek biting
Infection	Thrush (acute hyperplastic candidosis) Chronic hyperplastic candidosis (candidal 'leukoplakia')
Lichen planus and similar conditions	Lichen planus Lichenoid reaction (topical and systemic) Lupus erythematosus
Idiopathic or smoking	Idiopathic keratosis (*leukoplakia*) including: Sublingual keratosis Smoker's keratosis Speckled leukoplakia Stomatitis nicotina (smoker's palate)
Neoplasia	Squamous cell carcinoma

■ ***Which of the above lesions would you include in the differential diagnosis for this particular lesion?***

1. Squamous cell carcinoma
2. Idiopathic white patch with or without dysplasia including speckled leukoplakia
3. Chronic hyperplastic candidosis
4. Lichenoid reaction.

■ ***Justify this differential diagnosis.***

The most important consideration in differential diagnosis for all oral white patches is that squamous carcinoma or a premalignant lesion may be the cause. This is especially so when lesions are red and white or speckled.

Squamous carcinoma is a likely diagnosis and the most significant diagnosis. Although this patient is young for a squamous carcinoma, cases are seen in the fourth decade of life and the incidence in younger patients appears to be increasing both in the UK and elsewhere. The patient drinks and smokes heavily and these are the main risk factors for oral squamous cell carcinoma. She drinks 14 units of alcohol per week (maximum recommended intake 14 units female, 21 units male). These maximum intakes are considered 'safe' in terms of liver and cardiovascular disease risk but no safe limit is recognized for cancer. There is no safe intake for tobacco and the combined relative risk for this patient to develop carcinoma is at least 5–10 times higher than for a nonsmoker or occasional drinker. The presence of the lesion in a high-risk site, its speckled appearance and association with smoking are very worrying regardless of the patient's age. This lesion should be considered a carcinoma until proved otherwise.

A premalignant lesion would be the next most likely diagnosis. Option 2 in the differential diagnosis covers all white patches of unknown aetiology, some of which carry a risk of malignant transformation and show dysplasia on microscopic examination. The risk of malignant transformation is higher in those with a red component which may be either a speckled area or in a separate, usually adjacent, site. The risk factors are the same as those for carcinoma, and if this lesion is not a carcinoma it is almost certainly premalignant.

■ ***Which lesions are less likely possibilities? Explain why.***

Candidal infection should always be considered as a cause of white patches, particularly when red areas are associated. It is very common. The combination of red and white is most likely to signify thrush (acute hyperplastic candidosis. However, lesions of thrush are usually more widespread than in the present case and at least some of the white plaques may be removed by rubbing. Chronic hyperplastic candidosis (candidal 'leukoplakia') forms a discrete white plaque that is sometimes associated with red areas. Although it is normally found on the buccal mucosa and dorsal surface of the tongue, it is a possible diagnosis for the current lesion. It should also be remembered that almost any white patch in the mouth may be susceptible to infection by candida simply because of the increased thickness of keratin on the surface of the epithelium. Thus the presence of candidal infection does not preclude an underlying carcinoma, dysplasia or a lichen planus like condition.

Lichen planus and similar conditions are relatively common causes of intraoral white lesions. Lichen planus, lichenoid reactions and lupus erythematosus are usually readily identifiable by virtue of a presence of lacy white striae, association with atrophic areas and/or desquamative gingivitis and their symmetrical bilateral distribution. In smokers, both lichen planus and lichenoid reactions may present as discrete white plaques but these *plaque-type* lesions are not usually associated with red areas. Localized single white lesions may also result from topically induced lichenoid reactions such as those to dental restorative materials. However, these are all most unlikely to be responsible for the current lesion because their clinical appearance and distribution are distinct.

■ ***What features might indicate that this lesion is already malignant? Which are early and which are late signs?***

Feature	Early	Late
Red or speckled areas	*	*
Nonhealing ulceration	*	*
Rolled everted ulcer margin		*
Induration of surrounding tissues		*
Bleeding from the surface		*
Fixation of the tissues		*
Destruction of adjacent bone		*
Enlarged hard lymph nodes		*
Size	Small carcinomas are probably those which have been diagnosed early but there is great variation in rate of growth and this is only an assumption	
Pain	Unpredictable, often absent, sometimes the presenting complaint	

Investigations

■ ***What special investigations are indicated?***

A biopsy is generally considered mandatory for any oral white lesion. This is especially important if no cause is apparent. When malignancy or significant dysplasia is suspected, as in the present case, the biopsy should be performed as soon as possible because early diagnosis is a major factor for successful treatment of oral squamous carcinoma.

■ ***Would you perform this biopsy in general practice?***

No, definitely not. Although removing a sample of the tissue is well within the capability of the general dental practitioner, it would be unwise to do so. The patient will return for the result and dental practitioners are not usually the appropriate person to break the news of malignant disease. There is also a theoretical risk that biopsy of the wrong site or removal of the whole of a small lesion might compromise subsequent treatment but this is a largely theoretical problem. In a practice environment the patient should be referred urgently, preferably the same day, to the centre where definitive treatment is likely to be provided. This will allow the most appropriate biopsy to be performed. No other special investigations are indicated at this stage.

UK treatment centres operate a 'two week wait' referral pathway for suspected malignancy. To use this fast-track process the dentist must usually FAX a specific referral form direct to a central office at their local Cancer Network treatment centre.

■ ***Which part of the lesion should be removed for biopsy?***

The specimen should include those areas most likely to be malignant, the red and speckled parts. Some normal tissue should also be included and the sample should be about

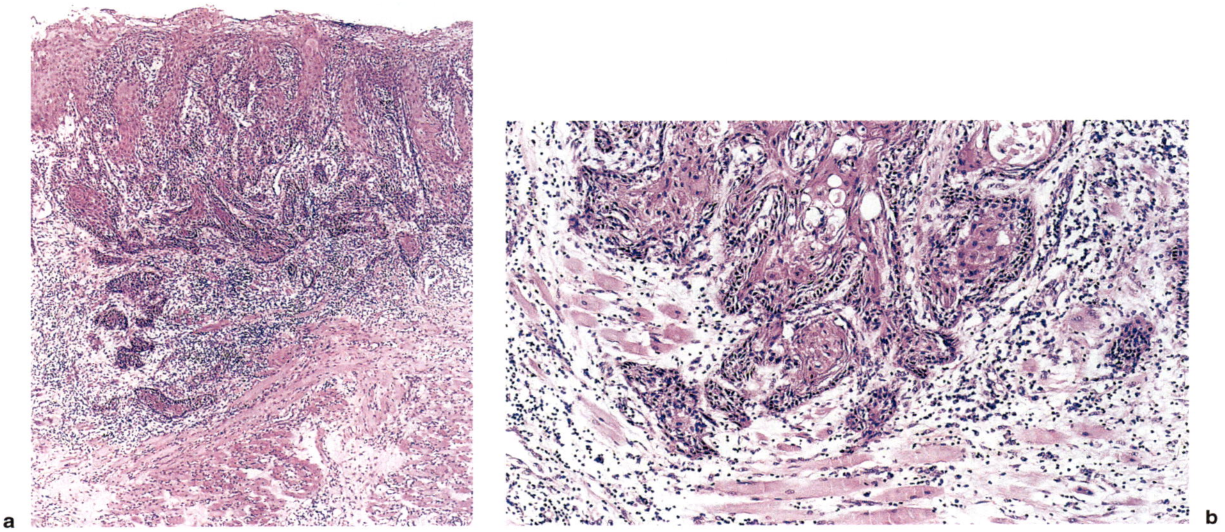

Fig. 46.2 The histological appearances of the lesion, **a** Lower power view; **b** higher power view.

1cm long, 4–5 mm wide, and an even depth including underlying muscle. Larger malignancies are often friable and if the specimen is too small it may disintegrate on removal. No attempt should be made to excise the whole lesion until a diagnosis is obtained.

■ ***The biopsy specimen is shown in Figure 46.2. What are the microscopic features and how do you interpret them?***

The lower power view (Fig. 46.2a) shows tongue mucosa with underlying muscle. The overlying epithelium is very irregular and instead of being an even and well organized layer it forms an irregular series of rete processes which penetrate deeply into the underlying tissue. The deepest epithelium is breaking off into apparently separate islands and strands and these extend deeply between muscle bundles. The higher power (Fig. 46.2b) view is taken from the deep surface and shows the deepest epithelium invading muscle. The epithelium is disorganized, with keratin forming in the centre of islands and an irregular darkly stained basal cell layer around the edge. This epithelium has lost its ordered maturation and stratification and is invading the underlying muscle. Invasion indicates malignancy and the malignant epithelium shows squamous differentiation.

Diagnosis

■ ***What is the diagnosis?***

The patient has a squamous cell carcinoma. It is only superficially invasive and probably an early lesion.

Treatment

■ ***What types of treatment are possible and what is the prognosis?***

The lesion appears to have been diagnosed at a much earlier stage than most oral carcinomas. Treatment may be by radiotherapy (implant or external beam), by surgery or both in combination. The final decision will depend on the results of investigations to stage the carcinoma (determine its size and extent of metastases to lymph nodes and distant sites). In the absence of metastasis, treatment is likely to be surgery alone and a 5-year survival rate of 85% or better can be achieved. If the lesion were larger, implant radiotherapy might well be suggested. If the patient survives 10 years she is likely to be cured. However, 10% of oral carcinoma patients develop a second primary lesion in the mouth or upper aerodigestive tract. The chances of developing a second lesion are assumed to be reduced by stopping smoking and the patient should be encouraged to do so. Smoking-associated cardiovascular disease, if severe, may also compromise treatment.

Further details of the treatment of oral carcinoma are given in Case 57.

Mobility should be assessed. Mobility is increased slightly if there is inflammation of the periodontal ligament. If a periradicular abscess or acute inflammation is present, the tooth may be raised in the socket. You must exclude increased mobility caused by periodontal disease, root fracture, recent trauma, and premature occlusal contact.

Periodontal probing to detect loss of attachment or exposed dentine. Dentine hypersensitivity would not cause such severe, long-lasting pain. However, pocketing or previous periodontal treatment could have exposed a lateral canal or canal in the furcation, allowing bacteria access to the pulp.

Search for a sinus. This would indicate periradicular infection. Sinuses may heal and present as a small fibrous nodule indicating past or intermittent infection. The search must include lingual alveolar mucosa because the apices of lower molars lie closer to the lingual than buccal cortex.

On examining the patient you find that no teeth are mobile, tender to percussion or have apical tenderness. There is no detectable sinus. Inflammation appears limited to the pulp. No periodontitis is present.

Investigations

■ ***What investigations would you perform?***

Tests of pulp vitality are required to increase confidence in your assessment of the status of the pulp. Electric, and hot and cold thermal testing are available and a stimulus that usually provokes the pain is recommended. If tests give equivocal responses, a test cavity without local analgesia should prove conclusive.

A periapical radiograph of the first and second molar teeth is required.

■ ***What are the limitations of tests of vitality?***

Tests of vitality do not measure pulp vitality but test for a continuous sensory nerve pathway from the pulp to the brain. For this reason they are sometimes referred to as sensitivity tests.

It is assumed that pulp without sensory innervation is devitalized but this is not necessarily so. Inflammation can alter sensation and sensation may be incorrectly localized (see Case 1). Conversely, a positive response does not guarantee the health of the pulp.

Tests sometimes indicate a hypersensitive pulp and this is a more useful piece of information because detection of hypersensitivity is not prone to false results.

■ ***What are the causes of misleading electric pulp test results?***

Both false positive and false negative sensitivity responses can occur. Causes are listed in the table at the bottom of the page, together with precautions that minimize the risk of a spurious result.

On performing these tests you discover that the lower second molar gives a hypersensitive response to hot gutta percha. The pain lasted until a local anaesthetic was given.

■ ***The periapical radiograph is shown in Figure 47.1. What do you see?***

The lower premolar teeth are unrestored and there is no caries. The molar teeth show several changes:

First molar	Second molar
The tooth is crowned and the distal margin is defective and carious. Caries extends into the furcation.	The tooth has a disto-occlusal restoration with a large ledge distally.
The mesial root has a root canal filling present, short of the radiographic apex and a periradicular radiolucency.	There is also a large carious lesion mesially that extends close to the mesial pulp horns.
There is no evidence of a root canal filling in the distal root. The canal is not visible radiographically and may be sclerosed.	No periradicular radiolucency is visible.
There is a suggestion of periradicular radiolucency within the furcation.	

Cause of error	Possible precautions to minimise
False positive response	
Patient's anticipation of pain/sensitivity	Test control teeth first, several times if unsure, raise tester setting slowly
Multirooted tooth with one or more canals containing necrotic pulp tissue, the remainder vital tissue	Test at several sites, over each root, on exposed dentine if possible
Sensation originates in the gingiva because the tooth is not electrically isolated	Ensure teeth are dry, keep electrode away from amalgams that extend subgingivally
Sensation originates in an adjacent tooth because the tested tooth is not electrically isolated	Keep electrode away from amalgams that contact adjacent teeth, dry teeth, isolate teeth with a small piece of rubber dam
C nerve fibres within the pulp tissue can still function for some time after loss of their blood supply	None possible
False negative response	
Poor contact between electrode and tooth	Ensure good contact surface area and use conductive jelly to bridge surfaces
Inadequate electrical access to tooth tissue because of insulating nonmetallic coverage	None possible unless restoration is to be replaced, access can be cut in crown
Advanced age. Pulp insulated by thick physiological secondary dentine	None possible
Heavily restored or worn tooth with a pulp insulated by thick reactionary, tertiary, dentine	Place electrode close to root canal rather than occlusally if this is suspected
High pain/sensation threshold	None possible, not usually a problem

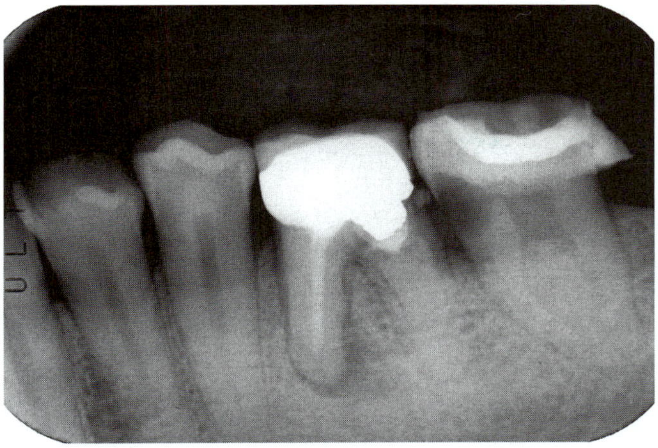

Fig. 47.1 Periapical radiograph on presentation.

Diagnosis

What is the most likely diagnosis?

Irreversible pulpitis in the lower left second molar tooth caused by the large mesial carious lesion. When the pain started 8 months ago the carious lesion would have been smaller and the pulpitis reversible.

Treatment

What emergency treatment would you provide at the first appointment?

The first molar is unrestorable because caries involves the furcation. This tooth will require extraction but this is not an immediate problem. The periradicular lesion is chronic and painless and the second molar, as the cause of the pain, is the first priority.

Loss of the first molar makes it desirable to conserve the second if possible. Caries is extensive in the second molar and extension down the mesial root is a potential problem. Definitive restoration will require either a deep subgingival restoration or a crown lengthening procedure. The possibilities will become clearer after excavating the caries, but it is possible that extraction will be required or requested by the patient.

Assuming the tooth is to be conserved, the priority is relief of pain. Having assessed the pulpitis as irreversible, extirpation of the pulp is the only appropriate treatment and this will require cleaning and shaping of the root canals to ensure no remnants remain. Extirpation with barbed broach alone risks leaving fragments of inflamed vital pulp that could cause pain after treatment. A root canal dressing of calcium hydroxide will inhibit bacterial growth. This must be sealed from the mouth with a suitable temporary dressing material to prevent bacterial ingress pending definitive treatment.

Pulpotomy, with removal of the coronal pulp, or partial pulpectomy, with removal of pulp from the widest canal, is sometimes advocated in multirooted teeth but should be avoided. The apical extent of inflammation in the pulp is unknown and pain relief cannot be guaranteed.

What definitive treatment does the patient require for the second molar?

The patient should return for obturation of the root canals and a definitive coronal restoration. A cuspal coverage indirect restoration should be considered to give protection against occlusal forces, either an onlay or core with a full coverage crown. Post crowns in molar teeth are to be avoided because of the incidence of perforations and root fractures. Retention should be sufficient from the undercut shape of the pulp chamber and the remaining coronal tooth structure (see Case 1 and Case 9).

After discussing the possibility of restoring or extracting the second molar, the patient opts for root canal treatment. You carry out the first stage of treatment successfully. However, the patient fails to return to complete the treatment for 6 months. When he returns you discover that the tooth has remained asymptomatic but the coronal temporary restoration has been lost and the lingual cusp has fractured off. The pulp chamber is open to the oral cavity but the tooth is still restorable.

What effect will this have on the long-term prognosis for this tooth?

Loss of the coronal seal will have allowed microbial invasion of the root canals and dentinal tubules. Bacteria and their metabolic and breakdown products are major irritants and will penetrate apically and along lateral canals to induce or maintain periradicular inflammation. In addition, the flora in the canal will change and a more mixed oral flora with anaerobes will become established in the canal. This may be more difficult to eradicate and be more likely to penetrate through the apex and induce an acute abscess. Fracture of the lingual cusp further weakens the tooth and complicates building up a core to support a definitive restoration.

What should be the next stage of treatment?

Root canal treatment must be recommenced as soon as possible. The tooth should be isolated with rubber dam and the root canals cleaned and shaped, using appropriate files and copious irrigation with sodium hypochlorite. Sodium hypochlorite is antibacterial but some bacteria may survive in lateral canals and dentinal tubules that are blocked by the smear layer produced by instrumentation. The smear layer must be removed by occasionally irrigating with either citric acid or EDTA solution. Hypochlorite will then be able to penetrate the dentine and lateral canals. It is important that coronal root canal preparation is carried out first to reduce the bacterial load and improve access to the apical portion of the root canal. The working length can then be determined and confirmed with a working length radiograph (Fig. 47.2).

The working length radiograph is shown in Figure 47.2. What do you see and what does it mean?

There is a large periradicular radiolucency that was not present in Figure 47.1; the lesion has developed as a result of the canals being left open. This is almost certainly a

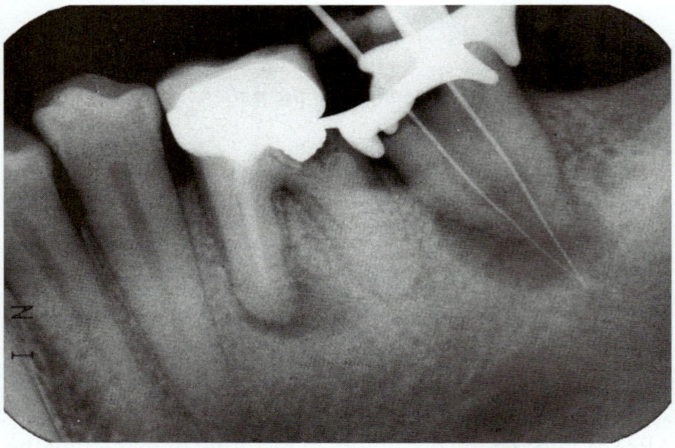

Fig. 47.2 The working length radiograph.

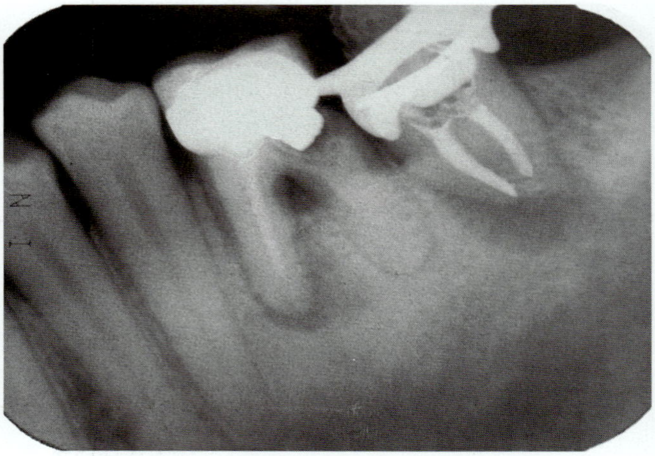

Fig. 47.3 The completed root canal filling.

granuloma rather than a radicular cyst, as cysts take some time to develop.

The working length files have been placed beyond the root apices. This should be avoided as debris, irrigants, medicaments or bacteria can be introduced into the periradicular tissues, delaying the healing process.

A further film is required to confirm the working length using larger ISO-size files. Determining the working length has clearly been a problem and an apex locator may help locate the apical constriction, which is 1–2 mm short of the radiographic apex and often not visible on a periapical film.

A further dressing of nonsetting calcium hydroxide paste for 1 week is required to kill any bacteria remaining within the root canal system. If the tooth remains asymptomatic, obturation can be carried out at the following visit. The definitive restoration should be placed without delay to prevent coronal leakage and to avoid further fracture of tooth structure. The final appearance after obturation is shown in Figure 47.3.

■ ***How long should this tooth be reviewed after completion of root canal treatment? What are the criteria for success?***

Root canal treatment should be reviewed for at least 4 years because complete healing may require considerable time.

Outcome must be evaluated clinically and radiographically. The radiographic assessment must be made by comparing the appearances with previous films, taken under as near standardized conditions as possible.

Criteria for success and failure are shown below:

Success	No symptoms No tenderness on percussion or increased mobility No sinus Width and contour of periodontal ligament normal Slight radiolucency around excess filling material allowable
Uncertain	No symptoms No tenderness on percussion or increased mobility No sinus Residual radiolucency at 4 years that is smaller than seen on completion of root canal filling. Some authorities suggest that under these circumstances a further period of 3 years' healing time should be given
Failure	Symptoms Tenderness on percussion or increased mobility Sinus Unchanged or enlarged periradicular radiolucency Development of new radiolucency at another site on the tooth

Case • 48

An endodontic problem

SUMMARY

A 60-year-old female patient has pain from a root-treated tooth. What will you do?

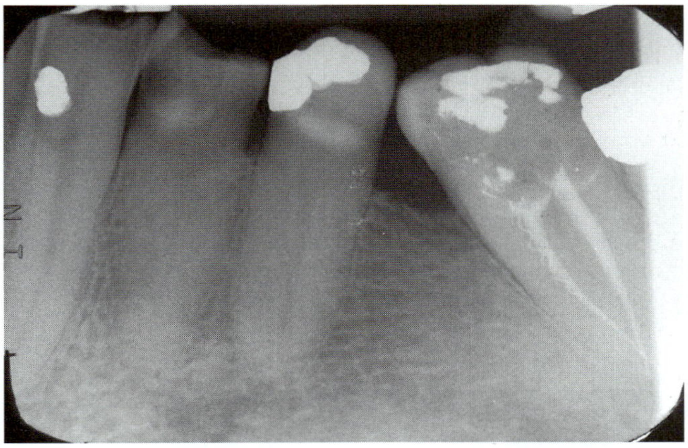

Fig. 48.1 The preoperative radiograph.

History

Complaint

The patient presents complaining of discomfort from a lower left back tooth. The filling was lost from the tooth about 4 months ago.

History of complaint

She has suffered intermittent problems since the tooth was root canal-treated 2 years ago. Pain is triggered by biting on the tooth and changes in temperature have no effect. The symptoms have remained similar in intensity ever since the root canal treatment was completed.

Dental history

The patient has always attended regularly for dental treatment, requiring occasional treatment for failed restorations over the last 10–15 years.

The lower left second permanent molar was originally treated endodontically because the patient developed acute pulpitis. Two attempts at root canal treatment were carried out before the intense pain subsided, with the root canal filling being placed at a third appointment. An endodontic instrument fractured in one of the root canals at the second appointment and the patient was informed of this by the dentist. A temporary restoration was placed to allow a period to assess resolution of symptoms but the patient preferred not to return to the same dentist, feeling that the treatment had gone wrong.

■ ***How do you assess the case so far?***

Several features of the history are significant.

Pain on biting and well-localized pain indicate periapical periodontitis and the cause is almost certainly failure of the root canal treatment.

There was a fractured instrument. This probably means that no apical seal would have been achieved in that canal, reducing the chances of successful treatment.

The provisional restoration was lost 4 months ago. This indicates a complete loss of coronal seal to the root canal system that would allow microleakage of bacteria and their toxins along the length of the root filling. The extent to which this will have occurred is time-dependent. As a general rule, if the root canal filling has been exposed to the oral cavity for 3 months or more, retreatment should be considered even in the absence of clinical signs or symptoms.

Examination

Extraoral examination

There is no facial swelling or tenderness associated with the tooth.

Intraoral examination

You examine the patient following the procedure outlined in problem 47. The lower second molar has a large cavity distally with obvious caries and exposed gutta percha root filling in the pulp chamber. It has tilted mesially and is tender to percussion. The third molar has a large, poorly contoured amalgam restoration.

Investigations

A radiograph is necessary and a periapical view of the teeth in the lower left quadrant is the most appropriate.

■ ***What information do you wish to obtain from the radiograph?***

- **What is the nature and quality** of the previous endodontic treatment?
- **Are any root canals detectable?** Failure of treatment may be caused by failure to detect or fill all canals. Any remaining canals in teeth that have large carious lesions, restorations, marked toothwear or suffered trauma may be sclerotic as a result of tertiary dentine formation.
- **Is there periradicular radiolucency?** This would indicate persistence of infection or inflammation.

- **What is the estimated working length?** This can only be estimated from a periapical radiograph, which is always slightly magnified even when taken with a paralleling technique.
- **What is the root morphology?** The number of roots and their orientation can be identified. Root curvatures and diameters can also be observed; however, it is important to remember that radiographic images are two-dimensional representations of three-dimensional structures. Canals are often much wider buccolingually than can be appreciated in a conventional radiograph.

The preoperative radiograph is shown in Figure 48.1. What do you see?

The canine and premolars are restored and no caries is present, though there is significant toothwear anteriorly. The tilted second molar is root-treated and the fractured instrument is visible in one of the mesial canals.

The film is not of adequate diagnostic quality. The packet or sensor has not been placed far enough posteriorly to include the third molar and the periapical tissues are not visible. The collimator has coned off the distal part of the film because the tube head has been positioned too far anteriorly. Using a paralleling technique with a film holder has produced a true parallel projection, but this has superimposed the mesial canals. It is not possible to determine which of the two canals contains the fractured instrument and it will be necessary to determine exactly where the instrument is, if an attempt is to be made to remove it.

How will you locate the fractured instrument?

By using the parallax technique. A second radiograph must be taken at the same vertical angulation, but at a different horizontal angle, usually from the mesial.

The original and second parallax view are shown in Figure 48.2. What do you see and where is the instrument?

The film on the left in Figure 48.2 is the original film and that on the right is taken from the mesial. The second film is better positioned and shows clearly the presence of a fractured instrument and that there is no periapical radiolucency. The poorly contoured amalgam in the third molar can now be assessed.

Using the MBD (mesial, buccal, distal) rule, when the X-ray beam moves to the *mesial*, the *buccal* canal will appear to move to the *distal*. The broken instrument appears to move mesially and so it must be in the mesiolingual root canal.

What endodontic instruments are prone to fracture and what has fractured in this tooth?

The broken instrument is a spiral root canal filler, recognized by its tapering helical shape and broad pitch.

Instruments prone to fracture are shown in Figure 48.3.

How can instrument fracture be prevented?

In the past, reuse and heat sterilization of instruments weakened them but the current guidelines recommending single-use instruments should largely overcome this problem. Instruments that jam in a root canal during use may become distorted, weakening them, and should be immediately discarded. All files should be inspected throughout use for signs of distortion, as shown in Figure 48.4.

Otherwise, the most important factors are correct use of instruments and correct access cavity design. Rotary nickel titanium files in particular must be used in an electric torque-controlled motor at the correct setting and with minimal apical pressure.

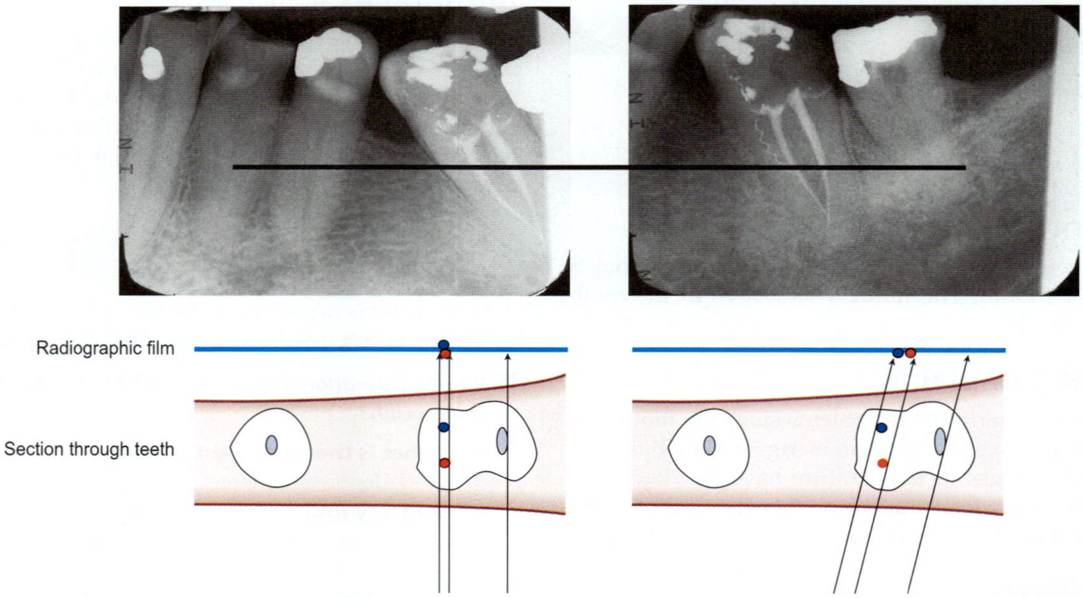

Fig. 48.2 The original film, top left and parallax view, taken from the mesial, top right. The black line across both films shows the level of the cross-section shown below from the occlusal aspect. On the left the beam angle superimposes both mesial molar root canals. On the right, the angled beam produces separate images of the two canals.

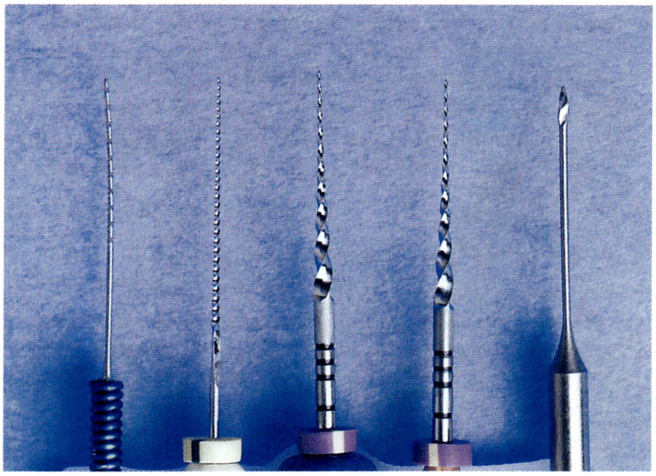

Fig. 48.3 Instruments prone to fracture in root canals. From left to right: a barbed broach, used to extirpate pulp tissue; stainless steel, hand and rotary nickel titanium files used to prepare and shape the root canal; and a Gates–Glidden bur, used for preparation of the coronal root canal.

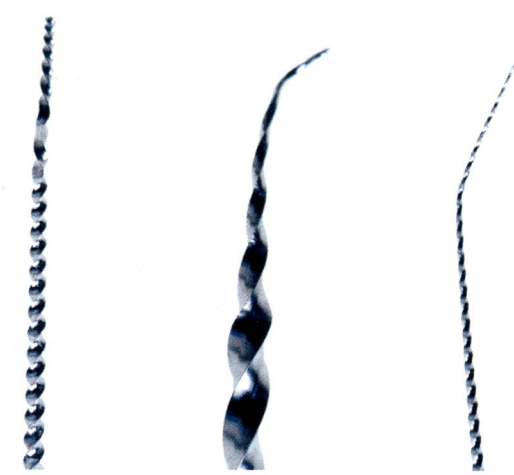

Fig. 48.4 Examples of distorted files which should be disposed of to avoid fracture within the root canal.

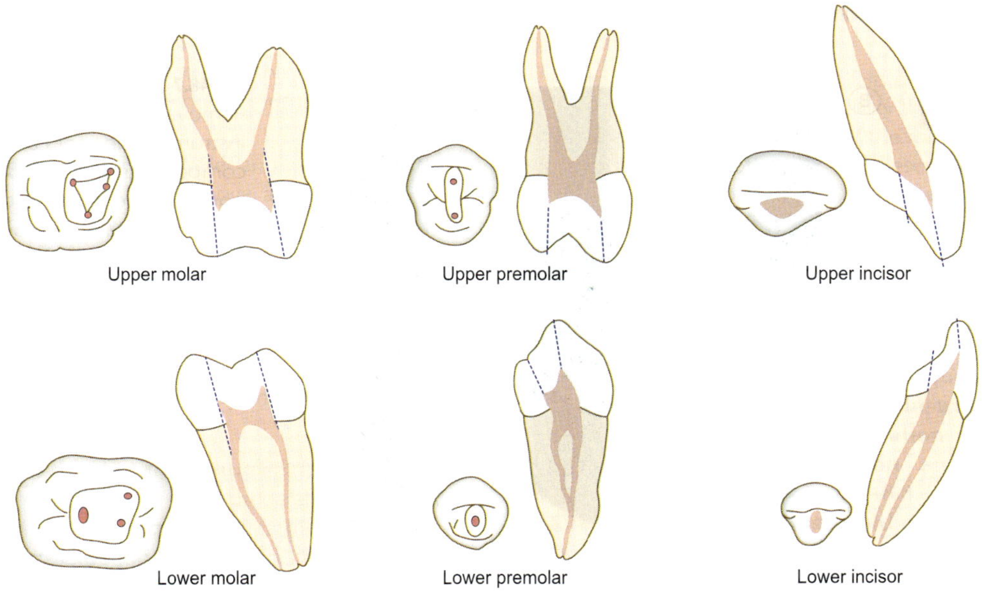

Fig. 48.5 Correct outline for access cavities.

Correct access cavity preparation underpins the success of root canal treatment. The cavity should allow straight-line access for instruments to the root canals. If not, instruments will be overstressed in use and develop weak points. Figure 48.5 outlines the ideal access cavity preparation for all tooth types.

Some instruments prone to fracture can simply be avoided. Gates–Glidden burs can lead to overpreparation and nickel titanium orifice shapers are a better option. Spiral root fillers are mainly used to place nonsetting calcium hydroxide paste between appointments. However, this is largely unnecessary because alternative applicators are available, as shown in Figure 48.6.

Treatment

■ ***How will you remove the fractured spiral filler?***

Magnification is an essential aid to treatment, both to locate canals and to identify the fragment.

Initially, try simple techniques. Sometimes an ultrasonic scaler tip applied to the fractured instrument can transmit sufficient energy through the instrument to break down the dentine jammed against it, loosening it. The main disadvantages are the potential for excessive root dentine removal and that often the end of the fractured instrument disintegrates. Where there is space alongside the instrument, it may be

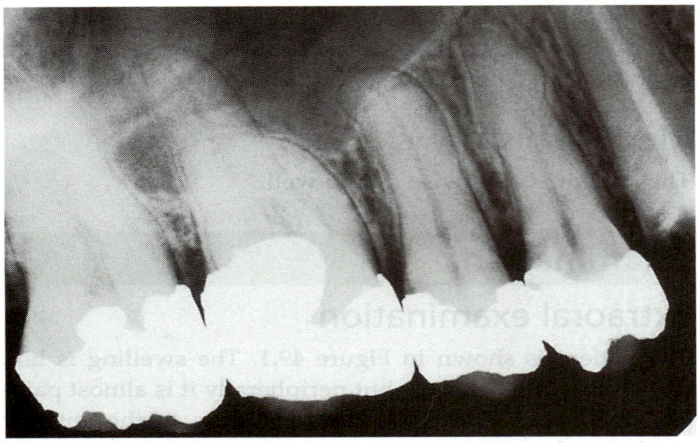

Fig. 49.2 Periapical radiograph showing the causative premolar.

Diagnosis

What do these findings tell you?

The combination of inflammation, the nonvital tooth and adjacent probable abscess indicate an odontogenic soft tissue infection. The history of severe toothache which suddenly resolved suggests pulpitis subsequently relieved by necrosis of the pulp. The subsequent pain of a different character with a tender tooth suggests an apical abscess. The patient points clearly to the second premolar and this is almost certainly the cause of the pain because pain involving the periodontal ligament is well localized.

Trismus is an important sign, indicating that infection or inflammation has spread to involve muscles of mastication. However, trismus is not severe and probably results from inflammation and oedema of the buccinator and the anterior fibres of the masseter which lie at the posterior border of the swelling.

The infection has induced minimal systemic effects and the patient is not significantly pyrexic. Luckily, the infection appears to be localized. The firm centre to the swelling and the swelling in the sulcus will contain pus.

What types of soft tissue infection arising from teeth cause facial swelling? How may they be distinguished and what is the relevance of doing so?

Facial swelling may be the result of oedema, abscess formation, cellulitis or their combination.

It is important to determine which of these types of infection are present because the treatment and sequelae are different. Abscesses require drainage. Cellulitis requires aggressive treatment, usually including antibiotics, and oedema requires no direct treatment but resolves when the causative tooth is removed or the pulp treated.

Despite the fact that these terms are convenient, in practice most odontogenic soft tissue infections are caused by a mixed microbial flora and do not fall neatly into one category or another. It is not unusual to find an abscess with a surrounding zone of cellulitis and a degree of oedema is always present. Which type of infection develops is determined by the virulence of the pathogens (and synergy between species in the mixed flora), the resistance of the host and the anatomical constraints on the infection.

Cause of swelling	Features
Oedema	Soft, not very red or hot, not tender on palpation and not painful. Compressible with slow continuous pressure. Often accounts for much of the facial swelling in children with odontogenic infection.
Abscess	Localized collection of pus which feels hard if small, tense or covered by a thick layer of tissues. If large it may be softer and exhibit fluctuance. Pointing to the skin or mucosa indicates abscess formation.
Cellulitis	Brawny, poorly localized swelling with marked tenderness and dusky redness. May contain small collections of pus but no large localized abscesses. Spreads, sometimes rapidly, through tissues. Usually associated with systemic symptoms, pyrexia, malaise, leucocytosis and lymphadenitis.

If infections are not easily characterized, what are the important features on which treatment must be based?

The critical factors which must be determined are whether:

- an abscess cavity is present (palpation, eliciting fluctuation)
- there is evidence of systemic effects (malaise, pyrexia, a toxic-shocked appearance)
- the infection is spreading rapidly (judged by the history and observation during treatment)
- the patient is predisposed to infection (from the medical history).

Which type of infection is this?

This appears to be primarily an abscess with surrounding oedema.

In what tissue space(s) is the infection tracking/ localizing? What are the boundaries of this space?

This abscess appears to be in the upper part of the buccal space. This is a potential space between the buccinator muscle and the facial muscles and parotid fascia, filled normally with loose connective tissue. Posteriorly it communicates with the masseter muscle and around the front of the ramus to the pterygoid space. Oedema spreads beyond the buccal space to involve the lower eyelid and anterior cheek in the canine fossa. The abscess is not yet pointing to the skin.

Why has the infection localized here? Will it remain localized here?

Abscesses arising from the canine, premolar and molar teeth which perforate the buccal plate of alveolar bone will spill out into the soft tissues either above or below the attachment of the buccinator. The attachment of the buccinator usually runs below the apices of the upper teeth so that infection is likely to pass superficially to the buccinator and into the cheek. If it passes below the attachment, an alveolar abscess or sinus will develop. Paths of spread of infection from an upper premolar are shown in Figure 49.3.

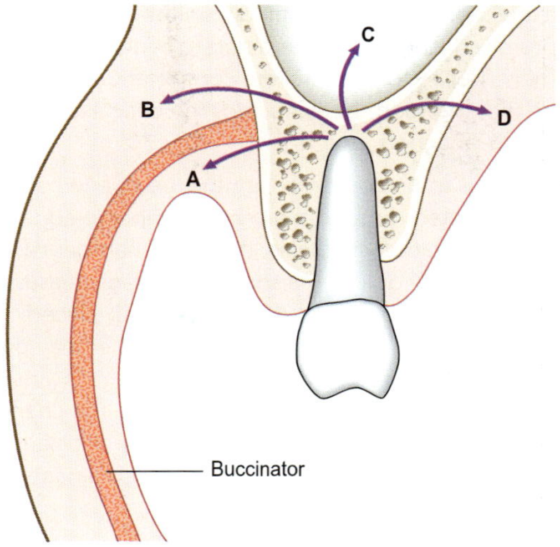

Fig. 49.3 Coronal section showing the paths of spread of infection from upper molars and premolars. Infection may pass buccally below the buccinator muscle into the sulcus or cheek intraorally (A), above the buccinator into the buccal space (B), into the sinus (C) or into the palate (D).

Despite being a thin muscle, the buccinator is a significant barrier to the spread of infection. It is unlikely that the infection would be able to perforate the muscle and develop a sinus into the mouth. Several sequelae are possible. Pus would be most likely to gravitate and spread through the whole buccal space down to the lower border of the mandible; it could point and then drain to the skin or spread laterally around the buccinator to involve other areas of the face, tissue around the masseter muscle or the pterygoid space. Its future course cannot be predicted.

■ ***Is this a potentially life-threatening infection? If so, why?***

Not yet. Infection appears localized, the spread is not particularly rapid and there are no significant systemic symptoms. If a more spreading infection developed, the situation would change.

Involvement of the tissues around the eyelid is worrying. At present the swelling here is caused by oedema, but if infection were to spread to the upper lid or medial canthus of the eye the patient would be at risk of cavernous sinus thrombosis. This is a very rare but potentially fatal complication.

It would also be possible for the infection to spread posteriorly into the pterygomandibular space and infratemporal fossa. From here the infection could spread via veins to the cavernous sinus or middle cranial fossa.

■ ***What is cavernous sinus thrombosis and what are its features?***

Thrombosis of the cavernous sinus follows spread of odontogenic infection along two main venous pathways. Bacteria and infected emboli travel posteriorly from the upper lip and face via the anterior facial vein. This connects via the ophthalmic veins to the cavernous sinus without valves which might otherwise prevent this retrograde flow. Alternatively, infection may spread from the pterygoid space via the pterygoid plexus of veins which connect directly to the cavernous sinus via the foramen ovale.

The local features are seen on one side at first but the signs become bilateral as the thrombus grows. The features are:

Local effects	Marked oedema of the eyelids Pulsating exophthalmos caused by venous obstruction A dilated facial vein Inhibition of movement of the eye Papilloedema and retinal haemorrhage
Systemic effects	Rapid pulse Marked pyrexia Severe malaise

In addition to treatment for the infection, thrombosis requires anticoagulation. The mortality rate is high.

Treatment

■ ***What are the general principles of treatment for all odontogenic infections of the soft tissues?***

Treatment should be started rapidly. Infection may spread quickly and in some cases progress to a life-threatening situation with great rapidity. Identify patients with a risk of significant complications. Those at risk of airway obstruction, cavernous sinus thrombosis or showing toxaemia, suffering malaise or with a high temperature should be treated immediately, possibly even with parenteral antibiotics pending definitive diagnosis, and admitted to hospital for treatment.

Pus must be drained as soon as possible. With most infections causing swollen faces, effective drainage of pus and removal of the cause are the only treatment required. To ensure success, a drain may need to be placed in the incision.

Remove the cause as soon as possible. Removal of the causative tooth both prevents continuing infection and also drains the intraosseous abscess. The exception to this rule is when the cause is pericoronitis. In this case the soft tissue rather than the tooth is the cause and extraction can be detrimental (see Case 32).

Provide antibiotic treatment if necessary. Antibiotics provide little benefit over drainage and removing the cause, but are often used and occasionally required. Pus should be collected on drainage and submitted to microbiology for culture and sensitivity investigation, in case a change of antibiotic is required subsequently.

Provide supportive measures. Ensure that the patient can eat, maintain a good fluid intake and rests. Consider admission to hospital until recovery has started and provide appropriate analgesia.

Review progress regularly. Daily review is appropriate for those treated on an outpatient basis. Those whose infection is serious enough to merit admission require more frequent review, between every hour and 6 hours depending on their status. If signs and symptoms do not improve progressively, further investigation and treatment is probably required.

What are the principles of obtaining drainage? How will you drain the pus in this case?

The principles of incision for drainage are:

- Take the anatomy into account and avoid incising near important structures.
- Incise only when pus has localized, unless rapidly increasing swelling is threatening the airway, in which case it should be drained as quickly as possible.
- Incise where the abscess is pointing or at the point of maximum fluctuation.
- Incise along the most direct route to the pus.
- If incision does not release pus, deepen the incision using blunt forceps, not a scalpel. Open the forceps blades to break open the abscess wall (Hilton's method).
- After incision explore, identify and open all locules of pus.
- Provide dependent drainage if possible.
- Place a drain if the abscess is large, deep or if the incision might close before the abscess resolves (e.g. if the incision penetrates layers of muscle, fascia or skin that can move independently). Leave the drain in place for at least 12–24 hours, or until drainage stops.
- If possible, drain intraorally to prevent facial scarring and skin contraction.
- On the skin incise along Langer's lines or in a skin crease.
- On the skin, try to incise healthy skin. It will scar less.

In this case the pus lies between the buccinator muscle and skin. It is not pointing and is palpable in the upper buccal sulcus. Incision at this site under ethyl chloride spray anaesthesia is perfectly appropriate. However, the incision must extend through the buccinator to be effective, and some might prefer to obtain drainage with the patient under a short general anaesthetic.

Should drainage ever be delayed?

Occasionally drainage must be delayed until pus is properly localized into an abscess. If no pus can be identified on examination, incision will be futile. Waiting a day and providing antibiotics may induce pus to localize. Such a decision must be carefully considered.

Will a drain be required?

Quite probably. The abscess is not very deep but the incision must pass through a muscle. On the other hand, drainage will be dependent: the incision is being made below the pus and gravity will favour drainage. It may not be possible to decide in advance. If pus drains freely on incision and a cavity in the tissues is present, it would be sensible to place a drain, preferably a strip of corrugated rubber or, as a second choice, gauze. This should be sutured to the edge of the incision to prevent displacement. In this case a drain would be as easily placed under local as general anaesthetic.

Can the tooth be conserved after soft tissue infection? How might you remove it?

A soft tissue infection does not mean that the tooth has to be extracted and almost all could, in theory, be preserved. However, most such cases arise through neglect; the tooth is often badly broken down and is best extracted. Occasionally, when infection is spreading rapidly or if the airway is compromised the tooth is extracted to avoid delaying treatment, but even these severe complications do not require that the tooth be extracted. The critical factor is that drainage is obtained.

If the tooth is to be conserved, it must be opened and drainage effected through the pulp chamber in addition to draining pus by incision. Ideally the pulp chamber can be closed again fairly quickly. As soon as drainage ceases, the pulp chamber can be cleaned and a dressing placed. If pus continues to drain for some time, the chamber may be left open for up to 24 hours. After this period there is a risk that the oral flora may enter the tissues, reducing the chances of subsequent successful root treatment. Many clinicians will prescribe antibiotics because they consider drainage to be less effective when the tooth is retained.

Extraction is the more usual treatment. If local anaesthesia can be obtained and trismus is not severe, the tooth may be extracted at once. Infiltration anaesthesia is often difficult to achieve because of the low pH of inflamed tissues. Injection into infected tissue also carries the risk of spreading the bacteria more widely. Block anaesthesia is required.

A general anaesthetic may be necessary. If so, it will be convenient to admit the patient to hospital and complete all the surgical treatment at the same time. An anaesthetic may take some time to organize and in the meantime it would be appropriate to try to extract the tooth under local anaesthetic. A general anaesthetic should not be used in an attempt to overcome trismus. Forcing the jaws open will spread the infection.

If a surgical extraction is required, it may be delayed. As a general principle, surgery should be avoided if the surgical field is infected. However, this rather old rule is often not followed now, because of the availability of very effective antibiotic treatment. Some operators will perform a surgical extraction immediately, and the risk of spreading infection or inducing osteomyelitis seems to be extremely small.

In this case anaesthesia could not be obtained and so drainage and extraction were performed under a general anaesthetic. A short corrugated rubber drain was inserted.

When should antibiotics be prescribed for odontogenic soft tissue infection?

The attitude to antibiotic treatment varies between different centres. Antibiotics are unnecessary for the treatment of the majority of localized soft tissue abscesses and this is particularly so when pus collects superficially in the buccal sulcus or on the palate. Drainage and removal of the cause are much more important. However, in practice, many patients who require incision and drainage tend to be given antibiotics by clinicians, without a clear rationale.

Antibiotics should be prescribed if:

- the patient is prone to infection, for instance is diabetic or immunosuppressed
- there is spreading infection (cellulitis)
- the airway is compromised
- there is significant malaise, pyrexia or toxaemia

- the tooth is to be preserved rather than extracted (the cause is not immediately eliminated)
- cavernous sinus thrombosis is possible.

Antibiotics prescribed for spreading infection may cause pus to localize, and drainage of abscesses may be possible a day or so later.

Antibiotics should never be provided as an alternative to draining pus.

What microorganisms cause odontogenic soft tissue infections?

Odontogenic soft tissue infections are mixed infections. The microbial flora usually contains about 25 species derived from the oral flora, of which about half are cultivable. Anaerobes outnumber aerobes by 10 or 100 to 1 and commonly isolated species are *Porphyromonas* sp., *Prevotella* sp., *Peptostreptococcus* sp. and *Fusobacterium* sp.; however, facultative anaerobes are usually present, often members of the *Streptococcus milleri* group. Although numerically a minor component of the flora, these organisms are important when selecting antibiotics.

If you decided to do so, which antibiotic would you prescribe initially? Explain why.

Almost all the organisms in odontogenic soft tissue infections are sensitive to penicillins. There is a small but increasing proportion of resistant strains but these do not seem to contraindicate penicillins. It is not necessary to prescribe penicillinase-resistant drugs just because one member of the microbial flora shows resistance and they are of no proven benefit in odontogenic infection. Penicillin V or G is sufficient provided drainage can be achieved.

Metronidazole is effective against the anaerobic species and is often prescribed. However, metronidazole should be used as an adjunct to a penicillin and never alone. It will kill the anaerobes but leave facultative anaerobes such as the *Strep. milleri* group unscathed. These organisms are capable of causing a spreading soft tissue infection as a monoculture. Removing their anaerobic microbial competitors with metronidazole risks turning a relatively well-localized, mixed infection into a spreading streptococcal infection. In the wrong site this could be fatal.

In this case the patient received a single dose of 500 mg amoxicillin and 400 mg metronidazole intravenously during the anaesthetic. The same doses were prescribed orally three times a day for 5 days afterwards and this is an appropriate regimen for most odontogenic soft tissue infections. However, as noted above, it may not have contributed greatly to the patient's recovery.

Why bother to take a specimen for culture and sensitivity testing?

As noted above, empirical treatment with penicillin with or without metronidazole is almost always effective. However, in some cases the infection stabilizes but fails to resolve. This may be due to inadequate drainage but a change of antibiotic may be considered a sensible precaution. The result of sensitivity testing may be helpful in selecting another antibiotic and identifying any unusual pathogens present. As culture and sensitivity testing takes about 3 days it must be requested as soon as a sample of pus can be obtained and before antibiotics are administered.

In order to be useful, the sample obtained for culture must be taken in such a way as to favour the growth of anaerobes and fastidious organisms. Ideally it should be taken directly from the abscess through a needle or through a sterile skin incision and transported anaerobically to the laboratory. Samples on swabs contaminated with oral flora are unlikely to be useful and may even provide a misleading result.

When interpreting the results of culture and sensitivity tests obtained from a simple swab of pus it must be remembered that the organisms isolated are unlikely to be representative of the flora. Routine culture methods in most hospitals will detect only a few species, probably not the main component of the flora. Unless a change to a different antibiotic is clearly justified, it would be better to consider changing the dose and route of administration.

How quickly should the swelling resolve?

Patients may often feel much better within a few hours and a noticeable reduction in swelling, trismus, pain and pyrexia should be observed within 24 hours. By this time drains do not usually show pus and are removed and dressings placed over the site if extraoral. If there has been no resolution, the diagnosis, antibiotic treatment and effectiveness of drainage must be reviewed. Almost complete resolution should follow in 3–6 days, as in the present case.

Case 50

Missing upper lateral incisors

SUMMARY

A 15-year-old boy presents to you in general dental practice requesting closure of the spaces between his upper front teeth. What is the cause and how can a better appearance be achieved?

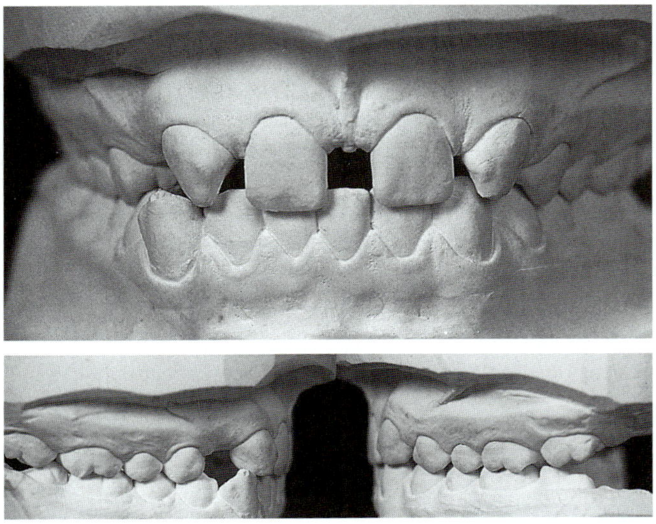

Fig. 50.1 Study models taken at presentation.

History

Complaint

The patient does not wish to have gaps between his upper front teeth.

History of complaint

His permanent teeth erupted at a normal age with large spaces between them. The primary predecessors had all been present and were exfoliated normally. None of the permanent teeth has been extracted.

Medical history

The patient is fit and well.

Family history

The patient's mother had a number of teeth missing. They had been replaced with a partial denture at an early age.

Examination

Extraoral examination

The patient has a skeletal class I appearance without facial asymmetry. There is a slight deviation of the mandible to the patient's left-hand side on opening, but no limitation of opening, temporomandibular joint clicks or crepitus or masticatory muscle tenderness.

Intraoral examination

The patient's soft tissues are healthy and his oral hygiene is good, with no calculus deposits, gingival inflammation or bleeding on probing. The teeth appear sound, with the exception of a buccal amalgam restoration in the lower left first molar.

Study models taken for treatment planning are shown in Figure 50.1.

■ ***What features relevant to treatment do the study models show?***

Both upper lateral incisors are absent. From the front the upper central incisors are upright and separated by a large midline diastema. There is a mild class III incisor relationship, with a normal overjet but a reduced and complete overbite. The upper canines are mesially inclined and mesiolabially rotated, that on the left being more prominent. The lower right canine is labially placed, slightly distally inclined and in crossbite with the upper canine. There is mild lower labial crowding. The posterior teeth are well aligned and the first molars on the right-hand side are in a class I relationship and on the left-hand side in a half a unit class II relationship.

■ ***What are the possible causes for the absent lateral incisors? What is the cause in this case?***

Missing	Developmentally absent, possibly associated with cleft lip or palate or other craniofacial syndrome Extracted Avulsed
Failure to erupt	Dilaceration and/or displacement as a result of trauma Scar tissue preventing eruption Supernumerary tooth preventing eruption Insufficient space as a result of crowding Pathological lesion (e.g. cyst or odontogenic tumour) preventing eruption

In this case the most likely cause for the missing lateral incisors is genetic absence. Genetic absence of some teeth is found in 3–7% of the population. The teeth most commonly missing are, in descending order of frequency, third molars, maxillary lateral incisors and second premolars. The absence of maxillary lateral incisors is a hereditary trait in about 1–2%

of the population. The fact that the patient's mother wore a denture to replace missing teeth from an early age suggests a possible familial aetiology. Trauma or extraction and their related sequelae are readily excluded by questioning. The other causes are discussed in Case 5.

Investigations

■ ***What investigations are required? Explain why for each.***

Investigation	Reason
Tests of vitality of the upper anterior teeth	To exclude incidental loss of vitality, to ensure that endodontic treatment is not required and that unsuspected loss of vitality does not compromise the subsequent treatment plan.
Radiographs	To determine whether the lateral incisors are present and unerupted and to exclude underlying lesions such as supernumerary teeth or cysts. Examination for this case should include a panoramic radiograph to provide a survey, exclude significant periodontal bone loss and confirm the presence or absence of third molars. In addition periapical views or an upper standard occlusal view are required for detailed analysis of the incisor region which suffers from superimposition in the panoramic view. Further films may be required to define the caries status.
The study models should be mounted on an articulator	To assess the occlusion and produce a diagnostic wax-up if required.

In this case all the upper anterior teeth responded to tests of vitality by ethyl chloride and an electric pulp tester.

■ ***The panoramic radiograph is displayed in Figure 50.2. What does it show?***

The dental panoramic radiograph shows that the upper lateral incisors are missing with no evidence of supernumerary teeth or other lesions in this region. All other teeth are present including the unerupted third molars. This confirms the diagnosis that the upper lateral incisors are developmentally absent.

Treatment

■ ***What are the main treatment options? What are their advantages and disadvantages?***

Option	Advantages and disadvantages
Space closure with adhesive restorations	Composite restorations added to the approximal surfaces of the central incisors and canines could reduce the spaces. This is the most conservative option, technically straightforward and might be acceptable as a provisional solution. However, complete closure could not be achieved with such wide diastemas and each tooth would look unacceptably wide.
Orthodontic space closure	This would bring the canine into the position of the lateral incisor requiring the shape of the canine to be modified by selective grinding of the tip and placement of composite to disguise it as a lateral incisor. However, the darker colour of the canine would be difficult to conceal, as would the gingival contour because of the canine eminence. The palatal cusp of the first premolar tooth is frequently visible and compromises the appearance. When the difficulty of complete space closure is taken into account, it is clear that this option is rarely ideal. It frequently produces a poor result despite being a time-consuming and costly procedure.
Create space for lateral incisors	Space creation by orthodontic treatment followed by provision of lateral incisors with a prosthesis involves a protracted phase of orthodontics and is costly. However it would produce the best appearance.

■ ***The patient's main concern is his appearance. How would you demonstrate the possible results to him?***

The patient is considering committing himself to a long and complex treatment so the result of each of the treatment plans should be assessed with study models and diagnostic wax-ups. The possibility of the orthodontic treatment can be

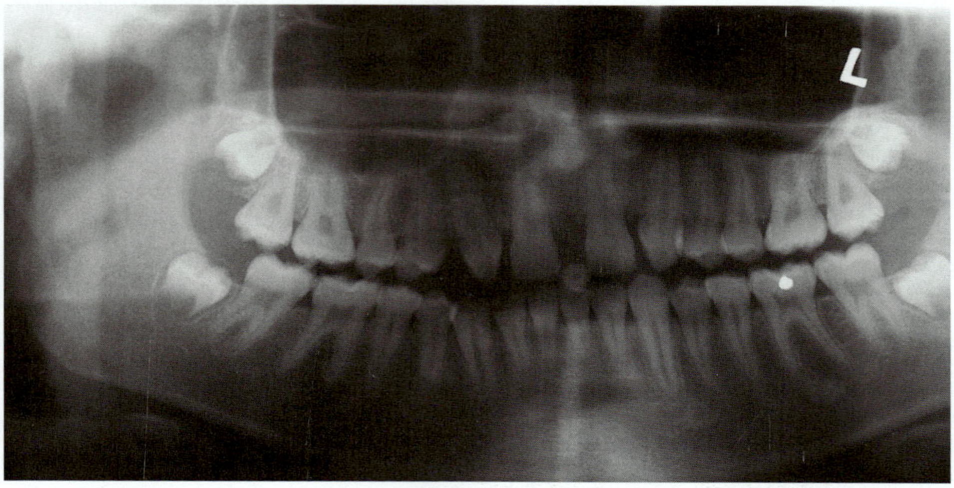

Fig. 50.2 Panoramic radiograph.

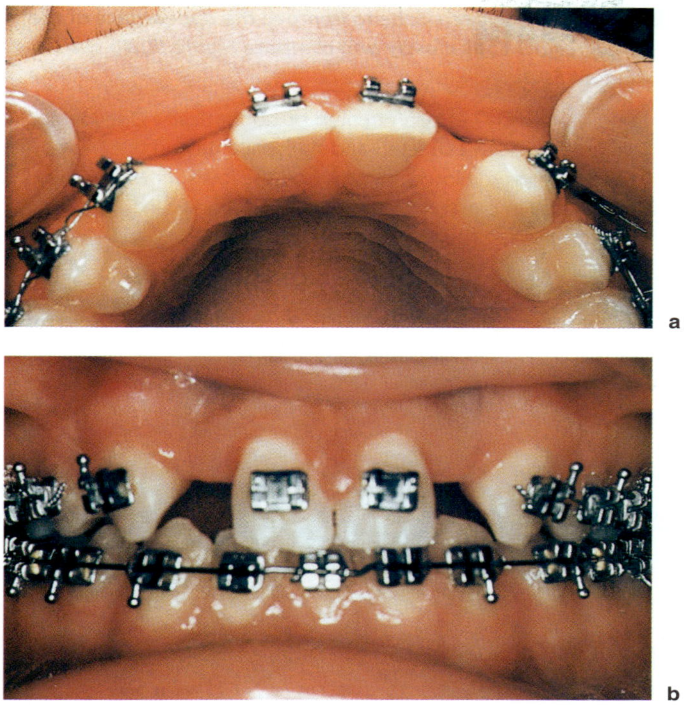

Fig. 50.3 The final orthodontic result.

visualized by cutting the teeth off duplicate study models and fixing them in an orthodontically achievable position, the so-called Kessling set-up. Patient and dentist can then see what might be achieved by each treatment option.

Following discussion, the patient opts for the third treatment plan.

■ *How would you carry out the orthodontic treatment?*

The tooth movement demands fixed appliance treatment. Tooth tilting using a removable appliance would result in a poor appearance in the midline and produce spaces which are difficult to fill with a prosthetic replacement. If a fixed appliance is used the incisors may be more accurately positioned and derotation of the canines is possible. The orthodontic result for this patient can be seen in Figure 50.3.

■ *How would you now replace the missing lateral incisors?*

Prosthetic treatment should be as conservative as possible because the upper anterior teeth are vital and sound, and the patient is young. The teeth can be replaced with fixed or removable prostheses but the treatment of choice would be a minimum preparation bridge or bridges. Possible designs are shown in Figure 50.4.

Normally a fixed–fixed design in a minimum preparation bridge should be avoided. This is because debonding of one retainer will create an area of stagnation below it and risk caries. A typical minimum preparation bridge to replace a lateral incisor would be a cantilever design retained on the canine or central incisor.

However canine abutments (option A) would have a major disadvantage in this case. The canines were originally

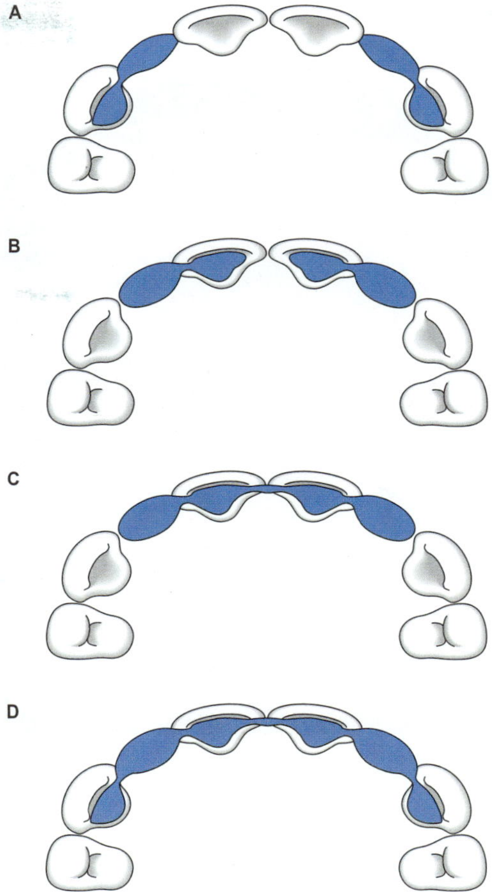

Fig. 50.4 Possible designs for minimum preparation bridge(s).

mesiolabially rotated and the orthodontic result is potentially unstable. Relapse would result in the pontics swinging out labially. An alternative might appear to be a cantilever design retained on a central incisor (option B) which has the advantage of a greater enamel area for bonding. However, two separate cantilever bridges retained on the central incisors would also enable the orthodontic result to relapse and the midline diastema to reappear. Linking the central incisors together (option C) would prevent this but could not prevent the canines from relapsing to their original position.

A degree of orthodontic retention must be designed into the prosthesis and only a fixed–fixed bridge extending from canine to canine is suitable (option D). The potentially unstable orthodontic result may in itself favour debonding of one of more of the wings. Regular recall will be essential to detect this early. If debonding is a repeated problem, replacement with a conventional bridge may have to be considered. The need for orthodontic retention is the main reason that an implant retained solution is not appropriate.

The final bridge design and appearance are shown in Figure 50.5. Note how the orthodontic treatment plan must take into account the occlusal clearance required to cover the palatal surfaces of the canines.

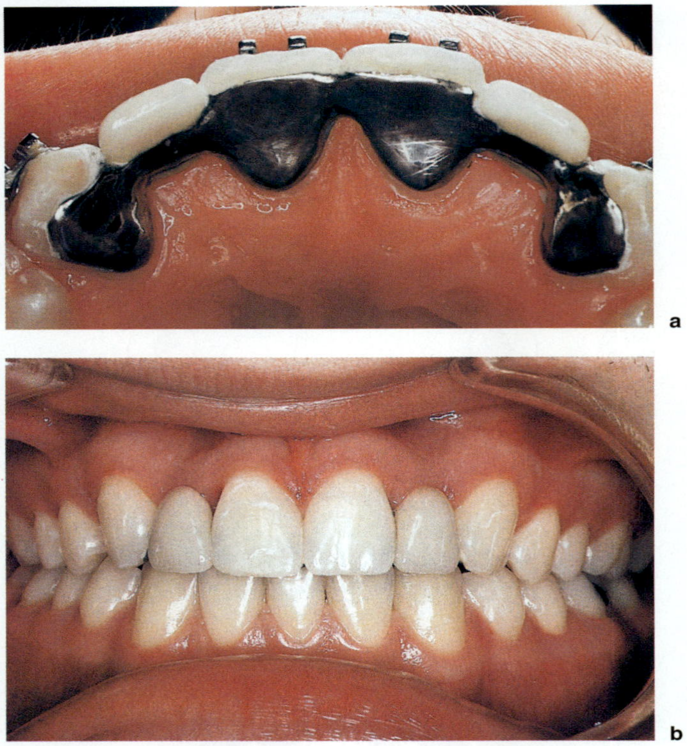

Fig. 50.5 The final result.

■ ***What else has been done to improve the appearance of the final result? Look closely and compare Figure 50.5b with Figure 50.1.***

The lower arch has been treated orthodontically. One lower incisor has been extracted and the space gained has been used to align the lower incisors and the lower right canine, which was in crossbite. This has made a significant contribution to the final appearance.

Case • 51

Anterior crossbite

SUMMARY

An 8-year-old girl is referred to you for an orthodontic opinion. She has an anterior crossbite. What is the cause and how would you treat it?

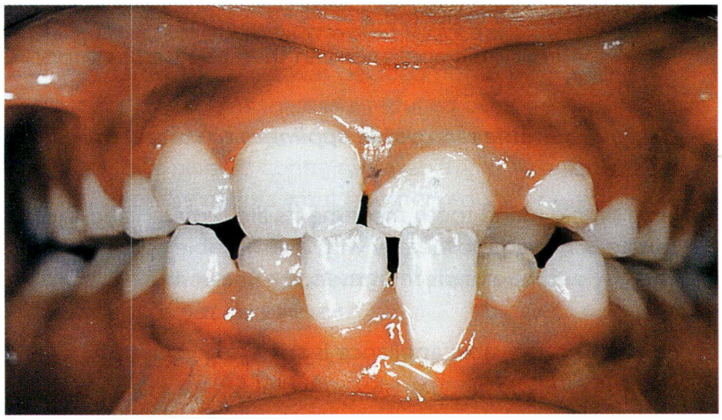

Fig. 51.1 The patient's appearance on presentation.

History

Complaint

The mother of the patient noticed the crossbite and is very anxious about her daughter's appearance. She requested a referral from the family's general dental practitioner.

History of complaint

The incisors erupted into their present positions and there is no history of trauma.

Medical history

The patient is fit and healthy.

Examination

Extraoral examination

There is no facial asymmetry and no clicks, locking or crepitus are present on examination of the temporomandibular joints.

Intraoral examination

- ***The appearance of the teeth on presentation is shown in Figure 51.1. What do you see?***

The patient is in the early mixed dentition stage and the teeth present are:

6EDC21	12BCDE6
6EDC21	12 CDE6

The upper and lower incisors are crowded and the upper left central and lateral incisors are in crossbite. The lower left central incisor is labially placed and there is gingival recession and loss of attached gingiva to the mucogingival junction on its labial aspect. The oral hygiene is reasonable though mild interdental gingivitis is present around the poorly aligned incisors. The dental health is good.

- ***What specific feature would you check in your examination? Explain why for each.***

See Table 51.1.

Diagnosis

- ***What is your diagnosis?***

The diagnosis of crossbite has already been made by the patient's mother. The incisor crowding, gingival recession and anterior displacement of the mandible are the other significant factors requiring recognition.

Table 51.1 Features to be examined

Feature	Reason
Can the patient achieve an edge-to-edge incisor relationship when closing on hinge axis?	On closing in a retruded position the patient makes initial contact on the lower left central incisor. If left untreated this could result in continued excessive occlusal loading on this tooth, causing further loss of support. The ability to achieve incisal contact is regarded as favourable because it indicates that minimal tooth movement should be required to correct the crossbite.
If so, is there an associated forward displacement of the mandible?	The initial contact on the central incisors displaces her mandible forwards into the intercuspal position shown in Figure 51.1. Early correction of the displacement activity may prevent possible temporomandibular joint dysfunction in later life. There is not yet significant wear faceting on the incisors. However, if they are left untreated, considerable attritional wear may develop.
How mobile is the lower left central incisor? Are probing depths increased?	Mobility is limited (grade 1) and probing depths are less than 2 mm. This would suggest that the prognosis for the tooth is good. If there were significant mobility or periodontal destruction, extraction of the incisor might have to be considered as part of an orthodontic treatment plan.
How might space be provided to relieve the incisor crowding?	At the present stage of dental development, sufficient space would be provided by the extraction of deciduous teeth.

Table 52.1 Conditions, diseases and lesions that may mimic plaque-induced gingivitis and periodontitis

Condition	Typical features	Diagnostic tests
Conditions that mimic gingivitis		
Hereditary gingival fibromatosis	Presents in childhood or adolescence. Generalized fibrous enlargement of gingiva in presence or absence of infection. May cover crowns of teeth. Solitary or associated with several different syndromes. Family history	Family history, identification of other features in syndromes. Biopsy
Deposition diseases and inborn errors of metabolism	Presents in newborn or children. Gingiva enlarged by deposition of various metabolic end products such as abnormal glycogen or mucopolysaccharides	Biopsy, biochemical analysis, family history
Granulomatous gingivitis (caused by orofacial granulomatosis, oral Crohn's disease, Melkersson–Rosenthal syndrome and sarcoidosis)	Presents from childhood to middle age. Lumpy granular gingivitis, more marked in areas of plaque retention. Tags and flaps of redundant gingiva may develop. Shrinks slightly but does not respond completely to plaque control. Tissue contains granulomas. Sarcoidosis may be associated with raised serum calcium, raised serum angiotensin-converting enzyme and lymphadenopathy, especially hilar. Bowel disease may be present in those with orofacial granulomatosis or Crohn's disease	Biopsy. Evidence of bowel, lung or other sites involved. Investigations depend on any associated conditions
Wegener's granulomatosis	Presents in middle age. The classical gingival presentation is unusual, a rare presentation but striking. Overgrowth of granular or red and white speckled 'strawberry gums'. May grow to cover teeth in a few weeks. Renal involvement may be fatal rapidly	May be evidence of disease in nose, sinuses or elsewhere, especially kidney. Circulating antineutrophil cytoplasmic antibodies present
Leukaemia	Usually presents in children with acute myelomonocytic or monocytic leukaemia or in elderly patients with chronic myeloid leukaemia. May be a lumpy gingivitis with few suspicious features, a very inflamed maroon or greenish gingivitis or one or more ulcerated growths from the gingival margin	Biopsy, blood film, history
Foreign-body gingivitis	May present at any age. Usually caused by impaction of abrasive particles from prophylaxis paste into the gingiva. Tends to occur in those with very frequent or overzealous professional cleaning. The particles elicit a foreign-body reaction and the gingiva looks duskily inflamed but plaque control has no effect. May be painful	Biopsy
Fungal infection	South American blastomycosis (paracoccidioidomycosis) causes lumpy granular inflamed gingival swellings but this is an endemic disease and is not seen in the UK. May extend beyond the gingiva	Biopsy
Conditions that mimic periodontitis		
Odontogenic tumours	Occasionally odontogenic tumours form in the gingiva rather than in bone. Most cause a small mass or erode superficial bone and are easily excised without problems. The commonest odontogenic tumour to occur extraosseously is the calcifying odontogenic cyst. Squamous odontogenic tumour merits special mention because it sometimes arises in the periodontal ligament or gingiva and mimics periodontitis or even localized juvenile periodontitis	Biopsy
Langerhans' cell histiocytosis	Solitary or multifocal destructive lesion that often affects the skull and jaws. May arise at almost any age and then destroys bone around teeth. In late disease the teeth appear to be 'floating in air' radiographically as no bone remains	Biopsy
Squamous carcinoma of gingiva	Gingiva is a very rare site for carcinoma and it usually presents in those aged more than 50 years. Destroys soft tissue and bone	Biopsy
Metastatic malignancy	Most metastatic malignant neoplasms of the jaws grow in the medullary space of the posterior mandible. However, metastases may also seed to the gingiva to produce solitary or multiple masses, often ulcerated	Biopsy, history
Hypophosphatasia	Teeth exfoliate with forming roots almost immediately after eruption. No cementum present. Caused by mutation of the tissue nonspecific alkaline phosphatase enzyme required for bone mineralization	Serum alkaline phosphatase, family history

The appearances are typical of Langerhans' cell histocytosis. Sheets of neoplastic Langerhans' cells infiltrate the tissues and attract eosinophils, which tend to cluster together and degranulate externally. Bright red eosinophil granules can be seen lying between cells on the right-hand side of the second panel.

Although the diagnosis is clear, it is necessary to identify the Langerhans' cells specifically. Macrophages can also look similar. In the past this has been done by electron microscopy to show the characteristic Birbeck granules in the cell cytoplasm, tennis racket-shaped vesicular organelles. Immunocytochemical staining for the cell surface molecules CD1a or langerin is easier and faster. The third panel shows a low-power view in which brown stain labels CD1a on the Langerhans' cells. At high power in the fourth panel, the stain can be seen to localize around the cell, forming a dark ring at the cell membrane.

Diagnosis

The diagnosis is Langerhans' cell histiocytosis.

What is a Langerhans' cell?

A dendritic cell found in epithelium. They develop in the bone marrow from the monocyte lineage, migrate to the epithelium of skin and mucosa and reside there to present external antigens to the immune system.

What is Langerhans' cell histiocytosis?

A clonal proliferation of Langerhans' cells that presents as a spectrum of disease severity (Table 52.2).

All types have a predilection for the skull bones and jaws. Lesions may be painful or asymptomatic and may be accompanied by soft-tissue swelling. This patient has multifocal single-organ system disease because only bone is affected.

Table 52.2 Langerhans' cell histiocytosis

Presentation	Typical features
Multifocal multiorgan disease (acute form)	A malignant neoplasm of Langerhans' cells affecting infants and young children below 3 years of age. Affects skin, liver, spleen, lymph nodes and bones and requires aggressive treatment with chemotherapy. Bone marrow is involved. Half of patients die before 5 years of age
Multifocal single-organ disease (chronic multifocal form)	Usually causes multiple bone lesions in the skull and jaws. When the pituitary is involved diabetes insipidus develops and this, with exopthalmos and bone lesions, is called Hand–Schuller–Christian triad or syndrome. Occasionally fatal but usually treatable by curettage of lesions, sometimes with chemotherapy
Unifocal disease (chronic unifocal form)	The commonest type, usually involves bone. Solitary lesions with a relatively benign course. Curettage is usually curative

Treatment

What treatment would you recommend?

A radiographic survey of the skull is required, together with a bone scan or skeletal survey to identify any lesions elsewhere. Medical examination and a detailed history are required in case of soft-tissue involvement.

Lesions in chronic multifocal disease and solitary eosinophilic granulomas usually respond to curettage. This will require removal of the upper right first and second molar to gain access and ensure complete removal. All involved soft tissue must be excised. There will be a risk of oroantral communication.

The lower right premolar lesion may be curetted without tooth loss but the surrounding presumed affected soft tissue must be removed and this may necessitate tooth loss. A more conservative approach may be possible if the patient accepts a risk of recurrence. Any recurrence could be re-curetted.

The lower left molar lesion could be due to periodontitis and requires a biopsy for treatment planning.

Long-term follow-up is required. Lesions may recur and new lesions may develop over a period of many years.

Case 53

Unexpected findings

SUMMARY

A 14-year-old boy presents with toothache and a slightly swollen left cheek. What is the diagnosis and how will you treat him?

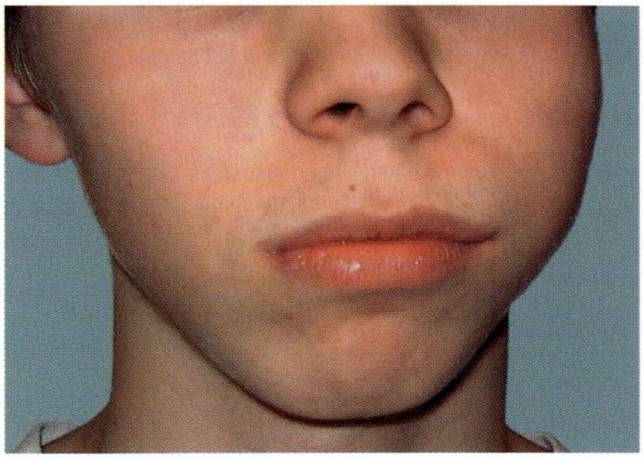

Fig. 53.1 The patient's appearance on presentation.

History

Complaint

The patient complains of intermittent toothache on the left side of his face, which he feels is coming from an upper tooth.

History of complaint

He has been aware of intermittent pain and discomfort from an upper back tooth when eating, especially anything very hot or cold, for several months. The pain is gradually getting worse.

Medical history

The patient is otherwise fit and well.

Dental history

He has never been to a dentist before.

Examination

Extraoral examination

The patient is a fit and healthy looking boy. His left cheek appears slightly swollen but there is little extraoral asymmetry. The cheek is not tender or inflamed and both the patient and his parents say that he has always looked like this. No lymph nodes are palpable and his temporomandibular joints appear normal.

Intraoral examination

The upper left first molar has heavily stained fissures and the whole crown is discoloured. The other teeth appear sound. The alveolus in the upper left quadrant is enlarged, with reduction of depth of the buccal sulcus. The swelling affects the buccal and palatal aspects, is smooth, uninflamed and is not tender to palpation.

In addition, the upper left second premolar appears missing and there is a small space between the first premolar and molar tooth. Several supernumerary teeth are evident.

■ ***How do you interpret the history and examination so far?***

There could be several explanations for the presentation. The history of the pain, exacerbated by hot and cold, and poorly localized almost certainly indicates pulpitis. The obvious cause would appear to be caries in the upper first molar. The whole crown is discoloured and there may be extensive caries despite the intact occlusal surface.

The enlargement of the alveolus has expanded into the buccal sulcus and could account for the slight extraoral swelling. The commonest cause of smooth uninflamed expansion of the alveolus is an odontogenic cyst. Further investigation is required.

The absent second premolar may be unerupted or absent. Missing premolar teeth is a relatively common developmental anomaly but the patient also has supernumerary teeth and it would be unusual to have missing and supernumerary teeth in the same patient. In addition, if the premolar had never developed, the space between the first premolar and molar would have been likely to have closed completely. The tooth is probably unerupted and relatively superficial in the alveolus, holding the teeth apart.

Investigations

■ ***What investigations would you now undertake and why?***

Vitality tests. The vitality of the upper first molar needs to be determined and on testing it you discover that it appears vital, as are the adjacent teeth.

Radiographs. Right and left bitewings for caries assessment and a panoramic radiograph to assess the overall dentition are indicated. These views should provide sufficient information to explain the missing upper left second premolar, assess any further unerupted supernumerary teeth and to investigate the swelling of the left maxilla. If required, further views including periapicals, oblique upper occlusal views or antral views may be required later but are not indicated at this stage.

■ ***The panoramic radiograph is shown in Figure 53.2. Look carefully. What do you see?***

The panoramic radiograph shows:

- a large carious cavity in upper first molar
- right and left supplemental maxillary canines
- peg-shaped supernumerary overlying upper right lateral incisor and right canine
- upper left second premolar present, unerupted and inverted
- developing third molars in all four quadrants
- increased opacity in the region of the left maxillary sinus.

■ ***What terms are used to describe extra teeth? What do they mean?***

Term	Definition
Supernumerary tooth	Any tooth over and above the normal complement of teeth.
Supplemental tooth	Supernumerary tooth with the morphology of a normal tooth, usually an additional tooth in a series, for instance additional lateral incisor, third premolar or fourth molar.
Mesiodens	Supernumerary tooth in the upper midline, may be conical (forms early and rarely interferes with eruption of incisors) or tuberculate (with a wide crown with cusps, forms late and often interferes with eruption). See Case 5.

■ ***What is the cause of supernumerary teeth?***

The cause is unknown but some clues are available. Supernumerary teeth can be caused by mutations in single genes, for instance the CBFA-1 gene. Mutations of this gene cause cleidocranial dysplasia, in which multiple supernumeraries are a prominent feature. More is known about congenitally **missing** teeth and only a single gene mutation is sufficient to cause teeth to be absent. For instance, mutations in the skeletal patterning gene MSX-1 are associated with missing second premolars and third molars and mutations in PAX-9 are associated with missing molars and lower incisors. It seems likely that supernumerary teeth in normal patients will turn out to have similar relatively simple genetic causes.

■ ***The section of the panoramic radiograph showing the left maxilla is enlarged in Figure 53.3. What else does it show?***

There is loss of the thin radiopaque (white) line of the maxillary cortex forming the bony floor of the maxillary antrum. This is clearly visible on the patient's right side in Figure 53.2. A domed relatively radiopaque lesion occupies most of the maxilla and antrum. It has a very thin radiopaque margin at its upper limit.

The panoramic radiograph is shown again in Figure 53.4 with the features including the supernumerary teeth and the margin of the lesion in the left maxilla indicated.

Differential diagnosis

■ ***What is the cause of the patient's pain?***

Pulpitis. As noted above, the symptoms fit pulpitis. The first permanent molar is the most likely source; it is vital and has extensive caries. Periapical periodontitis can be eliminated as a cause because the pain would be well localized and because there are no nonvital teeth in the quadrant.

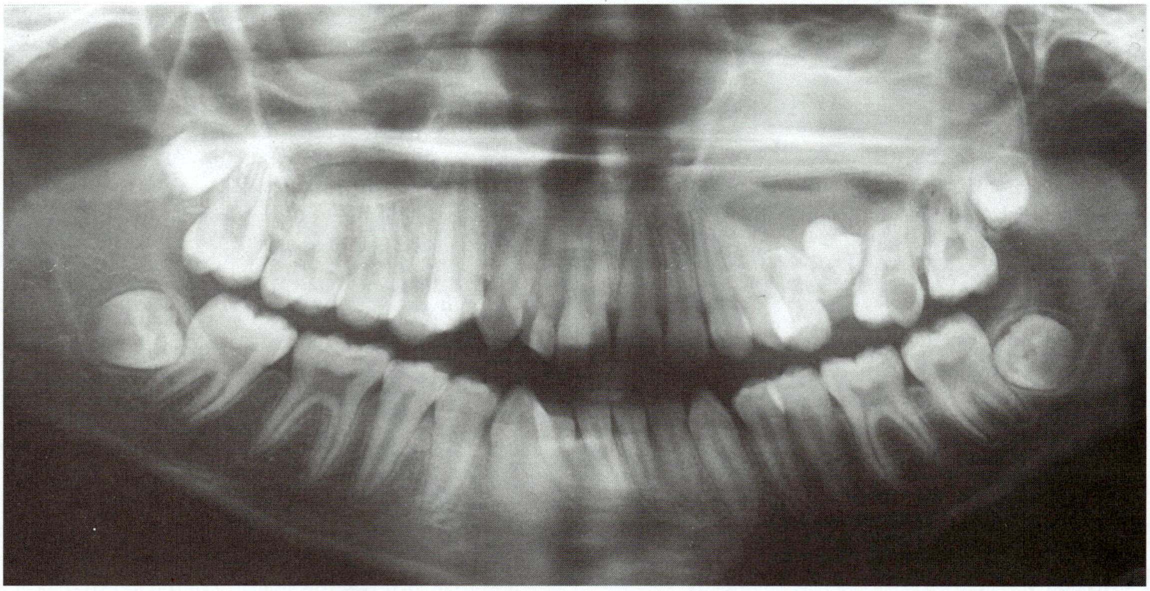

Fig. 53.2 Panoramic radiograph.

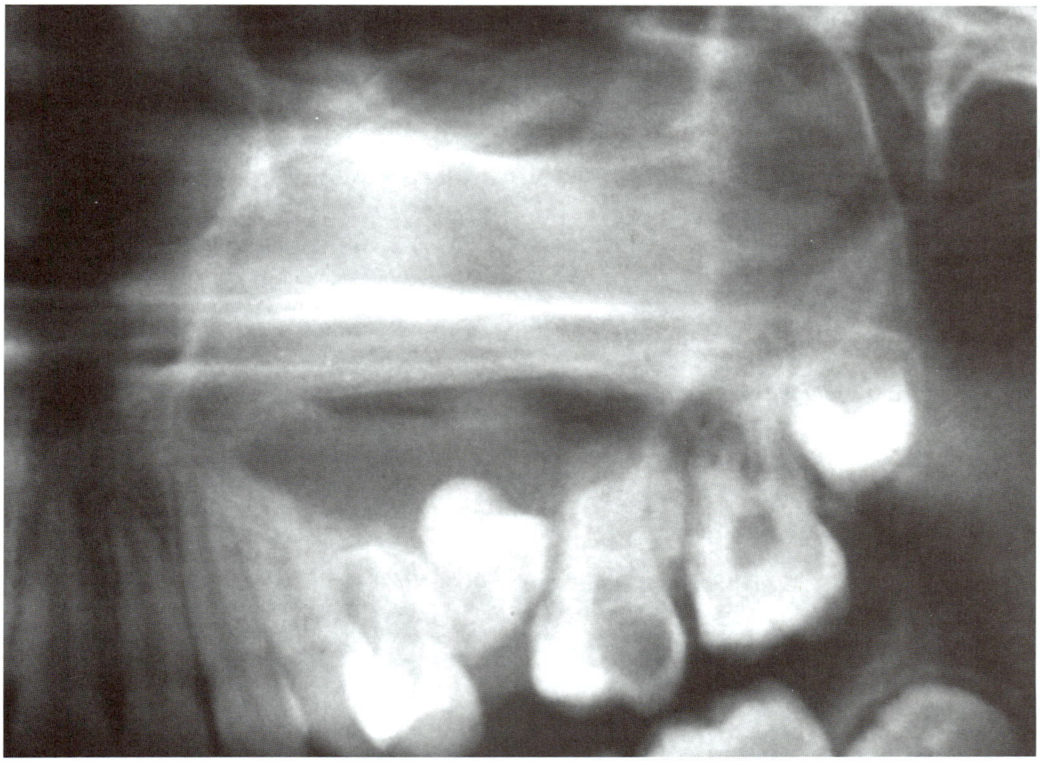

Fig. 53.3 Left maxilla enlarged from Figure 53.2.

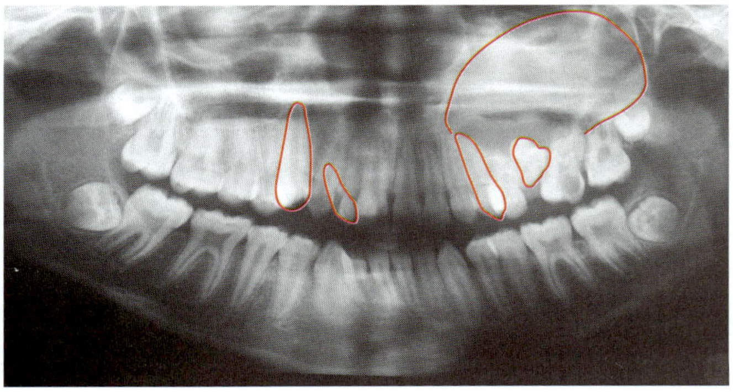

Fig. 53.4 The panoramic radiograph with the features outlined.

■ ***Give a differential diagnosis for the lesion in the left maxilla. Explain which cause is most likely and why.***

The unilocular dome-shaped lesion with a thin bony margin of expanded periosteal new bone and the overall round shape are highly suggestive of a cyst. The commonest cysts in the alveolus and maxilla are odontogenic. There are no radiological features of malignancy.

Dentigerous cyst. Relatively common and found in children. Dentigerous cysts arise around the crown of an unerupted tooth and the cyst lining is attached to the tooth at the amelocemental junction. This cyst is certainly closely associated with the crown of the unerupted second premolar but the radiographic views are not clear enough to see whether the edge of the cyst joins the tooth at the amelocemental junction. This would have been almost conclusive but even without this information, this is the most likely diagnosis.

Odontogenic tumour. A less likely possibility. The lesion is not multilocular to suggest ameloblastoma but in theory an odontogenic tumour is possible. The odontogenic tumours to consider in children are usually ameloblastic fibroma and ameloblastoma. However, these are solid, less radiolucent and cause more expansion.

The adenomatoid odontogenic tumour can present as a dentigerous cyst and might be considered if mineralization was detected in the cyst on radiographs. This lesion usually arises on upper lateral incisors in females but, while unlikely, is a possibility.

Radicular cyst. The commonest odontogenic cyst but it would have to arise at the apex of a nonvital tooth. The first molar tooth with caries and all other teeth in the quadrant are vital, excluding this diagnosis. This will only turn out to be the diagnosis if the vitality test result is incorrect.

Antral cyst. These cysts arise in the antral mucous glands (*antral inclusion* or *retention cysts*) but would be unlikely to cause such marked expansion. Also, they would not have a bony margin because they arise within the antral mucosa rather than in bone and so do not expand the alveolus as they enlarge.

■ ***Do you need to make a definitive diagnosis before treatment?***

No, a dentigerous cyst is almost certainly the cause. Dentigerous cysts and the alternatives can be treated in the same way. Therefore treatment can be planned on this basis and the final diagnosis confirmed later.

Treatment

■ *What treatment would you recommend for the pain?*

The caries in the first molar should be removed and a sedative temporary dressing placed. The details of the final restoration will depend on the findings after excavation of the caries and the effectiveness of the dressing in reducing pain.

■ *What types of treatment are available for cysts?*

Cysts are usually enucleated, i.e. the bony cavity is opened, the cyst lining separated from its inner bony surface, removed and the cavity allowed to fill with blood clot and reorganize.

Alternatively the cyst may be decompressed and marsupialized. Decompression involves opening the cyst to the exterior to relieve the internal pressure. Radicular, dentigerous and many other cyst types enlarge through hydrostatic pressure and so decompression prevents further enlargement. Marsupialization is the method by which decompression is ensured. The cyst is opened and the lining sutured to the overlying mucosa to convert the cyst into a pouch communicating with the mouth (or sometimes the nose or antrum). Without its internal pressure to cause enlargement, the cavity slowly shrinks and reorganizes from its periphery.

Procedures are slightly different for odontogenic keratocysts because of their risk of recurrence. The lining is thin and easily torn on removal making enucleation difficult. Access to the cavity needs to be good to ensure all the lining is removed and the lining is sometimes treated with a fixative, Carnoy's solution. This can be dabbed onto the lining to make it tougher and also to kill the epithelium, so that any small fragments left behind cannot seed recurrences.

■ *What are the advantages and disadvantages of decompression and marsupialization in the treatment of cysts?*

Surgical procedure	Advantages and disadvantages
Enucleation and primary closure	Complete treatment in one episode In very large cysts the clot may break down and become infected, though this is largely a theoretical disadvantage
Decompression and marsupialization	The cyst cavity reduces in size only slowly, months of follow up may be required It is difficult to keep the cavity clean – it requires regular washing The opening will also shrink, making access difficult Complete resolution is unlikely A period of shrinkage may allow enucleation without damage to adjacent structures such as the inferior dental nerve Shrinkage may allow more teeth to be preserved Usually ineffective for odontogenic keratocysts because they enlarge by growth of the lining, not hydrostatic pressure

Because marsupialization has several disadvantages it is usually used only for a short period for specific reasons. The cyst can be enucleated when it has shrunk to a more manageable size or away from important structures.

■ *What treatment would you recommend for this particular cyst?*

The inverted second premolar cannot erupt and needs to be removed. The cyst extends around the apices of adjacent teeth and marsupialization would have the advantage that their vitality could be preserved. However, washing out the cavity after marsupialization would be difficult and in a child it would be better to perform enucleation and complete the treatment in one episode. If adjacent teeth were devitalized they would require root treatment, unless orthodontic assessment for the crowding suggested gaining space by extraction. In practice it will probably prove possible to enucleate without devitalizing the adjacent teeth.

A further possibility when enucleating the cyst is to break down the bony wall separating the cyst from the antrum, remove the cyst lining and extract the unerupted tooth. This effectively reforms the antrum immediately. A nasal anterostomy (opening from the sinus through the lower part of the lateral wall of the nose) would be required to ensure drainage from the sinus until the antral healing is complete.

Whichever procedure is carried out, a sample, preferably all, of the cyst lining should be taken for histological examination to confirm the diagnosis.

Further investigations

■ *Figure 53.5 shows the histological appearances of the cyst after enucleation. What do you see and how do you interpret the appearances?*

The left-hand figure shows a length of fibrous cyst wall (W) lined on its inner aspect by epithelium of regular thickness (E). In the bottom right-hand corner there is a focus of inflammation, seen as dark nuclei of inflammatory cells (I), and above it a large pink mural nodule of cholesterol clefts in loose tissue (C) protruding into the lumen. The cholesterol elicits a foreign body giant cell reaction and, although they are not clear at this magnification, the very dark angulate areas among the cholesterol crystals are foreign body giant cells. Haemorrhage (H) is present in and around the mural nodule, visible most easily as red cells on the left of the nodule between it and the epithelial lining. The cholesterol is derived from breakdown of cell membranes of erythrocytes and inflammatory cells that die in the cyst. Two less inflamed areas are shown on the right. The rest of the cyst was lined by similar nonkeratinizing epithelium, often very thin and without rete processes.

Taken together with the radiological features the appearances indicate dentigerous cyst. Dentigerous cysts are lined by nonkeratinizing stratified epithelium, though this is not in itself a diagnostic feature. In the early stages the epithelium is characteristically only two cells thick because it is reduced enamel epithelium that has separated from the tooth crown.

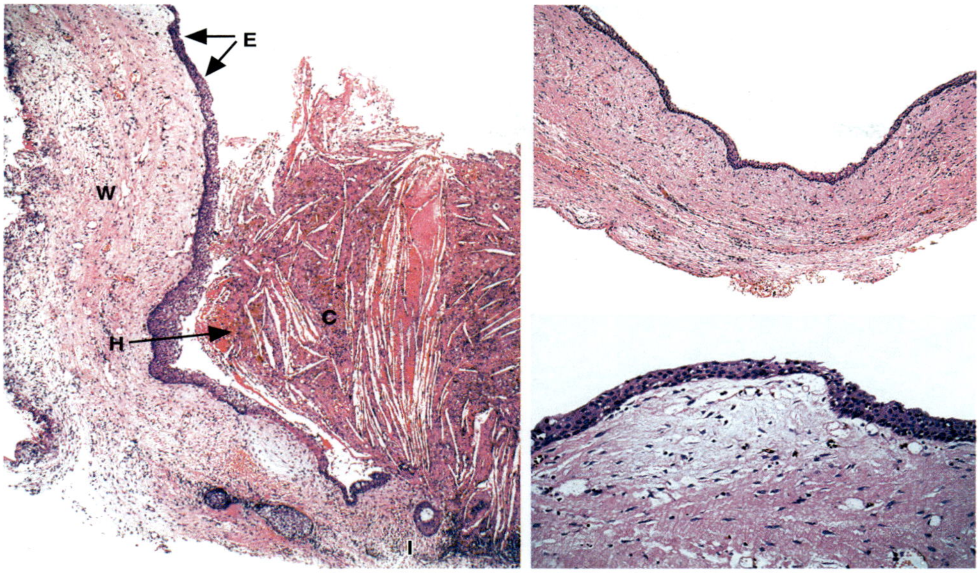

Fig. 53.5 Appearances of the cyst lining after removal, sections stained with haematoxylin and eosin. The width of the cyst wall is 1–1.5 mm.

As the cyst enlarges and impinges on mucosa or the antrum it becomes inflamed. The inflammation causes the epithelium to undergo hyperplasia, thicken and develop rete processes. Inflammation causes haemorrhage and release of cholesterol to form crystals in the wall, which ulcerate into the lumen to form the mural nodules. The appearances can then be very like a radicular cyst and the histopathology is not diagnostic. Therefore, the main reason for submitting the surgical specimen for examination is to exclude an unexpected diagnosis such as odontogenic keratocyst or ameloblastoma. These alternatives have characteristic histological appearances that are not present here.

The definitive diagnostic criterion is that the epithelial lining and cyst wall join the unerupted tooth at the amelocemental junction. This might be seen only by the surgeon at operation.

Case • 54

A gap between the front teeth

SUMMARY

A 35-year-old man has noticed a gap appearing between two incisor teeth. What is the cause and how can you treat him?

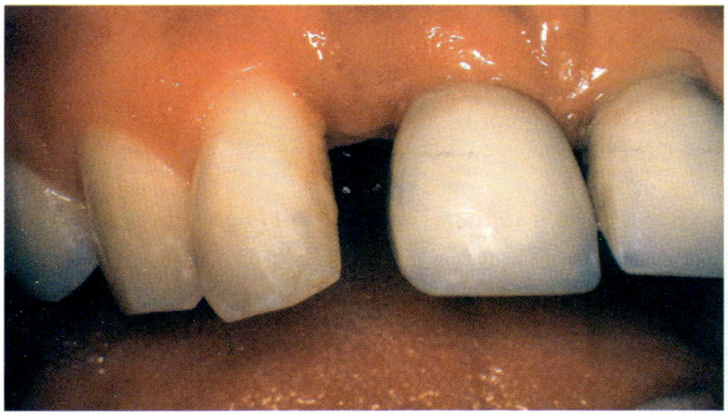

Fig. 54.1 The patient's anterior teeth on presentation.

History

Complaint

The patient is concerned about the gap between the crowned upper right central incisor tooth and lateral incisor.

History of complaint

He noticed the gap about 9 months ago and feels that it has enlarged, that the teeth have drifted forwards and that the crowns are now loose. He has had no symptoms from these or any other teeth.

Medical history

He has mild asthma controlled with an inhaled steroid and salbutamol. He does not smoke.

Dental history

The patient is new to your practice. He attended the dentist regularly, previously going every 6 months but now less frequently. The crowns are approximately 6 years old and were fitted to replace some unsightly fillings.

■ ***The patient's anterior teeth are shown in Figure 54.1. What do you see and how do you interpret the appearances?***

The upper right lateral incisor is rotated mesiolabially and the central incisor distolabially. There is recession on both central and lateral incisors. The gingival tissues have some rounding of the margin and no obvious gingivitis, though there is loss of stippling and contour. The appearances suggest labial drifting as a result of loss of periodontal support. Pocketing is probably present even though it is not obvious.

Examination

Extraoral examination

There is no lymphadenopathy and no temporomandibular joint signs. The two crowns, although prominent and rather light in shade, are under control of the lower lip associated with a competent lip seal. The patient has a broad smile and moderately high lip line.

Intraoral examination

The oral mucosa is healthy, there is no caries and only a few amalgam restorations but there is focal marginal inflammation and plaque lying interdentally. The metal ceramic crowns on the two upper central incisors have good margins but there is 3 mm recession palatally and both teeth are grade 2 mobile. A further diastema is present in the opposing arch between the lower right canine and first premolar (Fig. 54.2) and the adjacent lateral incisor has grade 3 mobility.

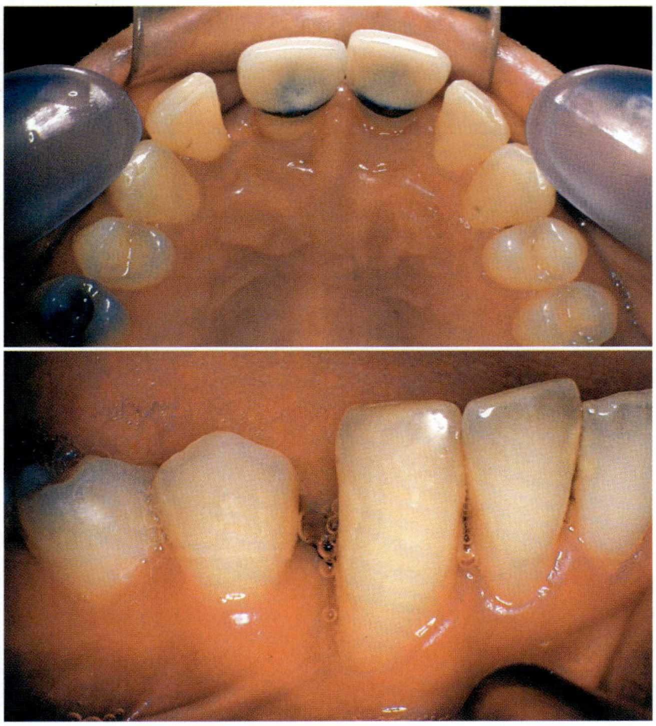

Fig. 54.2 Further views showing the appearances on presentation.

The gap between the upper central incisor and the lateral incisor is at least 3 mm and on gently probing the area there is profuse bleeding. The gingival tissue in that area is red, inflamed and has lost any contouring or stippling. There are deep probing depths on several teeth and mobility. Probing depths and gingival bleeding are shown in Figure 54.3. For details of indices and periodontal examination see Case 38.

The crowns of the upper incisors are rather bulky palatally, probably as a result of inadequate tooth preparation. On closing to intercuspal position the lower teeth occlude on the crowns in premature contact and displace the teeth labially. In both instances the entire tooth is loose, not just the crown.

Investigations

All teeth are vital.

The choice of radiographs for periodontal diagnosis is reviewed in Case 38. Periapical radiographs for this patient are shown in Figure 54.4.

Diagnosis

What is your diagnosis?

The patient has chronic gingivitis and localized periodontitis. The periodontitis has reduced the bony support for the upper and lower right anterior teeth and they have drifted labially. Bone loss extends close to their apices and they would have drifted further had they not been retained by the high lower lip line and competent lips. Recession is also the result of the periodontitis (see Case 4).

However, the pattern of periodontitis is unusual. The patient is only 35 years old but has severe localized attachment loss.

What causes severe localized periodontitis?

The causes are usually local factors affecting the distribution of chronic periodontitis, such as:

- food packing and diastemas
- overhanging and poorly contoured restorations
- subgingival calculus
- destructive habits and self-inflicted injury
- perio-endo lesions
- root fractures
- high fraenal attachment
- localized aggressive periodontitis.

Can any of these explain this patient's pattern of disease?

Primarily the incisors and first molars are involved. The pattern of localized destruction and the shape of the deep infrabony pockets suggests *localized aggressive periodontitis*. This is the currently accepted diagnostic term for this presentation following the International Workshop for the Classification of Periodontal Disease in 1999. Previously this pattern would have been labelled *localized juvenile periodontitis* and in an adult might have been referred to as *postjuvenile periodontitis*. The new name has been chosen to reflect the fact that both adults and adolescents may be affected.

Although the crowns have good margins they are in traumatic occlusion and the jiggling forces on closing would increase the mobility of the teeth.

Treatment

Is this patient suitable for treatment in general practice?

The severity of the complaint and the age of the patient indicate that there is a predisposition to periodontitis and so

							1	2	2								Mobility
	3 2 3	6 8 10	4 2 3	3 2 3	3 2 3	3 5 7	7 6 5	10 2 7	5 2 2	2 2 3	4 2 3	3 2 3	6 3 3	3 2 3		Buccal (Attachment loss)
	4 2 3	7 9 9	3 3 3	3 3 4	3 2 3	3 3 9	9 7 4	8 7 8	5 4 3	3 2 3	3 2 3	3 2 3	7 2 3	2 2 3		Palatal (Attachment loss)
8	7	6	5	4	3	2	1	1	2	3	4	5	6	7	8	Tooth
8	7	6	5	4	3	2	1	1	2	3	4	5	6	7	8	Tooth
	3 2 4	3 3 3	3 2 3	3 2 3	5 5 3	3 2 3	2 2 3	2 3 2	7 3 9	3 3 4	3 2 4	3 2 5	3 2 5	2 2 3		Lingual (Attachment loss)
	3 2 3	3 2 2	2 2 3	3 2 4	7 4 3	4 2 3	2 2 3	3 2 4	6 4 8	2 2 2	3 2 3	3 2 4	4 3 5	3 2 2		Buccal (Attachment loss)
									2							Mobility

Fig. 54.3 The probing depths (in mm) at six points, bleeding sites (ringed in red) and mobility (grade), recorded for each tooth.

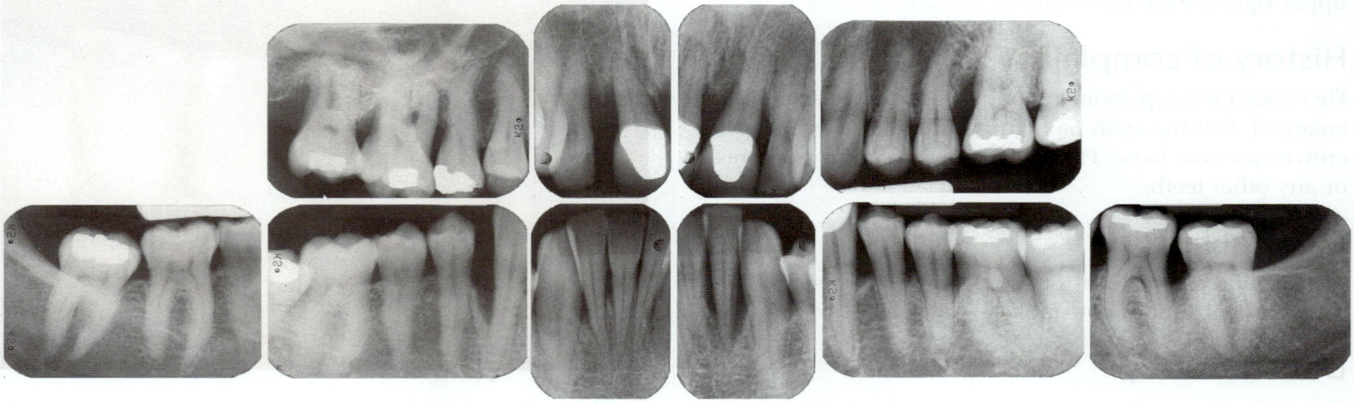

Fig. 54.4 Periapical radiographs of the patient on presentation.

it may progress despite treatment. Initial phases of treatment could be carried out in general dental practice but some teeth already have a very poor prognosis. This is a complex case and unless you have a special interest or are a specialist in periodontology, the case might be best referred for treatment.

What would you include in your letter of referral?

- Patient's name, title, age and address including full postcode.
- Short dental history including pattern of attendance and past treatment needs.
- Relevant medical history.
- Your clinical findings including any special test results or study models you have.
- Anything else that you feel is relevant or will save time or a misunderstanding at the time of consultation.
- Whether you are referring for advice, a single aspect of treatment or comprehensive treatment to be undertaken.
- The radiographs or digital images should be sent with the letter so that repeat radiographs and the consequent radiation dose can be avoided.

What treatment plan would be appropriate?

The prognosis for the three worst affected upper anterior teeth is hopeless as a result of loss of bony support, drifting and poor appearance. Additionally, if the teeth were to be saved, they would require new crowns. The upper right first molar has furcation involvement and bone loss to the apex and must also be extracted. The anterior teeth are symptomless and do not require immediate extraction but should be extracted in the near future to preserve what alveolar bone remains. An immediate replacement denture is the treatment of choice because no definitive restorations can be planned until the periodontitis is brought under control and the longer term prognosis for the other teeth is clear.

In the lower arch the left lateral incisor has bone loss to the apex and probably requires extraction. The long-term prognosis for the lower right canine remains to be determined but, at least initially, it is worth taking a conservative approach and assessing the response to root planing under local analgesia.

The ideal treatment plan would include:

- patient education
- instruction in plaque control, tooth brushing and interdental cleaning
- subgingival scaling
- extraction of both upper central, right upper lateral and lower left lateral incisors and the upper right first molar
- immediate replacement prosthesis
- root planing all severely affected teeth under local analgesia, particularly the lower right canine
- a maintenance phase to assess the response
- continued care of the remaining dentition including caries prevention
- extraction of further teeth as required
- assessment for permanent prosthetic replacement.

The details must be discussed with the patient including the time commitment and cost of treatment. The patient must be given a written treatment plan to consider and agree.

The patient indicates that he would rather attempt to preserve the lower right canine than have it extracted, even though there is no guarantee of success.

What are the options for an immediate replacement prosthesis in the upper arch?

Immediate insertion removable acrylic denture using wrought stainless steel clasps for direct retention. The denture must be kept clear of the gingival margins as much as possible so as not to compromise the periodontal health. The patient already has inadequate oral hygiene and has never experienced a denture before. Once the anterior ridge remoulds, the denture will not fit well in this region and a chairside reline will be necessary. Acrylic has the advantage that further teeth can be added should the periodontitis progress.

Immediate insertion minimal preparation bridge. This is much more complex and success is less predictable. The span is long and the occlusion unfavourable.

Implant solutions. Again, success would be unpredictable with the complex techniques required. There is little residual bone and implants would require autogenous bone grafts or guided regeneration techniques with membranes. Immediate insertion implant techniques have a lower chance of success that delayed placement and would not be recommended.

What are the options for an immediate replacement prosthesis in the lower arch?

Immediate insertion removable acrylic denture. In the lower arch this is a less advantageous option. A simple partial denture will be relatively bulky and could not be designed to avoid gingival margins. It would therefore be much more likely than an upper denture to compromise plaque control and risks being poorly tolerated.

Immediate insertion minimal preparation bridge. This could comprise a cantilever pontic retained on the central incisor or the canine. The canine is the obvious choice because of its more favourable crown:root ratio but you will need maximum wrap-around to maximize retention. The quality of laboratory work will be critical because the restoration cannot be temporized if the fit is not satisfactory; if the immediate replacement does not fit after the extraction, the patient will be left with an unsightly gap. In the immediate insertion option, moisture control and haemostasis will be of critical importance if the bond is to be sufficiently strong. The design of the pontic must be optimized to favour plaque control in view of the patient's susceptibility to periodontitis. Probably the best option if a replacement is required.

No replacement. In the short term it is quite possible that the patient might accept the appearance of the gap. This would be the best option for the periodontal treatment and the situation could be reassessed when the prognosis of the lower teeth becomes clearer.

The patient opts for an upper immediate insertion removable acrylic denture and extraction of the lower left lateral

- These changes may be infections. Enquire whether he knows of any reason why he might be particularly prone to infection.
- Point out that there are several possible reasons for being prone to infection and that it would be worthwhile investigating further to find the cause. Proffer examples such as anaemia, immunosuppression as a result of steroid therapy or viral infection. Patients who know that they are at risk of HIV infection may often use the prompt of a viral infection to discuss the possibility.
- If the patient indicates that they are HIV positive, ask whether you might have their clinic address so that if necessary you may make contact for medical advice relating to dental treatment.
- If the patient gives no indication that they are HIV-positive, they should be referred to their general medical practitioner or to a specialist oral medicine or oral surgery unit for further investigation.

It is inappropriate to ask questions about lifestyle or sexuality. Even pointing out that HIV infection is one potential cause of the oral signs may not be well received in a dental setting. It would be reasonable to check the medical history questionnaire, including whether the patient has recorded coming into contact with someone with HIV infection or AIDS.

If the patient discloses HIV infection you should respond positively and acknowledge that you will respect the confidentiality of this sensitive information.

■ ***What other oral signs may be associated with HIV infection?***

Diseases strongly associated with HIV infection
Candidosis
Erythematous
Pseudomembranous
Hairy leukoplakia
Periodontal disease
Linear gingival erythema
Necrotizing ulcerative gingivitis
Necrotizing ulcerative periodontitis
Kaposi sarcoma
Lymphoma
Lesions less commonly associated with HIV infection
Mycobacterial infections
Melanotic pigmentation
Necrotizing (ulcerative) stomatitis
Cystic salivary gland disease
Thrombocytopenic purpura
Nonspecific ulceration
Viral infections including *Herpes simplex*, *Herpes zoster* and human papilloma virus infection

In addition a wide variety of unusual infections may be found more rarely.

■ ***Which of these signs are specific for HIV infection?***

None. All may be seen in other types of immunosuppression and many can be found in normal patients, albeit very rarely.

Diagnosis

The patient readily informs you that he is HIV-positive and has only recently been diagnosed. He is aware of the Kaposi sarcomas, which were the presenting sign of HIV infection. He has just started on therapy with a combination of three antiretroviral drugs.

The lower left second premolar has a periapical abscess draining via a sinus.

Treatment

Extraction of the tooth is indicated.

■ ***Is it appropriate that the tooth should be taken out in a general practice surgery?***

The General Dental Council (GDC) advocates that patients with HIV should be treated in general practice. Denying this patient treatment on the grounds of having HIV infection alone would put you in breach of the GDC and British Dental Association (BDA) guidelines and might lay you open to a legal case under the Disability Discrimination Act 1995.

However, when a patient has late or symptomatic HIV infection, their medical history may become so complicated that a referral to a specialist dental clinic is appropriate. Referral may not be possible in an emergency situation and treatment, including extraction, may need to be carried out in a general practice setting.

■ ***You will need medical advice. How will you obtain it?***

People with HIV usually attend outpatient hospital clinics. The patient's general medical practitioner may not have the most up-to-date test results but the clinics are usually extremely helpful if telephoned for information. However the patient's right to confidentiality must be respected at all times. Firstly, the patient's permission must be obtained to telephone and secondly, it is enough to explain to the clinic what you propose to do and to request the results without mentioning the patient's disease status or irrelevant information.

■ ***What additional information would you require from the patient's HIV management clinic? Why?***

See Table 58.1.

CD4 T lymphocyte counts and the viral load, a measure of HIV viral RNA in the blood, are often known to the patient or may be given by the clinic. These indicate the level of immunosuppression and infectivity, respectively, but are not directly helpful in predicting whether a patient is likely to bleed or be at risk of infection after an extraction.

■ ***Should the tooth be taken out without this extra information?***

No, in a general practice situation that would be unwise.

■ ***Would any special infection control precautions be required for the extraction?***

No, the patient should be treated normally. It is assumed that all patients have the potential to carry an infectious disease and dental practices should have one level of infection

Table 58.1 Further information needed from HIV clinic

Information	Reason
Is the patient prone to infections?	Antibiotics may be prescribed in immunosuppression when they would not normally be considered necessary, but should be reserved for patients with known susceptibility to infections. This is because the risk of adverse effects such as candidosis and diarrhoea resulting from disturbance of the normal flora is increased in HIV infection.
Neutrophil count	Patients may be neutropenic. Neutrophils provide the first line of defence against infection and if the circulating count is less than $1\text{–}1.5 \times 10^9$/l, postoperative antibiotics may be appropriate.
Platelet count	Bone marrow suppression in late HIV infection causes thrombocytopaenia. The normal number of platelets is $150\text{–}400 \times 10^9$/l, but they do not usually fall to a low enough level to cause bleeding problems until late disease. However, this patient has signs of late disease (Kaposi sarcoma) and the red spots on the palate are probably petechial haemorrhages.
Does the patient have co-infection with hepatitis B or C?	These infections are not uncommon in HIV-positive individuals. Liver damage may cause a coagulation defect that could complicate the extraction. It also disturbs drug metabolism.
The names of the drugs that he is taking	Some of the retroviral drugs have significant interactions with other classes of drugs (see below). The patient is taking efavirenz, tenofovir and emtricitabine.

Table 58.2 Interactions with antiretroviral drugs and drugs commonly used in dental practice

Drug	Antiretroviral drug	Effect
Metronidazole	Atazanavir, darunavir, lopinavir, tipranavir, ritonavir	Antiretroviral formulations may contain alcohol so causing a disulfiram reaction.
Clindamycin	Ritonavir	Increase in clindamycin levels.
Erythromycin	Darunavir, fosamprenavir, indinavir, lopinavir, sauinavir, tipranavir, ritonavir	Large increase in erythromycin levels.
Diazepam, midazolam	Protease inhibitors, non-nucleoside reverse transcriptase inhibitors	Oral administration of many benzodiazepines is contraindicated due to their altered metabolism. This leads to an increase in their sedative effects. Oral midazolam is particularly to be avoided. Note that intravenous midazolam, as used in dentistry, is titrated to the patient's response and this is not contraindicated. However, great care needs to be taken in the titration to avoid oversedation. Proceed slowly. There remains a possibility of prolonged sedation although this does not appear to be a problem in clinical practice. Reversing the sedative effect with flumazenil may later result in re-sedation. The time to discharge should be increased to monitor this.
Lidocaine (lignocaine)	Protease inhibitors, non-nucleoside reverse transcriptase inhibitors	There is a theoretical risk of impaired lidocaine (lignocaine) metabolism. The significance of this is unclear in the dental setting but it would be prudent to avoid approaching the accepted maximum dose.
Fluconazole	Tipranavir, nevirapine	Increase in levels of tipranavir, nevirapine.
Miconazole oral gel	Protease inhibitors, non-nucleoside reverse transcriptase inhibitors	Poorly absorbed but may be ingested with saliva. Potential to raise antiretroviral blood levels if used to excess.

A useful online tool for assessing the potential for interactions is: http://www.hiv-druginteractions.org/

control ('universal precautions') for all patients. Additional precautions are required for surgical procedures and not for routine dentistry.

What antiretroviral treatment might the patient be taking?

There are three main classes of antiretroviral drugs: Nucleoside/Nucleotide (NRTIs), Non-nucleoside Reverse Transcriptase Inhibitors (NNRTIs) and Protease Inhibitors. Recently, there have been developments in entry, integration and maturation inhibitors. These are mainly confined to those patients who have a high degree of resistance to the mainstream antiretroviral drugs.

Chemokine antagonist	maraviroc
Fusion inhibitor	enfuvirtide
NRTIs	abacavir didanosine emtricitabine lamivudine stavudine tenofovir zidovudine
NNRTIs	delaviridine efavirenz etravirine nevirapine
Integrase inhibitor	raltegravir
Protease inhibitors	amprenavir atazanavir darunavir indinavir lopinavir nelfinavir saquinavir tipranavir ritonovir
Maturation inhibitor	bevirimat (unlicensed)

Do these drugs interact with any likely to be prescribed in general dental practice?

Yes, and the interactions may be significant (Table 58.2). See also the notes on prescribing antibiotics in the table above on additional medical information.

■ *The clinic tells you that the patient has a platelet count of 45 × 10⁹/l and a neutrophil count of 1.9 × 10⁹/l. There is no co-infection with viral hepatitis. Will you take out the tooth?*

No. The platelet count is too low. Bleeding problems would be expected if the count is below 50×10^9/l. You arrange with the clinic for the patient to be treated in a specialist centre.

■ *The patient asks to return to your practice, for routine treatment. What is your reaction?*

Yes, he should be able to have routine dental treatment without problems though further extractions might require referral. Block analgesia is possible provided the platelet count remains above 30×10^9/l.

Antiretroviral combination therapy is usually very effective and his oral signs are likely to disappear with time and platelets rise in number. Antiretroviral drugs and HIV-associated salivary gland disease may cause dry mouth and this is a risk factor for caries. People with HIV are also more prone to periodontal attachment loss with gingival recession. The preventive aspects of dental disease will need to be emphasised and if there were evidence of continuing attachment loss or of excessively high levels of decay then a referral to a specialist centre would be appropriate. Otherwise, it would be appropriate to reduce the interval between recalls if there are risk factors for dental disease.

Case 59

Difficulty in opening the mouth

SUMMARY

A 40-year-old Indian man presents to you in your general dental practice with limitation of mouth opening. You must identify the cause and institute appropriate follow up.

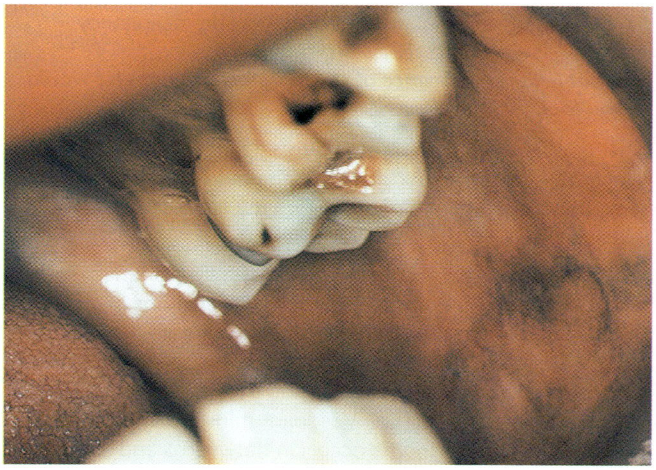

Fig. 59.1 Buccal mucosa, photographed at maximum mouth opening.

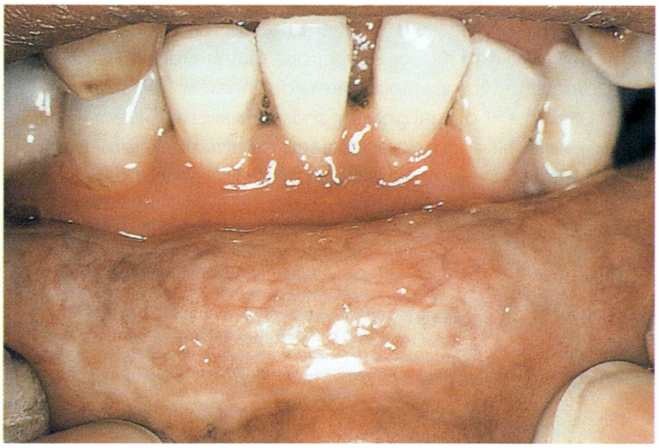

Fig. 59.2 The lower lip mucosa.

History

Complaint

The patient complains of difficulty in eating. He cannot open his mouth widely enough to place a proper mouthful of food inside and also has difficulty chewing.

History of complaint

He has noticed the reduction of his mouth opening over a period of several years but has never sought advice. It has not been painful though he has felt a burning sensation from his oral mucosa on eating during the same period. This varies in intensity.

Medical history

The patient is otherwise fit and well.

■ ***What are the causes of limitation of mouth opening and how may they be classified?***

Limitation of opening is most frequently caused by trismus. By definition, trismus is spasm of the muscles of mastication, though the term is often used loosely when opening is prevented by oedema or inflammation of the muscles or joint. Trismus is usually temporary.

Permanent limitation of opening may be caused by scarring of the soft tissues around the joint or mandible or by fusion of the condyle to the glenoid fossa (ankylosis). The causes may be divided as follows:

Trismus	Inflammation in and around the temporomandibular joint Trauma (fractures and/or soft tissue injury) Tetanus and tetany Temporomandibular joint (myofascial) pain dysfunction syndrome Soft tissue infection around the jaws or joint (usually dental in origin)
Permanent limitation of opening	A. *Extra-articular causes* Fibrosis due to burns or irradiation Oral submucous fibrosis Mucosal scarring (e.g. in epidermolysis bullosa) B. *Intra-articular causes* Congenital ankylosis Traumatic ankylosis Ankylosis following pyogenic arthritis Ankylosis following juvenile arthritis Neoplasms and other causes of enlargement of the condyle

■ ***What questions would you ask?***

The patient should be asked whether there has been trauma or irradiation to the skull, temporomandibular joint or face and whether there have been any episodes of swelling of the face or around the joint. He should also be asked whether he uses betel quid (pan or paan).

The patient gives no history of trauma, irradiation, inflammation or infection. However, he has been a betel quid chewer for more than 20 years.

Examination

Extraoral examination

The patient looks mildly anaemic. There is no facial asymmetry or evidence of scars or inflammation around the joint. No tenderness can be elicited from the muscles of mastication. There are no clicks or crepitus or tenderness associated with the temporomandibular joint and no mandibular deviation on opening the mouth.

■ ***What measurement would you take?***

The maximum voluntary mouth opening. The normal interincisal opening in an adult is approximately 30–40 mm. Measurement will provide a baseline reading against which to judge treatment or progression. It will also indicate the feasibility of dental and other intraoral treatment.

This patient can achieve an interincisal opening of 17 mm.

Intraoral examination

■ ***The oral mucosa is shown in Figures 59.1 and 59.2. What do you see?***

The buccal and soft palate mucosae are paler than normal though some mucosal pigmentation consistent with the patient's skin colour makes this less obvious. When the mouth is opened fully, thin white hard bands run vertically just below the buccal mucosa. These are just visible in the picture and are much more readily felt as hard ridges. Some of the less pale areas are red and atrophic.

The same changes are found on the labial mucosa where bands of hard pale scar-like tissue are visible below the epithelium when the lip is everted. The gingival mucosa has lost its stippled appearance and there is oedema and rounding of the gingival contour consistent with gingivitis or periodontitis. There is some dark red/brown betel quid stain on the teeth.

If you were able to examine the patient you would find that he also has some reduction in mobility of the tongue and cannot protrude it very far. Most of the mucosa feels firm.

Diagnosis

■ ***What is your diagnosis?***

The presentation and features are characteristic of oral submucous fibrosis. There has been gradual limitation of mouth opening and restriction of tongue movements in a betel quid user who shows typical mucosal blanching and fibrosis as bands down the buccal mucosa. None of the alternative causes would produce these signs and symptoms.

■ ***What other features of oral submucous fibrosis might be seen?***

In the early stages some patients complain of vesiculation of the mucosa. In severe cases with extensive tongue involvement the filiform papillae are lost.

■ ***What is betel quid chewing?***

A habit practised by many people in the Indian subcontinent, much of south-east Asia and some parts of Africa. The basic quid comprises pieces or paste of areca nut and slaked lime, wrapped and tied into a packet in a vine leaf. A variety of other components is usually added; the combination varies between regions, but tobacco is almost always included together with flavouring agents such as cinnamon, cloves and ginger. The areca nut contains alkaloids which have a psychoactive effect and make the habit addictive. The quid is not chewed continuously but placed in the buccal sulcus and occasionally chewed. Many users have a quid in their mouth all day and some sleep with a quid. It has been estimated that 10% of the world's population use betel quid and chewing is a major health problem in many countries.

■ ***What are the possible effects of betel quid chewing?***

- Oral submucous fibrosis
- Oral and pharyngeal squamous cell carcinoma
- Periodontitis, recession and root erosion at the site of use
- Tooth staining
- Decreased taste sensation
- Possible worsening of asthma
- Possible association with diabetes and malignancy.

■ ***What is the significance of the diagnosis? What else would you look for?***

Oral submucous fibrosis is a premalignant condition. Tobacco and other carcinogenic agents in the quid make quid chewing one of the highest known risk factors for oral carcinoma.

The patient's oral mucosa must be carefully examined for carcinoma and premalignant lesions. The features of early carcinoma and potentially malignant lesions are discussed in Case 46. Approximately one-third of patients with submucous fibrosis have oral white patches and dysplasia is present in the mucosa of up to 16%. Malignant transformation to squamous cell carcinoma occurs in between 5 and 8% of cases.

The second significant feature is the restricted opening. This is often progressive and responds poorly to treatment. In the late stages of disease the patient may be unable to open the mouth at all and incisor extractions may be required to allow feeding. Limited opening is a major handicap for diagnosis and treatment of malignancy and premalignant lesions. It makes examination, detection and treatment extremely difficult and the prognosis for oral carcinoma in a patient with submucous fibrosis is very poor, mostly as a result of late diagnosis.

Investigations

■ ***What investigations are required? Explain why.***

Biopsy is required to assess dysplasia. If there are lesions suspicious of malignancy, red or white patches or areas of otherwise abnormal mucosa they should be sampled for

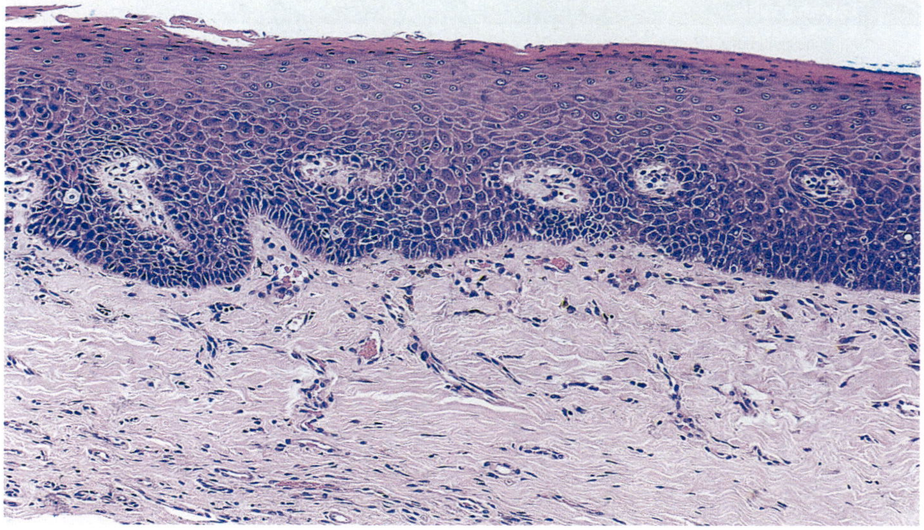

a

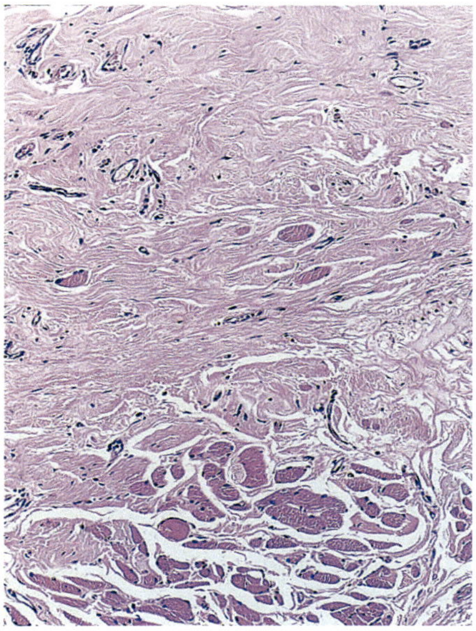

b

Fig. 59.3 Biopsy from the quid site: **a,** buccal mucosa; **b,** underlying tissue.

microscopy. More than one biopsy may be required. If no particular part of the mucosa is suspect, a sample should be taken from the area where the quid is held in the mouth.

The biopsy will probably also provide evidence to support the diagnosis of oral submucous fibrosis. However, in such a typical case biopsy for this purpose alone would not be justified. It might be considered in an early case where the diagnosis is in doubt.

■ ***Would you perform this patient's biopsy in a general practice setting?***

No. This patient is at high risk of developing an oral carcinoma and the biopsy and further recall should be carried out in a specialist centre. Further discussion about when to biopsy potentially dysplastic mucosa will be found in Case 45.

■ ***A biopsy from the quid site is shown in Figure 59.3. What do you see and how do you interpret the findings?***

The mucosa is covered by epithelium which is atrophic and parakeratinized. The thickness of the normal buccal mucosa is about twice the thickness from the surface to the dermal papillae in this specimen. It is normally nonkeratinized except for a thin layer near the occlusal line. The epithelium is largely well organized and stratification and maturation are not particularly disordered; the epithelial layers are easily differentiated. There is an expanded basaloid cell layer comprising rather disorganized small and darkly staining cells which show anisonucleosis (nuclei of different sizes) and irregularly shaped, often angular, nuclei. Towards the centre of the epithelium there is a cluster of prickle cells between two dermal papillae showing early and single cell keratinization. These features amount to mild dysplasia. Below the epithelium there is even fibrosis of the connective tissue and scattered lymphocytes.

The deeper tissue shows the fibrosis of the connective tissue more prominently. All the tissue between the epithelium and underlying muscle is replaced by relatively acellular dense fibrous tissue. The superficial muscle is atrophic and is being replaced by fibrous tissue. Occasional residual muscle fibres lie in the fibrosis. This deeper tissue is uninflamed.

The fibrosis involving deep muscle is consistent with the diagnosis of submucous fibrosis and the overlying epithelium shows mild dysplasia.

Treatment

■ ***What questions would you ask the patient about his betel quid habit?***

You need to know whether the patient includes tobacco in his quid, how many he uses each day and whether he sleeps with one in place. In addition you should check other smoking habits, because most quid users smoke as well, and some smoke traditional coarse unfiltered Indian cigarettes

Table 59.1 Treatment options

Option	Potential value
Habit intervention	Although areca nut is the main aetiological factor for oral submucous fibrosis, there are a number of other carcinogens. Therefore, cessation of the habit rather than altering the composition of the quid should be the aim. As a partial measure, discouraging tobacco in the quid would be valuable. This will reduce the chances of developing malignancy but limitation of opening may still worsen. Cessation is best but there would still be a risk of malignant transformation.
Regular review	The only reliable method for detecting dysplasia and early malignant transformation. Repeated biopsy may be required.
Muscle-stretching exercises	These appear to give good results in some patients. To be effective the muscle stretching must be frequent and prolonged. Bite wedges or a screw appliance may help produce the forcible opening required. Effective exercises are painful and patients must be highly motivated.
Intralesional steroids	These have been widely used, but the results are not encouraging in most patients and any benefit may not be maintained.
Surgical treatment	Occasionally used as a last resort. The fibrosis extends deeply into muscle and surgical excision of the scar tissue is rarely possible. Postoperative scarring replaces the original fibrosis and surgery is usually followed by relapse.
Nutritional supplementation	Many patients are deficient in iron and vitamins. Dietary supplementation with these and carotenes or vitamin A may be helpful in reducing progression but the effect is not marked.
Experimental methods	The lack of effective treatments has led to trials of many compounds, including interferon-gamma, but none has proved consistently useful.

consisting of a rolled uncut tobacco leaf *(bidi or beedi)*. Some users also practise a form of snuff dipping, placing ground quid constituents *(pan masala)* loose in the sulcus.

■ ***What are the available treatments or treatment options? What is the potential value of each?***

See Table 59.1.

No treatment regime is satisfactory and the aim is maintenance and prevention of complications. If patients are committed to opening exercises, they may be spared the worst effects of limited opening. However, if disease is advanced at diagnosis, progressive limitation is likely. The best results are seen in those who have relatively localized disease at diagnosis, perhaps limited to the site of quid placement.

The aims are best achieved by helping the patient to cease the habit and by detecting malignancy or dysplasia as early as possible. If suspicious lesions develop they may be treated using the same modalities of treatment as in other patients, trismus allowing. All abnormal mucosa must be regarded with the utmost suspicion and a biopsy performed.

■ ***What is the role of the general dental practitioner in such a case?***

Dental practitioners have an important role in the prevention of betel quid chewing just as in the prevention of smoking, primarily to prevent oral carcinoma rather than submucous fibrosis (a rarer effect of betel quid chewing). As noted above, most chewers also smoke and health workers need to address both tobacco habits.

The majority of those who regularly chew betel quid are from low socioeconomic groups and, at least in the UK, are often poorly informed of the health risks. Health education for chewers is most important and may need to be extended to other family members. The difficulty of convincing patients to give up should not be underestimated. The habit is addictive and is embedded in the cultural, social and religious customs of many ethnic groups. Many justify chewing on the basis of supposed health benefits that are accepted in their culture. The general dental practitioner can help the specialist centre to modify the risk behaviour, reinforcing the message to remove tobacco from the quid and encouraging patients to reduce the areca content and chew less frequently. The importance of prompt referral and regular mucosal examination for dysplastic lesions and carcinoma has already been stressed.

In the small number of patients who develop submucous fibrosis, dental treatment involves difficult choices and would be best carried out in a specialist centre. Initially treatment is not a problem and could be readily performed in general practice. However, some restorative treatment will be rendered impossible as restriction of opening progresses, and a thorough regime of effective preventive treatment must be adopted as soon as possible. Extraction of teeth with even small carious lesions or moderate periodontitis may become necessary, though it should be left until the last possible moment. It is still possible to restore and clean some teeth in late disease, though both activities are compromised. Every effort should be made to retain a stable occlusion to prevent progression to permanent overclosure.

■ ***This patient has a typical but late presentation. What are the earliest features?***

The earliest features are relatively subtle and nonspecific. There is typically burning of the mucosa and roughness, sometimes described as tiny vesicles. All or part of the lining mucosa may be affected and these symptoms associated with betel quid use should be regarded with the highest suspicion.

Case 60

Toothwear

SUMMARY

A 35-year-old policeman presents having noticed that his anterior teeth are becoming shorter. Identify the cause and outline options for management.

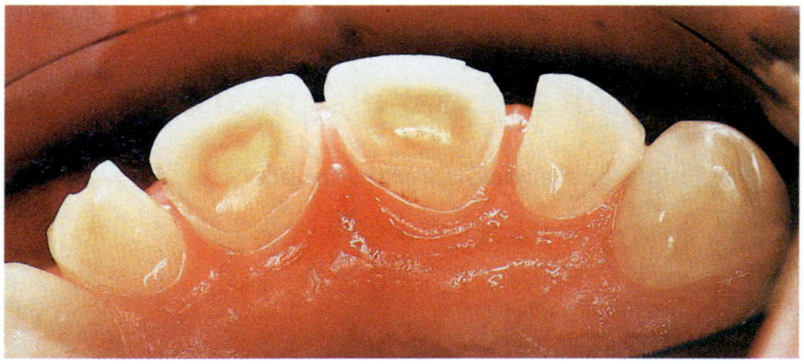

Fig. 60.1 Palatal view of the upper anterior teeth.

History

Complaint

The patient has become increasingly aware of his shortening front teeth. He is not greatly concerned about the appearance but feels that continued wear will eventually destroy the teeth completely.

History of complaint

He has noticed that his teeth have become worse over the last 3–5 years but cannot remember when he first noticed the signs. The patient has always attended a dentist regularly and has relatively few, small restorations and good oral hygiene.

Medical history

The patient is generally fit and well. He drinks about 10–20 units of alcohol each week.

Examination

Extraoral examination

The patient is a fit-looking man and slightly overweight. No submandibular or cervical lymph nodes are palpable. The temporomandibular joints appear normal and there is no evidence of hypertrophy of the masseter muscles.

Intraoral examination

■ ***The appearance of the anterior teeth is shown in Figure 60.1. What do you see?***

The palatal surfaces and incisal edges of the upper incisor teeth are worn. The wear involves the enamel and dentine but not the pulp. The palatal surfaces of the teeth appear smooth and unstained. The incisal edges are rough, small chips of unsupported labial enamel having fractured away.

If you were able to examine the patient, you would find that some of the upper and lower anterior teeth do not contact each other in the retruded contact and the intercuspal positions. All other teeth appear normal and the palatal surfaces of the upper posterior teeth are unaffected.

■ ***What does this appearance signify?***

This is toothwear, the loss of dental tissues through the processes of erosion, attrition and abrasion. Although each process may act alone, significant toothwear is usually the result of a combination of these processes and erosion is often dominant.

The smooth surfaces suggest that erosion is a factor in this case and the distribution of enamel loss suggests that regurgitation of gastric acid may be the cause. Dietary acids are usually associated with erosion on the buccal or labial surfaces of the upper anterior teeth but if the patient rinses or swills acidic drinks in the palatal vault prior to swallowing, the pattern of erosion is very similar to that seen when gastric acid is regurgitated. Either source of acid might be the cause.

■ ***Define erosion, abrasion and attrition.***

Erosion is the chemical dissolution of teeth by acids.

Attrition is the wear of tooth against tooth. Mild degrees of attrition are normal.

Abrasion is the wear of teeth by physical means other than the teeth.

Differential diagnosis

■ ***What is your differential diagnosis for this patient?***

1. Dental erosion caused by gastric acid combined with attrition
2. Dental erosion caused by dietary acids combined with attrition
3. Attrition alone
4. Industrial erosion.

■ ***Which of these causes would you exclude? Explain why.***

Attrition as a single factor is most unlikely to be the cause, because surfaces of the teeth do not contact in the intercuspal or retruded contact position. It would also be most unlikely that occlusal wear could affect the whole of the palatal surfaces of all incisors equally. Attrition is often associated with marked bruxism but there is no evidence of masseteric hypertrophy on examination.

Industrial erosion is now very uncommon. Acid present in the air of the working environment causes dental erosion but improvements in health and safety at work have almost eradicated this condition. Car battery acid workers used to suffer erosion, particularly affecting the buccal surfaces of the teeth. The patient's profession as policeman means he is unlikely to be exposed to an acidic environment though some patients may be exposed to volatile acids through hobby activities.

■ ***What specific questions would you ask? Explain why.***

Toothwear is often multifactorial and the patient must be questioned about all causes.

Do you suffer acid regurgitation from the stomach? Regurgitation of stomach acid can be noticed by the patient because of the taste. However, it may be unnoticed if it happens at night, and may or may not be associated with symptoms of gastric disease. Occasional mild reflux into the oesophagus or pharynx is relatively common.

What is your alcohol intake and what is the pattern of consumption? The patient has indicated an intake of 10–20 units of alcohol each week. Patients often under-represent their intake and it would be worth checking this with the patient. Many alcoholic drinks are acid, contributing to dietary acid (below), and binge patterns of drinking are often associated with vomiting. The possibility of a history of chronic alcoholism should be considered.

Do you have a high consumption of acidic foods or drinks? This is a common cause of dental erosion. The intake of both acid foods and drinks must be ascertained, together with the way in which they are consumed.

Do you grind or clench your teeth during the day or at night? Bruxism or other parafunctional habits are common causes of increased wear.

Have you ever suffered from an eating disorder such as anorexia or bulimia nervosa? These causes of gastric regurgitation need to be excluded. Such eating disorders are uncommon in males but their incidence is increasing.

In response to your questioning, the patient denies frequent acid intake, vomiting or bruxism. However, he indicates that he does suffer some acid regurgitation associated with his dyspepsia (heartburn) and that alcohol is sometimes associated with the attacks. He has had heartburn and regurgitation for 20 years but is not taking any regular medication to relieve the symptoms. He had not considered this significant enough to mention on his medical history questionnaire.

Investigations

■ ***What investigations would you perform?***

A thorough dietary record should be taken by the patient to determine the true consumption of acidic foods and drinks. Diet analysis sheets need to be filled in for 4 or more days, including a weekend, and it is emphasized that the patient should write down all the foods and drinks taken over that time, including between-meal snacks. Both frequency and amount need to be noted and the patient should be specifically told to note suspect foods such as carbonated drinks, citrus fruits and drinks, vinegar and white wine, to ensure that none is missed.

Study casts of the patient's teeth should be taken. These will provide a baseline record against which progression of erosion can be detected. Tests of tooth vitality and intraoral radiographs might be taken if it is suspected that the wear has compromised the vitality of the pulp in any teeth.

Diet analysis confirms the patient's statement that he has a low consumption of acidic food and drink. This excludes dietary acid as a cause, leaving gastric acid as the only other source. Regurgitation erosion occurs when the stomach juice passes from the stomach into the mouth. The pH of stomach juice is around 1 or 2, and if regurgitation occurs frequently the damage to teeth can be catastrophic.

Further differential diagnosis

■ ***How might gastric acid enter the mouth?***

1. Gastro-oesophageal reflux disease
2. Eating disorders
3. Chronic alcoholism
4. Rumination.

■ ***What features of these conditions might aid definitive diagnosis?***

Gastro-oesophageal reflux disease is usually associated with heartburn (intermittent retrosternal pain radiating along the oesophagus, worsened by lying down or a recent large meal), or epigastric pain (centred over the xiphisternum). When symptoms are related to meals, the term dyspepsia is sometimes used. In most patients symptoms of gastro-oesophageal reflux are self-limiting and little or no acid enters the mouth. In others complete regurgitation into the mouth is frequent, pain becomes persistent and patients seek medical advice. A small proportion of patients treat their pain with over-the-counter antacids and are unaware of the potential for damage to their teeth or oesophagus. A history of taking antacid preparations is a useful indicator for the activity of gastro-oesophageal reflux disease, and this patient has already indicated that he has noticed some regurgitation. This is the most likely cause.

Eating disorders are a cause of erosion in younger patients. Both anorexia nervosa and bulimia nervosa tend to affect young, adolescent, intelligent females with a history of overprotective parents. Anorexia is self-destructive. Sufferers lose body weight by starving themselves and/or vomiting to lose weight in an attempt to improve their body self-image. A small proportion of patients with severe anorexia die from the disorder. Unlike anorectics, bulimic patients usually have a stable body weight. They eat and drink in binges and vomit to control their body weight. There may be an accompanying history of drug and alcohol abuse.

Alcoholism. As noted above, alcoholism is associated with dental erosion, either through vomiting or the low pH of some alcoholic drinks.

Rumination is an unusual practice, being the habitual chewing of food, swallowing and then regurgitating it mixed with stomach acid to be chewed and swallowed again. It is considered rare but there is no accurate information on its prevalence and it is thought to affect young, healthy and mainly professional people. If the habit is continued it can cause significant damage to teeth.

The patient gives a clear history of regular heartburn and symptomatic regurgitation. He denies rumination and alcoholism and there is no suggestion of an eating disorder, an unlikely possibility in this age group.

Diagnosis

■ ***What is your diagnosis?***

The diagnosis is toothwear caused primarily by erosion. The cause of the erosion is gastric acid reflux secondary to gastro-oesophageal reflux disease.

Treatment

■ ***How will you manage the patient?***

The patient should be referred to a gastroenterologist or his general medical practitioner for further investigation of his symptoms. Reflux may be caused by a reduction in pressure around the lower oesophageal sphincter (as for instance in hiatus hernia) or abnormal oesophageal motility. Referral is necessary to detect such associated conditions and, if symptoms merit, to consider treatment with drugs which block acid secretion.

A conservative approach should be taken to treatment of the erosion. No immediate treatment is required if the erosion is relatively minor, as the patient is happy with the appearance of the teeth. If the cause is identified and treated, erosion will cease or progress more slowly. Study models taken at yearly intervals may be compared to those taken at the initial visit to assess progression, and if the toothwear progresses, restorations may be considered.

In the early stages of erosion provisional plastic restorations will protect the palatal surfaces from further damage. However the short lifespan of such restorations commits the patient to further treatment. Alternatively palatal veneers of porcelain, composite or metal provide a longer term restoration if there is sufficient space occlusally for the restorations.

■ ***What precautions must be taken to prevent iatrogenic damage when restoring worn teeth?***

Accurate diagnosis is essential. If attrition rather than erosion is diagnosed, occlusal splints might be prescribed. These would worsen erosion caused by gastric regurgitation because acid would be trapped beneath the splint away from the pH-neutralizing effect of saliva. There is also the potential for unglazed or unpolished porcelain to wear the enamel of the opposing teeth. This might become significant if there is an element of attrition causing the wear or if the restoration were allowed to occlude against dentine.

Case • 61

Worn front teeth

SUMMARY

A 60-year-old man presents at your general dental practice saying that his teeth have worn down. What is the cause and how should he be managed?

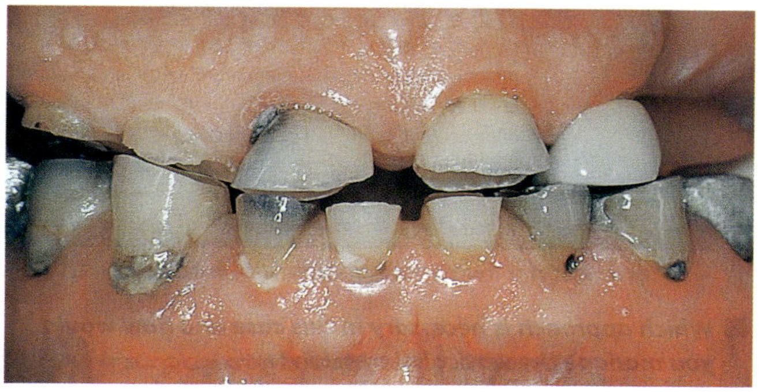

Fig. 61.1 The patient's appearance at presentation.

History

Complaint

The patient is unhappy about his short and discoloured upper anterior teeth. He is also finding that he has difficulty eating. The appearance of his teeth has recently become more important to him because he has taken a job in which he deals with the public. He wishes primarily to improve his appearance and appears to be sufficiently motivated to complete a course of complex dental treatment.

History of complaint

The patient has only recently started to attend his dentist regularly, after a 10-year period without treatment. Most of his posterior teeth were extracted before the age of 45 and he has worn his present upper partial denture for at least 12 years.

Examination

Extraoral examination

No submandibular or cervical lymph nodes are palpable, the temporomandibular joints appear normal and there is no tenderness around the muscles of mastication. Despite the anterior toothwear there is no evidence of loss of occlusal vertical dimension.

Intraoral examination

The oral mucosa is healthy. In the mandible all teeth between the left and right second premolars are present but in the maxilla there are only five anterior teeth remaining. The appearances are shown in Figure 61.1

Wear of the incisal edges of upper and lower anterior teeth has produced short clinical crowns and the upper right lateral incisor and canine are worn almost to gingival level. There are deposits of plaque around the cervical margins of his teeth and a number of teeth have cervical caries. Despite the plaque, there is only occasional interdental bleeding on probing and no significant increase in pocket depths. The upper ridges are not extensively resorbed and are broad and well defined. When asked to bite his teeth together the patient adopts the forward mandibular posture shown in Figure 61.1.

Both lower lateral incisors and the lower left canine and first premolar appear discoloured. Only the lower left second premolar fails to respond to an electronic test of vitality.

The patient produces his acrylic upper partial denture from his pocket. It is poorly retentive and of indifferent fit.

■ ***What is your differential diagnosis? What features suggest each possibility?***

The patient is suffering toothwear. This is usually caused by a combination of three basic underlying processes: erosion, attrition and abrasion. In this case it seems likely that the cause is predominantly erosion with attrition as a secondary factor.

Aetiological factor	Features
Erosion	Erosion is usually caused by excessive dietary acid or regurgitation. Both possibilities must be excluded by careful questioning and dietary analysis (see also Case 60). The appearance of the wear facets suggests erosion as the major cause. Although the teeth interdigitate on incisal enamel, the dentine has been lost from an area which is not in contact with the opposing teeth.
Attrition	Attrition is usually caused by occlusal wear and a minor degree is normal. Bruxism and other parafunctional habits may have caused increased attrition. There is no evidence of masticatory muscle tenderness or hypertrophy to suggest that such habits contribute.
Abrasion	Abrasion of the teeth is wear by an external agent and is seen when a coarse diet is eaten, as in developing countries, or as a result of toothbrush abrasion.There is nothing to suggest an unusual diet in this case, though the possibility should be excluded by questioning. The pattern is not consistent with a primarily abrasive process.

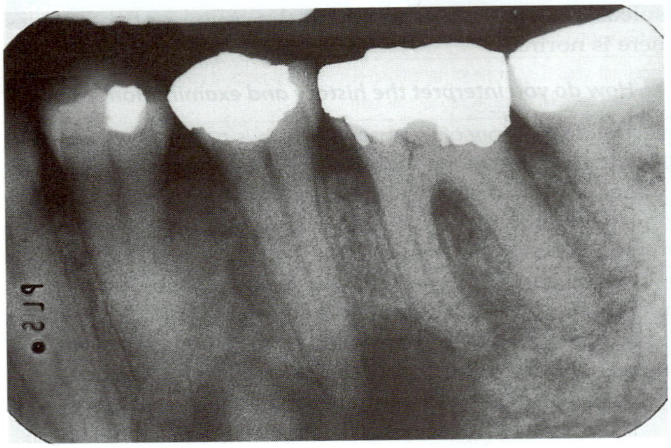

Fig. 62.1 Periapical of both lower premolars and first molar.

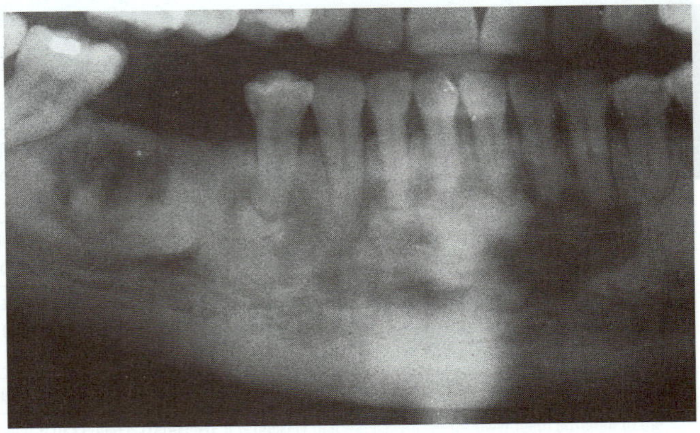

Fig. 62.2 Section from the dental panoramic radiograph.

- No radiographic evidence of dental caries.
- Early bifurcation bone loss associated with the first molar.
- A radiolucent area centred on the apex of second premolar which appears to extend to involve the mesial root of the first molar.
- Loss of lamina dura around the apex of the root of the second premolar and the first molar mesial root.
- An irregular but relatively well-defined radiopaque zone distal to the first premolar root.

What would you do next and why?

Further radiographic views are required. The radiograph has not aided diagnosis of the dental pain as no unsuspected cause for the pulpitis has been identified. However it has revealed an apical radiolucency on the second premolar and first molar which is not compatible with an uncomplicated periapical granuloma, infection or cyst. The presence of an apical radiolucency on the second premolar is also incompatible with the history and examination which indicate that this tooth is vital.

The presence of both radiopacity and radiolucency requires consideration of a wider differential diagnosis which would include fibro-osseous and cemento-osseous lesions, odontogenic tumours and a variety of bone disorders. The margins of the radiolucent lesion are not visible in the film and need to be defined before a more accurate differential diagnosis can be proposed. Because some fibro-cemento-osseous lesions may be bilateral, appropriate views would be a dental panoramic radiograph or right and left oblique laterals. These will also allow all the teeth and their supporting structures to be assessed because the patient is being seen in the practice for the first time. Bitewings to assess caries would also be appropriate in a new patient with several heavily restored teeth if there is clinical suspicion of caries.

Part of the dental panoramic radiograph is shown in Figure 62.2. What do you see?

The additional radiograph shows several features including:

- The lower right second premolar and first molar are absent, presumed extracted.
- A small occlusal restoration in the lower left second molar which has tipped slightly mesially.
- An extensive lesion of mixed radiodensity involving the central body of the mandible from the mesial root of the second molar across the midline to join that shown previously in the left.
- The lesion appears to be composed of several radiolucencies often with a central opacity centred on the root apices.
- There is little or no expansion of the bone despite the extensive lesion.
- The lesion has not displaced teeth or inferior dental nerve canal.
- There are no lesions in the maxilla (not seen in figure).

Diagnosis

What are the causes of a mixed radiolucency such as this in the jaws?

- Osseous dysplasias (Cemento-osseous dysplasias)
  - — periapical
  - — focal
  - — florid
- Chronic osteomyelitis
- Paget's disease of bone
- Fibrous dysplasia
- Metastatic malignancy.

What is the most likely diagnosis? Explain why.

One of the osseous dysplasias (cemento-osseous dysplasias) is the most likely cause of the patient's jaw lesions. The diagnosis may be made on the radiographic appearances alone. No other condition produces multiple lesions centred on the apices of the teeth, each with a central radiopacity and a variable and poorly defined radiolucent rim. As disease progresses this pattern may become less distinct, but it is clearly visible in several of this patient's lesions. This patient has the florid form of the disease in which one or more quadrants are affected. The periapical form affects a few teeth, usually the lower incisors, and the focal form gives rise to one large lesion but all are part of a spectrum of disease severity. The diagnosis is supported by the patient's race, these conditions being more prevalent in those of African or mongoloid racial stock. The lesion(s) are normally asymptomatic.

What diagnoses have you excluded? Explain why.

Chronic osteomyelitis produces a patchy mixed radiolucency but would give symptoms of dull boring central bone pain quite distinct from those reported. Sinuses or other signs of infection would probably be present. However, this diagnosis should not be completely excluded without a further consideration, because the sclerotic bone of fibro-osseous and cemento-osseous lesions such as florid osseous dysplasia is prone to infection, particularly dental infection, and in the past the condition was thought to be a form of osteomyelitis. A biopsy to confirm the presumed diagnosis is contraindicated because of the risk of initiating osteomyelitis.

Paget's disease of bone may be confidently excluded because it almost never affects the mandible without producing obvious lesions, signs and symptoms in other bones. If this were Paget's disease the maxilla would usually be more severely affected. Paget's disease affects predominantly elderly Caucasians.

Fibrous dysplasia might be considered as a cause of patchy and poorly defined radiolucency but presents with expansion of the jaw, usually the maxilla, during the first or second decade.

Metastatic malignancy might also be considered as a further cause. Most cancers cause purely radiolucent lesions but some, notably prostate and breast, may cause bony sclerosis and 'sun-ray' radiopacity. However the site is usually near the angle of the mandible, and the radiological appearances are sufficiently characteristic of florid osseous dysplasia to exclude this sinister diagnosis.

How might you confirm the diagnosis without biopsy?

Any previous radiographs should be reviewed to determine whether the lesion has been present and slowly progressing for several years. This would confirm the diagnosis.

A previous dental practitioner was contacted and provided the radiograph seen in Figure 62.3, which had been taken 11 years previously.

The radiograph shows the lower left quadrant. The lower left second premolar and first molar contain smaller restorations than at present and there is probable caries in the second premolar. However the first premolar appears to contain the same restoration as at present, and at its apex there is a lesion typical of early osseous dysplasia comprising a radiolucency with a central opacity at the root apex. This early stage of the lesion provides conclusive evidence for the proposed diagnosis.

What would you do about the patient's pain?

The causative tooth must be properly identified and the electric pulp test has suggested that the first molar is to blame. The increased sensitivity on electric and cold pulp testing may be accounted for by pulpitis or small vital pulp remnants in an otherwise nonvital pulp.

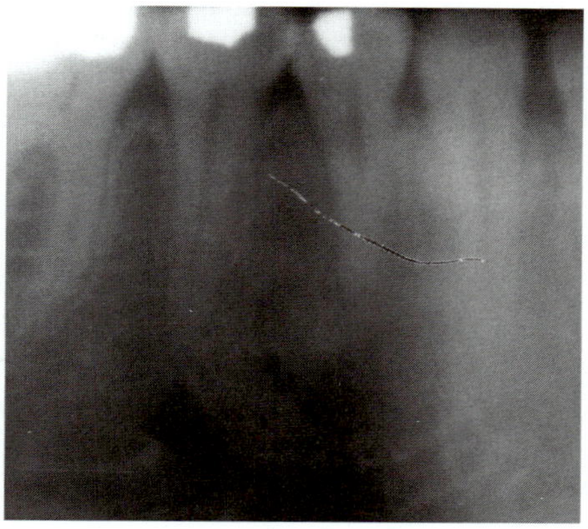

Fig. 62.3 Section from the dental panoramic tomograph taken 11 years previously.

When pulp tests fail to identify a definite cause, the most effective method is to perform a test cavity without local analgesia in the most likely tooth. This is not possible (or usually required) in a tooth with acute pulpitis, but works well for chronic low grade pain, if a pulp is completely or partially viable or when a patient's response to testing cannot be relied upon.

Alternatively, a diagnostic local analgesic injection may be given to abolish the pain, but this is not usually useful for first molars where a block is required for effective analgesia. Once the anaesthetic is given no further pulp tests are possible at that visit.

When a test cavity was performed the first molar was found to be nonvital, with vital pulp in one canal only. Either root canal treatment or extraction are required.

What about the apical radiolucency on the second premolar?

This is another early lesion of cemento-osseous dysplasia. Some years later radiographs revealed that the lesion had developed a zone of radiopacity centrally.

Does florid osseous dysplasia have any significant complications?

Yes. Precautions must be taken to ensure that the patient does not develop osteomyelitis in the sclerotic bone of the mandible. A preventive regime for caries and periodontal disease must be instituted to reduce the chances of future dental infection. The periodontal condition of the first molar is poor and extraction would be the preferred option. Other nonvital teeth should also be extracted if there are reasons to suspect that root canal treatment may not be successful. Antibiotics should be prescribed during the healing period for all extractions involving affected bone. Any surgery in the mandible should be similarly covered and would be best performed in hospital rather than general practice unless the practitioner has appropriate experience.

Case • 63

A child with a swollen face

SUMMARY

A 5-year-old boy has painless bilateral facial swellings. Identify the cause and recommend treatment.

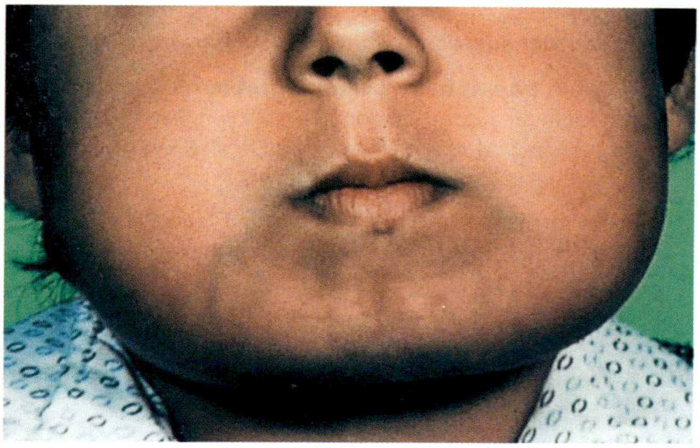

Fig. 63.1 The patient's appearance at presentation.

History

Complaint

The patient is brought by his parents who have noticed that his face has become fat. They are concerned about his appearance and say that he is being teased and bullied at school.

History of complaint

His parents say that the patient has had a chubby face since he was a toddler but that the swelling has become more noticeable over the last 2 years. He is in no pain.

Medical history

He is otherwise fit and well, has had all recommended immunizations and amongst the childhood illnesses has suffered only chicken pox. His medical practitioner has given him a general examination and found no systemic illness but has referred him to you for a further opinion.

Examination

Extraoral examination

The appearance of the child is shown in Figure 63.1. He appears healthy but has obvious bilateral enlargement of the side of the face. The temporomandibular joints appear normal on palpation. Some upper deep cervical lymph nodes are palpable bilaterally. They are only slightly enlarged, not tender and are freely mobile.

■ ***On the basis of what you know, what types of lesion would you consider?***

From this view alone it is difficult to tell whether the swelling originates in the salivary glands, mandible or soft tissues. Each site would have different possible causes:

Condition	Possible causes
Soft tissue enlargement	Masseteric hypertrophy is possible. Bruxism is common in children though significant masseteric hypertrophy is rare.
Salivary gland enlargement	Rare in children. HIV salivary cystic disease is seen in HIV infection. Mumps can be excluded. Mumps is acute and, in addition, the child would have had mumps vaccine with the rest of the routine childhood vaccinations.
Enlargement of the mandible	A few rare inherited disorders of bone could cause bilateral expansion of the ramus.
A developmental syndrome	Many syndromes have craniofacial signs and this is a possibility which should be borne in mind. There appear to be no associated features.

Intraoral examination

Intraoral examination reveals a minimally restored dentition and healthy oral mucosa. Palpation of the mandibular rami shows that they are the source of the enlargement. There is obvious rounded swelling of the posterior body and ramus of the mandible. The lower right second deciduous molar is missing.

Investigations

■ ***A radiograph is obviously required. Which view(s) would you choose?***

A dental panoramic radiograph is the investigation of choice as an initial view. The whole of the swellings will be visible and the left and right can be easily compared. A posterior–anterior view of the jaws would also be useful, providing a second view at right angles to the ramus in the panoramic view. It would allow mediolateral expansion to be assessed.

■ ***The radiographic appearance is shown in Figure 63.2. What are the radiographic features of the lesions?***

See Table 63.1.

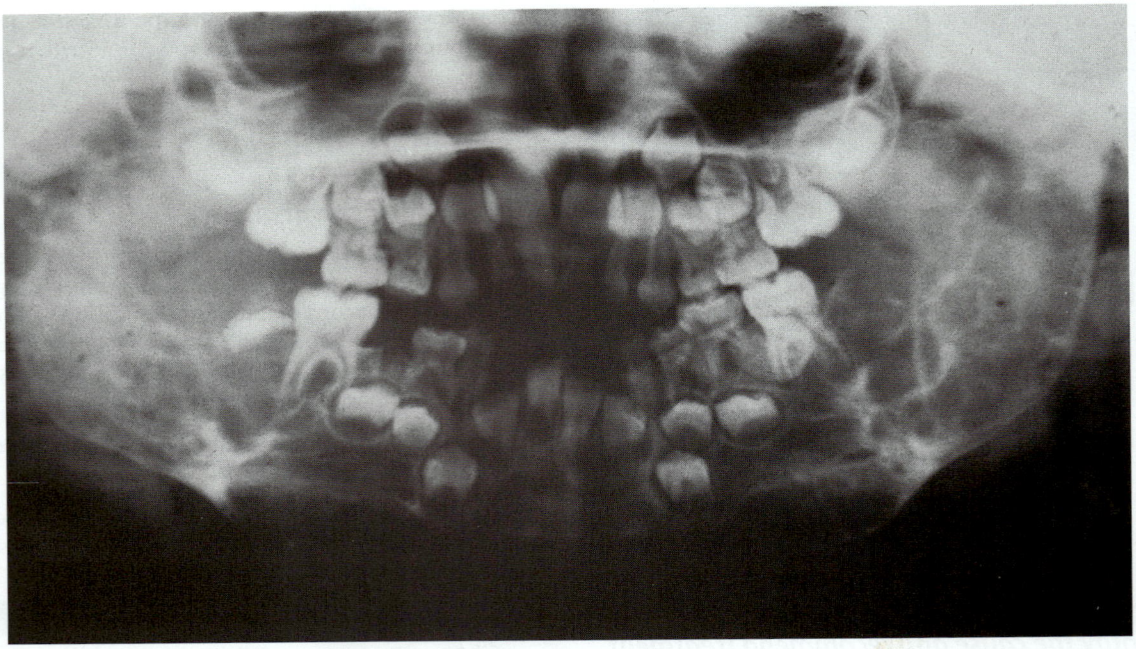

Fig. 63.2 Dental panoramic radiograph.

Table 63.1 Radiographic features

Site	Bilaterally in the posterior body, angle and rami of the mandible.
Size	Relatively large, about 5 × 8 cm.
Shape	Lesions on both sides are multilocular.
Type of outline/edge	Smooth, well defined and well corticated.
Relative radiodensity	Radiolucent with internal radiopaque septa producing a multilocular appearance. There are no dense radiopaque inclusions.
Effects on adjacent structures	Gross displacement of the developing permanent second molars. The lower right second primary molar has been lost, presumably by exfoliation. There has been extensive expansion of the height of the body of the mandible. The condyles are not affected.

Differential diagnosis

■ ***Give a differential diagnosis. Explain which is the most likely cause and why.***

Only a very short differential diagnosis is possible for this case.

Diagnosis	Similarity to present case
Cherubism	Causes bilateral radiolucencies in the mandibular rami and maxilla. Enlargement starts in children before the age of 5 years. The lesions appear multilocular and radiolucent and disrupt the dentition. The radiographic and facial appearances in this case are characteristic.
Other possible causes	There are a few very rare bone diseases and syndromes which may need to be considered if the most likely diagnosis of cherubism cannot be confirmed. Almost all other causes have prominent signs elsewhere in the body and none has been noted in this case.

■ ***What further questions might help confirm your diagnosis?***

Did either parent have a similar problem? Cherubism is inherited in an autosomal dominant fashion. Radiographs of both parents may reveal unsuspected healed lesions and this would aid diagnosis.

Are any brothers or sisters affected? For similar reasons, siblings would be expected to show similar signs.

How was the lower second deciduous molar lost? Cherubism may cause early exfoliation of teeth.

■ ***Would any further radiographs help confirm the diagnosis?***

More detailed radiographic examination with intraoral films would be helpful for the following reasons.

- To demonstrate involvement of the maxilla. More severely affected patients usually have lesions in the maxilla, usually centred on the tuberosity but sometimes extending to distort the orbit. These can easily be missed on extraoral films but, if present, confirm the diagnosis.
- To identify displacement or destruction of teeth. As noted above, cherubism often destroys tooth germs and displaces teeth.

■ ***Is a biopsy required?***

In a classical case of cherubism, the diagnosis may be made with certainty on the basis of family history, clinical and radiographic features. In a new case such as this, or if there were no family history, it would be prudent to confirm that the lesions are histologically compatible with cherubism.

■ ***A biospy specimen was removed from the expanded alveolar ridge. The histological appearances are shown in Figure 63.3. What do you see?***

The lesion is composed of cellular fibrous tissue which appears loose and oedematous with spaces rather than

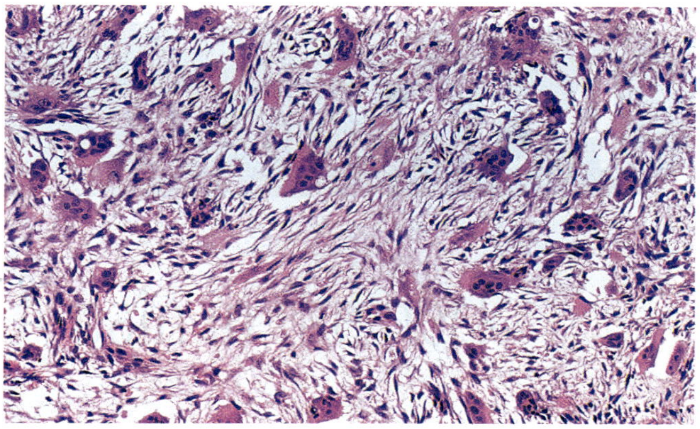

Fig. 63.3 The histological appearance of the biopsy specimen.

dense collagen between the cells. Scattered in the fibrous tissue are multinucleate giant cells. These are relatively small giant cells and have only 4–8 nuclei each.

■ *How do you interpret these appearances? Are they consistent with cherubism?*

Lesions with many giant cells fall into two broad categories, those with granulomas, such as tuberculosis, sarcoidosis and foreign body reactions, and the *giant-cell lesions*. No granulomas are present and these appearances indicate a giant-cell lesion, the causes of which are:

- central giant-cell granuloma
- brown tumour of hyperparathyroidism
- aneurysmal bone cyst
- cherubism.

These conditions cannot be distinguished from one another on histological grounds alone. However, the only one which matches the clinical and radiographic findings is cherubism.

Diagnosis

Taken together, the evidence supports a diagnosis of cherubism and this is a typical case.

Aetiology

■ *What is the cause of cherubism?*

Cherubism is caused by any one of several mutations in the SH3BP2 gene, a regulator of the C-Abl oncogene, a poorly understood signalling molecule involved in regulation of cell division and many other cell functions.

The condition is usually inherited in an autosomal dominant fashion. It would be expected that one parent would be similarly affected. Females are often less severely affected and cases may appear to be sporadic.

Treatment

■ *What treatment would you recommend? What other advice would you give to the parents?*

No treatment is required though the parents and child may need reassurance. The parents can be told that lesions of cherubism usually grow fastest before the age of 5. Although there will be further growth during the next few years, the lesions will stop growing spontaneously and start to regress around the age of puberty. The swelling should have completely resolved by the age of 25 and only radiographic changes will remain into the fourth decade.

Surgical intervention is not usually necessary but may be performed for cosmetic reasons if lesions resolve slowly. Some teeth will be lost through the disease process. The parents should also be warned that future children and siblings are likely to be affected. Genetic counselling would be appropriate.

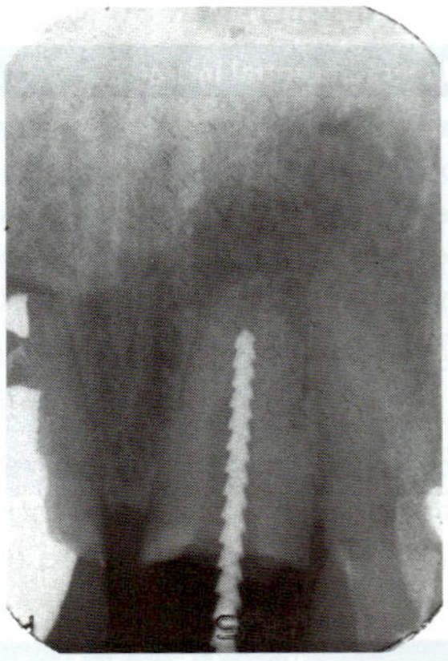

Fig. 65.4 Working length radiograph for the upper left central incisor. The rubber dam is retained on the premolar teeth for better access and no clamp is visible.

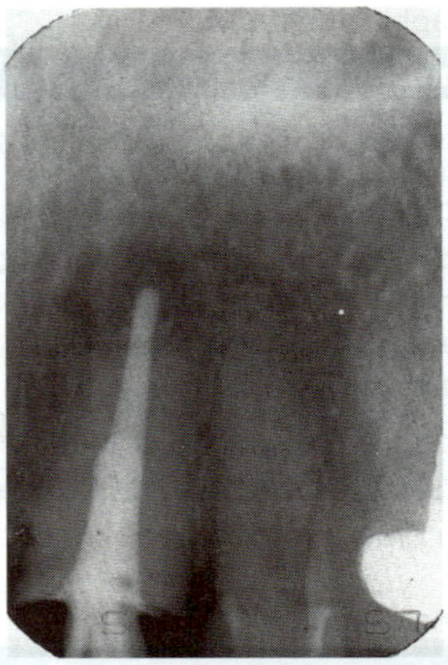

Fig. 65.5 Completed root filling in the upper left central incisor.

This tooth is therefore unrestorable and will require extraction. You continue to open the root canals of the other teeth under rubber dam. The single cone gutta percha root filling in the left central incisor was easily removed and, under copious irrigation with sodium hypochlorite, the working length was established.

■ ***The working length radiograph is seen in Figure 65.4. What can you deduce?***

The file used to take the working length radiograph is wide. This is because the previous root canal preparation was excessive and only a large file binds against the root canal walls. The file is approximately 2 mm short of the correct working length. The apical part of the root canal has been overprepared and this now poses a problem as the anatomical apical constriction has been destroyed and extrusion of the root canal filling through the apex is likely.

This is exactly what happened, as can be seen in Figure 65.5.

■ ***The teeth are now stabilized. What are the longer term options?***

The upper right lateral incisor has no active apical inflammation and a new post and temporary crown can be considered. However, the apical amalgam is less than ideal and the tooth is compromised as an abutment for a fixed bridge to replace the right central incisor.

The upper right central incisor is unrestorable and following extraction will need to be replaced with an upper acrylic immediate partial (removable) prosthesis for a 6 month period to allow for ridge resorption to take place. At this stage a definitive replacement can be considered.

The upper left central incisor may now be symptomless and the apical area may resolve. Attempts to remove the extruded material via the root canal are typically unsuccessful, pushing the material further into the tissues. Therefore it is advisable to place a new post and core straight away to establish a good coronal seal . A laboratory-made temporary crown can be placed for the 6 month observation period required for the right central incisor. Extrusion of gutta percha compromises the long-term prognosis and makes this tooth unsuitable as an abutment for a fixed prosthesis in its present state. If a removable prosthesis is the preferred option to replace the right central incisor, the prosthesis should be designed so that the other two compromised teeth can be added should treatment prove unsuccessful.

■ ***The patient expressed a strong wish to avoid a removable prosthesis. Are no fixed replacements possible?***

There are other possibilities but all involve expenditure of significant time and expense on severely compromised teeth. Assuming the root filling in the upper left central incisor is successful and that the root filling in the right lateral incisor remains so, posts and cores could be placed in both teeth and a fixed–fixed conventional immediate heat-cured acrylic bridge could be fitted as an interim restoration.

No more permanent restoration can be considered until the two root treated incisors are stable, and this can only be guaranteed by further periradicular surgery. This would allow removal of the poor apical amalgam reverse root filling in the lateral incisor and gutta percha extruded from the left central incisor. The chances of success reduce with each episode of apical surgery and normally a fourth attempt would be considered heroic. However, in this case there are clear reasons for failure of the previous surgery (inadequate orthograde root fillings) and so a further apicectomy does have some hope of success. The highest chance of success will be obtained with root end fillings of mineral trioxide aggregate (MTA).

Implants offer an alternative solution. The teeth could be replaced individually if and when the stabilization fails or replaced as a group with the intention of an implant-retained bridge or removable prosthesis. This could produce a faster result but would be significantly more expensive.

Case • 66

A pain in the head

SUMMARY

A 58-year-old female patient attending for routine dental care mentions that she has a severe headache and wishes to delay treatment. What should you do?

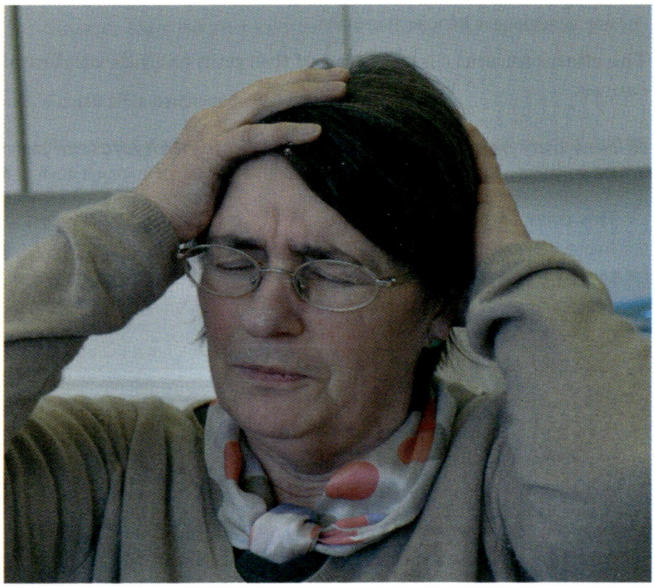

Fig. 66.1 The patient on presentation.

History

Complaint

The headaches affect her whole head, are short but severe, with dizziness, nausea and blurred vision (Figure 66.1).

History of complaint

The headaches started only 2 weeks ago. She has not been able to identify any causes. The only way she has been able to manage the pain is to lie still in bed until the pain is over. Over-the-counter painkillers have no effect. The present headache started on the way to your surgery.

Medical history

The patient is overweight, has smoked 15 cigarettes a day for 20 years and drinks 22 units of alcohol a week.

Dental history

The patient attends regularly and has no dental problems. You have noted attrition from bruxism but she has never complained of tenderness in the muscles of mastication.

■ ***How do you assess the history so far?***

Severe headaches with nausea and visual disturbance on an occasional basis would suggest migraine as a cause.

However, migraine usually has onset in young adult or middle age and would be unusual as a new diagnosis in a postmenopausal patient. The headache is not described as unilateral, as most migraines are, and there is no typical description of an aura. Dizziness, nausea and blurred vision, on the other hand, can be associated with migraine.

The bruxism is irrelevant. It may be associated with masticatory muscle tenderness but is usually asymptomatic.

■ ***What is the role of the dentist in headache diagnosis and treatment?***

It would be wise to consider this question before dismissing the complaint, referring to a medical practitioner or taking on analysis of the problem. A dentist would be expected to have a fairly broad knowledge of signs, symptoms and causes of craniofacial pain, but mainly for diagnostic and patient referral purposes.

The primary role of the dentist in headache is to exclude pain of dental or local origin. This is most important but not always easy.

The key causes of pain of dental origin that might present as headache are:

- Pulpitis and referred pain of dental origin
- Sinusitis
- Temporomandibular joint/myofascial pain dysfunction.

In addition some causes of head and neck pain can be misinterpreted by the patient as pain of dental origin and so present to the dentist. The key causes to consider are:

- Trigeminal and other neuralgias
- Giant cell arteritis
- Chronic idiopathic (atypical) facial pain.

The dentist should be very familiar with these causes of pain and should also be able to diagnose many others.

However, it is not the role of the dentist to undertake primary diagnostic responsibility for other causes of headache or facial pain. Craniofacial pain is usually managed by a multidisciplinary team, which may well include a dentist, and in such a setting the dentist may take on considerably more responsibility. In other settings the dentist will not have the necessary neurological knowledge or access to investigations.

E

F

P

Q

R

S

T

U

V

W

X

Z